STATISTICS IN MEDICINE

D. Pratt

STATISTICS IN MEDICINE

THEODORE COLTON, Sc. D. Associate Professor of Preventive and Social Medicine, Harvard Medical School, Boston, Massachusetts; Visiting Professor of Biostatistics, Dartmouth Medical School, Hanover, New Hampshire, and Memorial University of Newfoundland, St. John's, Newfoundland, Canada

Little, Brown and Company   Boston

Published November 1974

Copyright © 1974 by Little, Brown and Company (Inc.)

First Edition

Thirteenth Printing

Library of Congress catalog card No. 73-1413

ISBN 0-316-15249-8 (C)
ISBN 0-316-15250-1 (P)

Printed in the United States of America

HAL

To Carolyn, Andrew, and Joanna

Preface

This book enunciates the principles of statistics for the present or future practicing physician. I have tried to describe in terms meaningful to physician and medical student the structure and rationale of the most common, present-day statistical methods that pervade the quantitative evidence encountered in the medical literature. My aim has been to arm the reader with sufficient statistical expertise so that he can critically evaluate an author's presentation, analysis, and interpretation of data. *Statistics in Medicine* thus has, as one of its goals, prophylaxis, namely, the prevention of statistical wool being pulled over the medical reader's eyes.

Although focusing on the understanding and interpretation of statistics, I have not avoided the presentation of statistical methodology. The techniques are elaborated in sufficient detail so that the medical reader can, if he wishes, verify results for himself. I firmly believe that the act of performing these techniques will aid him in achieving better understanding and critical effectiveness when he must interpret and evaluate someone else's data analysis. Those chapters that deal with more quantitative and methodological matters contain a set of exercises (the answers are in the back of the book).

The medical researcher may find much of interest in this book, but he is not my intended audience. A number of excellent and comprehensive textbooks currently available (several of them are referenced in this text) display and guide the researcher through the armamentarium available in the statistical arsenal. I would hope that *Statistics in Medicine* appeals more to the physician who, although not primarily engaged in research, is faced with the task of assessing and implementing the proclaimed advances in knowledge of his researcher peers.

To illustrate principles and methods, I have utilized throughout the text real data extracted from the current literature, studies that suitably illustrate the pertinent statistical issues as well as contain intrinsic interest for the physician. In a number of these cited studies, my intent is to point out a misapplication of statistical technique or a misleading line of argument in the interpretation of numerical data. I clearly do not intend to embarrass or impugn the motives of the authors. My sole intent is to edify the reader by means of example regarding the pitfalls that befall the medical investigator as he presents, analyzes, and interprets numerical evidence. Although I could have contrived hypothetical data and situations to illustrate these points, this would have detracted from the educational impact achieved by confrontation with reality. Should any author thus cited read this text, I plead with him to try to contain his chagrin and bear with me in my educational effort. In a number of instances I may have cited data and statements that might appear somewhat out of context. If so, I apologize and offer not only the usual claim of space restriction, but the additional rationale of my goal to underscore and drive home a particular statistical lesson.

The book has developed from materials that I have collected over the past ten years, during which time I taught statistics to first-year students at several medical schools. Freshmen medical students vary greatly in their mathematical preparation. At Harvard, to cope with this variation, students have been offered alternative statistics courses at different levels. I have taught the large group of students that remains after the more mathematically curious and those keen on the potential use of statistics have been siphoned off into higher level courses. Thus, my course and this book omit mathematical justification. In several instances, I have outlined the rationale for many of the methods, but these clearly cannot be construed as proofs. The reader will find no trail-blazing techniques of data analysis; I have chosen those relatively simple techniques most frequently encountered in the medical literature.

Because of the better preparation in quantitative reasoning of present-day medical students, I have found it unnecessary to explain many of the very basic mathematical notions. For example, I assume the reader is familiar with the summation notation, so it is not necessary to explain the meaning of Σx or Σx^2. Likewise, I assume most readers can read and apply formulas and are capable of straightforward algebraic manipulations of equations. In a number of places there are suggested simple manipulations that the more mathematically inclined reader might wish to try in fleshing out some of the details. The section in Chapter 3 on probability distributions represents the book's upper limit of mathematical complexity. Mathematical development is not an essential aspect of the text; even the reader totally allergic to mathematics should be able to follow and pick up the main threads.

The text is divided into three main portions. Following an introductory chapter that sets the stage with the uses of statistics in medicine, Part I elaborates the basic building blocks of statistics: descriptive methods and probability. Part II sets forth the principles and methods of the process of statistical inference: drawing conclusions regarding populations based on evidence obtained from samples. The third portion (virtually devoid of formulas and algebraic symbols) expounds on the uses of statistics in medical research and contains chapters on clinical trials, medical surveys, and the common fallacies that abound in reasoning from medical data. The final chapter is a plea to the reader to synthesize whatever skills he has acquired in statistical reasoning with his medical knowledge and expertise as he critically evaluates what appears in print.

T. C.

Acknowledgments

Much of the manuscript was written while I was at the London School of Hygiene and Tropical Medicine; there I was supported by a National Institutes of Health Special Postdoctoral Fellowship (Number 1 FO3 GM51454-01) awarded by the Institute of General Medical Sciences. I am grateful for their support. Professors Peter Armitage and William G. Cochran kindly read the manuscript and made many useful suggestions and comments. I am indebted to them and to Dr. Alexander D. Langmuir for teaching me how to teach statistics to medical students. Thanks are due to my predecessor instructors at Harvard — Professor William G. Cochran and the late Professor Mindel C. Sheps — from whom I inherited a rich fund of teaching materials that formed the cornerstone for this book's development. Many fruitful discussions on medical statistics with Miss Rita J. Nickerson, my colleague, have helped enormously in the development of this book. My gratitude is extended to Dr. David D. Rutstein for his stimulus, encouragement, and support of my teaching activities over the years.

Mr. Nathan Mantel read a draft version of the first few chapters and pointed out a number of errors and inconsistencies. I hope that in detecting and removing inconsistencies in the later chapters, I have been as skillful as he was. I would greatly appreciate having readers call to my attention any residual errors and inconsistencies in the book, for which I assume full responsibility. Mrs. Charlotte Casler merits particular thanks for her patience, skill, and consistent good nature in the typing and retyping of the several draft versions of the manuscript. I am grateful to my wife Carolyn for her patience and encouragement. My children helped by keeping me well supplied with paper and pencils and providing me with the necessary long periods of uninterrupted concentration.

Finally, I am deeply indebted to the medical students whom I have instructed over the past years. Although I have never found teaching statistics to them an easy task, I have always found it challenging and personally rewarding. I have learned very much from my former students. I hope some of what they have taught me is reflected in this book.

T. C.

Contents

Chapter 1
Rationale for Statistics in Medicine

In comparison with the student of yesterday, the medical student of today may ask, "Why should I, as a practicing physician, know something about statistics?" There are several reasons why.

1. *Medicine is becoming increasingly quantitative.* As technology progresses, the physician encounters more and more quantitative rather than descriptive information. In one sense, statistics is the language of assembling and handling quantitative material. Even if one's concern is only with the results of other people's manipulation and assemblage of data, it is important to achieve some understanding of this language in order to interpret their results properly.

2. *The planning, conduct, and interpretation of much of medical research are becoming increasingly reliant on statistical methodology.* The following questions, some of which are faced nearly every day by the practicing physician, are to a great extent statistical in nature: Is this new drug or procedure better than that commonly in use? How much better? What, if any, are the risks of side effects associated with its use? In testing a new drug how many patients must be treated, and in what manner, in order to demonstrate its worth? What is the normal variation in some clinical measurement? How reliable and valid is the measurement? What is the magnitude and effect of laboratory and technical error? How does one interpret abnormal values?

   In fact, the two simple questions a patient can ask his physician—namely: "What's the diagnosis?" "What are my chances, Doc?"—are very frequently statistical in nature. In order to provide a sound answer, one often relies on the results of statistical analysis.

3. *Statistics pervades the medical literature.* As a consequence of the increasingly quantitative nature of medicine and its reliance on statistical methodology, the medical literature is replete with reports in which statistical techniques are used extensively. If the physician is to read these reports intelligently with the ability to evaluate critically the numerical evidence presented, he must have some understanding of statistics. Equipping the physician for the critical reading of the medical literature forms the central focus and theme for this book.

Underscoring the need for greater understanding of statistics in medicine is the fact that much of the statistical material in the medical literature is improperly conceived, executed, or interpreted. Schor and Karten document this point in a study in which all articles in three issues of eleven of the most frequently read medical journals were subjected to an intense biostatistical review [99]. The authors state:

Each communication was subjected to an abbreviated but intensive critical reading by a competent biostatistician with experience in reviewing scientific publications. The reviewers did not try to assess the relative merits of various methods of performing the experiment; they did not attempt to discover whether all the important information was extracted from the data. In short, they did not compare the actual experiment with the manner in which they, themselves, would have designed it if they had been consulted in advance.

The only requirement made was that the conclusions drawn were valid in terms of the design of the experiment, the type of analysis performed and the applicability of the statistical tests used or not used. . . .

The studies were grouped into three categories on the basis of the validity of the conclusions in terms of the design of the experiment and the type of analysis performed: those which were considered acceptable, those which should have been rejected because even major revisions could not make them acceptable, and those which should have been revised before publication on the basis of the errors found.

Among the 149 papers that were read and categorized as analytical studies (as opposed to case reports), only 28 percent were judged acceptable, whereas 68 percent were deficient but subject to revision, and 5 percent were totally unsalvageable. Accompanying this report, the editor of the *Journal of the American Medical Association* commented [33]:

The study is an indirect argument for greater knowledge and appreciation of statistics by the medical author, for a realization on his part that the biostatistician is not a worrisome censor, but a valuable ally, and that biostatistics, far from being an unrelated mathematical science, is a discipline essential to modern medicine—a pillar in its edifice.

It is the purpose of this book to provide a statistical foundation for the physician so that, at the very least, he will be able to distinguish some of the statistical wheat from its chaff in the medical literature.

SUBJECT-MATTER OF STATISTICS: DESCRIPTIVE STATISTICS AND STATISTICAL INFERENCE

A narrow view of the subject-matter of statistics is that it simply involves page upon page of numbers in volume upon volume stored on shelf upon shelf. In part, this is true. Also included in this view are the techniques for tabular and graphical presentation of data as well as the methods used to summarize a body of data with one or two meaningful figures. These aspects of organization, presentation, and summarization of data are labeled *descriptive statistics*. This was the main subject matter of statistics up to the 20th century.

One branch of descriptive statistics of special relevance in medicine is that of *vital statistics*. These statistics are derived from the official recording of vital events: birth, death, marriage, divorce, and the occurrence of particular diseases (e.g., for many communicable diseases, the law requires the attending physician to file an official report of each new case; in several geographical areas, reporting systems or registries have been established to record all cases of certain diseases, such as cancer). Coupled with results of periodic censuses and other special enumerations of populations, the data on vital events relate to an underlying population and yield descriptive measures such as birth rates, fertility rates, morbidity rates, mortality rates, life expectancies, and disease incidence and prevalence rates that pervade both the medical and lay literature. These *descriptive* statistics are used to characterize the health status of a population. Some aspects of vital statistics will be discussed in Chapter 2.

The branch of modern statistics that is most relevant to clinical medicine is *statistical inference*, the focal point of this book. Statistical inference concerns the logical basis by which conclusions regarding populations are drawn from results obtained in a sample. This process of inference from sample to population pervades the field of medicine as well as almost any other scientific discipline.

Consider the following examples of statistical inference in medicine:

Example 1.1.   *The analysis of a sample of blood or urine or the results from a biopsy of tissue.* From a sample obtained from a patient, one draws a conclusion regarding a larger "population," namely, the patient's *total* urine or blood volume, or his entire organ.

Example 1.2.   *The test of a new drug or a new medical or surgical procedure.* Based on the new drug's or new procedure's performance among a sample of patients with a disease, a conclusion is drawn regarding the drug's performance were it to be used among a population of patients with the disease. Clinical trials (i.e., experiments with new drugs and procedures on human patients) receive extensive consideration in this book as an illustration of various technical statistical procedures as well as a subject of great inherent interest to the biostatistician and physician.

Example 1.3.   *The United States National Health Survey.* This survey illustrates statistical inference from a survey rather than from an experimental viewpoint. From an ongoing sample of households throughout the United States, information is collected regarding illness, disability, the existence of chronic and acute conditions, and many other matters related to health. The analysis of results in these sample households permits inferences to be drawn regarding these characteristics in the total population of the United States.

This concept of inference from sample to population has, as its underlying foundation, the mathematical theory of probability; however, it does not mean that one must be acquainted with the mathematical theory in order to use the statistical methods effectively. It is sufficient to know the methodology, the basic assumptions by which the techniques may be used, and, most important, the proper interpretation of results. It has become somewhat of a cliché to draw an analogy with operation of an automobile. One need not know much, if anything, regarding internal combustion engines and how they function in order to drive a car. The attainment of several operational skills along with knowledge of the rules of the road suffices to enable one to operate an automobile safely and effectively in most terrain.

STATISTICAL INFERENCE: TARGET POPULATION VERSUS THE POPULATION SAMPLED

In drawing an inference, it is useful to distinguish between two populations: the target population and the population sampled. The *target population* is that population about which an investigator wishes to draw a conclusion. The *population sampled* is that population from which the sample actually was drawn and about which a conclusion can be made. As indicated in Figure 1.1, the methods of statistical inference enable an investigator to proceed from his sample results to conclusions regarding the population sampled. This process has its foundations in the mathematical theory of probability and the underlying concept of a random sample from a defined population.

Whether one can infer from the population sampled to the target population is quite another matter, a much more subjective issue that often involves considerable controversy. Sometimes the target population and the population sampled are identical. In such situations, there is no difficulty with the interpretation of the results of statistical inference applied to the sample data. More often, however, the target population differs from the population sampled. The way in which they differ is what is generally referred to as *bias*; the forces operating to distinguish the two populations are generally called *selective factors*. Extreme caution must be exercised when such a situation is likely to exist. Unfortunately, many investigators are often unaware of the existence of large biases and thus draw improper conclusions regarding their

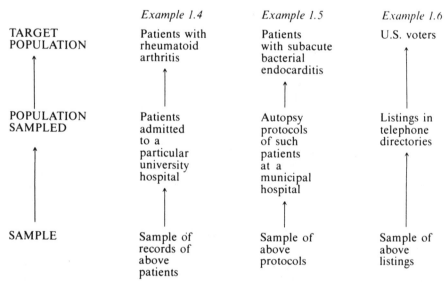

	Example 1.4	*Example 1.5*	*Example 1.6*
TARGET POPULATION	Patients with rheumatoid arthritis	Patients with subacute bacterial endocarditis	U.S. voters
POPULATION SAMPLED	Patients admitted to a particular university hospital	Autopsy protocols of such patients at a municipal hospital	Listings in telephone directories
SAMPLE	Sample of records of above patients	Sample of above protocols	Sample of above listings

Figure 1.1
The process of statistical inference.

target populations. The conclusions may be perfectly valid if applied only to the population sampled, whatever it may be. (Of course, in many situations one is unable to specify precisely what constitutes the population sampled.) Selective factors and biases, however, can completely vitiate the extension of results from the population sampled to the target population. These points are illustrated in the following examples and in Figure 1.1.

Example 1.4. *Rheumatoid arthritis in a university hospital.* Suppose an investigator is involved in some aspect characterizing the natural history of rheumatoid arthritis. He has chosen as his target population *all* patients with this disease. For his study, he arranges for the record room of the university hospital in which he is located to send him a sample of case records of patients with rheumatoid arthritis; for example, all such admissions during a one-year period. His statistical analysis and the resulting conclusions must be tempered by the consideration of what selective factors and biases distinguish his sample population—namely, all admissions with rheumatoid arthritis at his particular university hospital—from the target population of *all* patients with the disease. What are these factors?

Two selective factors immediately emerge. First, rheumatoid arthritis does not always require hospitalization. There is a sizeable proportion of patients with the disease who have not been hospitalized. Such patients could not possibly enter his study. Consequently, it may be entirely erroneous to draw conclusions regarding the natural history of rheumatoid arthritis in *all* patients when the only possible patients eligible for the study are those who were hospitalized. Second, even among hospitalized cases, the fact that the study is conducted in a university hospital indicates selectivity toward the more complex and serious cases. The characteristics of the patients in this hospital may be very different from those in other less highly specialized hospitals. Clearly, as further specifics regarding the nature of the investigation are delineated, additional selective factors and possible biases can be identified.

Example 1.5. *Bacterial endocarditis in an autopsy series.* A commonly occurring form of quantitative investigation consists of the analysis of the autopsy protocols of patients who have died from some disease. As an example, consider a series of autopsy reports on patients who died from bacterial endocarditis in a municipal hospital in Philadelphia. This particular disease at this institution was chosen because of the availability of published data that serve well to illustrate the selective nature of the autopsy study group. As shown in

Figure 1.1, application of the statistical techniques described in this book enables an inference to be drawn from the study sample to the population sampled, whatever that may be. However, to draw any inference regarding the target population of *all* patients with bacterial endocarditis is quite another matter.

Experience has shown that an autopsy group is determined by a host of selective factors, perhaps more so than almost any other form of medical investigation. Actually, an autopsy series is profoundly elite. To enter the group, one must first have the disease with sufficient severity as to require hospitalization. Second, the disease must be severe enough to result in death. Finally, only a portion of the deaths are selected for autopsy. All along this chain of entry to the study group, a host of selective factors operate to produce an atypical and unrepresentative group. Consider the last step alone, namely, the factors influencing who, among the deaths, arrives at the autopsy table. It is well known that autopsy rates vary according to demographic characteristics such as age, sex, and race. Furthermore, ethnic background and religious beliefs will often dictate whether or not the family will grant permission for an autopsy. As an additional factor, much depends on the physician's interest in seeking an autopsy and the diligence with which he persists in attaining it. Clearly, the physician tends to seek autopsies for the more interesting cases, namely, those that might involve some peculiar circumstances, those that are complex, and those that are associated with other diseases and complications.

Table 1.1. Characteristics of patients with bacterial endocarditis

Characteristic	96 autopsied patients	13 deaths, not autopsied	50 patients discharged alive
Mean age (years)	56	51	39
Over 65 years old	35%	31%	6%
Associated disease	60%	31%	21%
Mental aberrations	43%	47%	22%
Splenomegaly	12%	15%	38%
Murmurs	66%	100%	100%
Petechiae	35%	38%	54%

Data from Cooper et al. [22].

Some of these points are evident in the data presented in a study of bacterial endocarditis at a municipal hospital in Philadelphia [22]. These data, reproduced in Table 1.1, give several characteristics for three groups of patients with this disease: those on whom an autopsy was performed, those who died but were not autopsied, and those who were discharged alive from the hospital. The series are small but illustrate the point well. First, with respect to age, there are clear distinctions among the three series of patients. As expected, proceeding from those discharged alive to the deaths without autopsy to the autopsied deaths, the mean age rises and, correspondingly, the proportion of subjects over 65 years of age likewise increases. Similarly, the proportion with associated disease increases sharply as one proceeds along the chain of selection. There are sharp distinctions in the proportions of mental aberrations between the discharged-alive group and the two groups for deaths. It is clear from these data that the characteristics of autopsied patients differ from those of patients who died without autopsy which, in turn, differ from those of patients who were discharged alive. The extrapolation, then, of results among those autopsied to a broader group of all deaths or to an even broader group of all patients with the disease is fraught with danger.

Example 1.6.   *Sample of voters from telephone directories.* A classic example of the distinction between the target population and the population sampled can be found in a political poll of quite a few years ago that was aimed at predicting the outcome of a presidential election. The target population was all voters in the United States; the population sampled was obtained from listings in telephone directories. Parenthetically, it is worth noting that the magnitude of the sample size is relatively valueless in compensating for the factors of bias and selection; in this political poll there were over one million responses to the query! The time was 1936, the candidates were Roosevelt and Landon, and the poll was conducted by the *Literary Digest.* It is almost remarkable for the poll to have predicted a landslide victory for Landon, in view of the actual results which gave Roosevelt the largest margin ever achieved in a presidential election up to that time. Of course, in 1936 there were substantial numbers of people, mostly Roosevelt supporters, without telephones. The sample was over-represented by the more affluent who could, at that time, afford a telephone; these more affluent individuals tended to favor Landon.

With the political poll situation, population election results are available within a reasonable time to confirm or refute the consequences of the inferential procedure. Several hand-scorching gaffes such as this have led pollsters to be exceedingly careful and cautious in their choice of population frames for sampling. Perhaps more singed hands among medical investigators would be helpful in curbing the use of highly selected and atypical study groups as the basis for very broad and far-reaching medical conclusions.

Prospectus

This book emphasizes statistical inference. However, descriptive statistics form the building blocks for statistical inference. Hence, descriptive statistics are dealt with in Chapter 2. Since statistical inference is based on the mathematical theory of probability, some of the basic principles of probability follow in Chapter 3. Chapter 4 then begins the discussion of the details of statistical inference.

PART I
FUNDAMENTALS

Chapter 2
Descriptive Statistics

SCALES OF MEASUREMENT

A logical place to begin the discussion of descriptive methods is to consider the various forms in which medical data occur. The classification of various scales of measurement used in this section is based on examples from the medical literature.

Nominal Scale: Enumeration or Attribute Data

The simplest data consist of unordered, dichotomous, or "either-or" types of observations, i.e., either the patient lives or the patient dies, either he has some particular attribute or he does not. Mathematicians refer to this dichotomy as a *0–1 scale*.

Table 2.1. Nominal scale data: survival status of propranolol-treated and control patients with myocardial infarction

Status 28 days after admission	Propranolol-treated patients	Control patients
Dead	7	17
Alive	38	29
Total	45	46
Survival rate	84%	63%

Data from Snow [102].

Example 2.1.   Table 2.1 presents data from a clinical trial of the drug propranolol in the treatment of myocardial infarction [102]. There were two groups of patients with myocardial infarctions. One group received propranolol; the other did not and was the control. For each patient the response was dichotomous; either he survived the first 28 days after hospital admission or he succumbed sometime within this time period.

With *nominal scale data*, the obvious and intuitive descriptive summary measure is the proportion or percentage of subjects who exhibit the attribute. Thus, at the foot of Table 2.1, 84 percent of the patients treated with propranolol survived, in contrast with only 63 percent of the control group.

With regard to statistical inference, on the basis of the results obtained, the goal is to draw a conclusion concerning the drug's effects if used in a large population of patients with myocardial infarction. Does this experiment provide sufficient evidence that propranolol therapy will yield a higher survival rate for the first 28 days after hospital admission than with control therapy? The author concluded from analysis of these data that "Propranolol appears to be capable of significantly reducing the mortality from acute myocardial infarction." The statistical methodology for conducting this analysis is described in Chapter 5 (p. 166).

A nominal scale *need not* be dichotomous. Often there are more than two alternatives or classifications. For example, blood groups illustrate an unordered, multichotomous scale. There is no ordering among the classifications such that the blood groups O, A, B, and AB can be arrayed in any sequence.

Example 2.2.   Table 2.2 presents data on the blood group of two groups of women known to be taking oral contraceptives [60]. The

Table 2.2. Nominal scale data: blood groups of thromboembolic and healthy women taking oral contraceptives

Blood group	Women with thromboembolism		Healthy women	
	No.	%	No.	%
A	32	58	51	35
B	8	15	19	13
AB	6	11	5	3
O	9	16	70	49
Total	55	100	145	100

Data from Jick et al. [60].

first group consisted of 55 women discharged from the obstetrical and gynecological services of four Boston hospitals with a diagnosis of thrombophlebitis or pulmonary embolism. The second, the control group, consisted of 145 healthy, randomly selected women attending a Boston family-planning clinic. Inspection of the percentages by blood group suggests a deficit of O blood type among the thromboembolism group (16 percent) compared with controls (49 percent). The question involving statistical inference is whether oral contraceptive users of blood group O are less likely to contract thromboembolic disease than oral contraceptive users of other blood types. (See p. 179 for the analysis of these data.)

The analysis of these data and other similar series collected in the United States and abroad led the authors to conclude, "Our present findings provide substantial preliminary evidence that apparently healthy women of blood type O have a lower risk of developing venous thromboembolic disease . . . while taking oral contraceptives than women of other blood types."

Ordered Classifications

The distinction from the preceding situation is that there now exists a predetermined *order* among the response classifications.

Table 2.3. Ordered classification data: assessment of radiological appearance at six months as compared with admission in clinical trial of streptomycin for the treatment of pulmonary tuberculosis

Radiological assessment	Patients treated with streptomycin and bed rest		Patients treated with bed rest alone	
	No.	%	No.	%
Considerable improvement	28	51	4	8
Moderate or slight improvement	10	18	13	25
No material change	2	4	3	6
Moderate or slight deterioration	5	9	12	23
Considerable deterioration	6	11	6	11
Deaths	4	7	14	27
Total	55	100	52	100

Data from Medical Research Council [76].

Example 2.3. Table 2.3 illustrates ordered classifications with the results of a clinical trial of streptomycin in the treatment of pulmonary tuberculosis [76]. The data presented are the results of radiological assessment at six months after entry into the study for two groups of patients with documented pulmonary tuberculosis. The first group consisted of 55 patients who were treated with both streptomycin and bed rest. The second group, the control series, consisted of 52 patients treated with bed rest alone. With regard to the conduct of the radiological assessment, the authors state, "The films have been viewed by two radiologists and a clinician, each reading the films independently and not knowing if the films were of control or streptomycin cases." Thus, the assessment was "blind." (See the discussion on p. 262.)

Of course, the essential question is the comparison of streptomycin with bed rest alone in the treatment of tuberculosis. On the basis of these sample observations, what conclusions can be drawn regarding the comparison of streptomycin with bed rest alone in the treatment of a population of patients with pulmonary tuberculosis? The results suggest the superiority of streptomycin. Note that at the two extreme classifications there are substantially more patients exhibiting "considerable improvement" and there are fewer deaths in the streptomycin-treated group (compared with the bed rest group). Are the data sufficient to draw a conclusion regarding streptomycin's superiority?

This post–World War II study was among the pioneer controlled clinical trials that form the prototype for present-day therapeutic trials. The authors concluded, "The overall results . . . show differences between the two series that leave no room for doubt. The most outstanding difference is in the numbers who showed 'considerable improvement' in the radiological picture—i.e., those for whom at the end of the six-months period there was a reasonable prospect of recovery."

Note that with ordered classifications one need not assume equal distances between categories. For example, the difference between "considerable improvement" and "moderate or slight improvement" is not necessarily the same as the difference between "moderate or slight deterioration" and "considerable deterioration."

Ranks

A *full ranking scale* is one that arrays the members of a group from high to low according to the magnitude of the observations, assigns numbers to the ranks, and neglects distances between members of the array. For example, suppose patients with chronic headache participate in a clinical trial in which they receive four different analgesic preparations on four different occasions. Each patient may be asked to rank the preparations from high to low according to the degree of relief provided. If a patient felt that drug *A* was best and drug *B* second best, he would rank them 1 and 2 regardless of whether he felt drug *A* was far superior to *B* or whether *A* was just slightly better than *B*.

In previous years, medical students were familiar with ranks and they were the subjects for detailed ranking procedures. Grade-point averages, calculated for each student, formed the basis for ranking students from top to bottom of the class.

Example 2.4.   Table 2.4 illustrates a sample of rank data on medical students. These data are for 12 graduating senior medical students who had each undergone a one-hour oral examination by a team of three faculty members. After the team completed all their examinations, the members of the team ranked the students from high (rank 1) to low (rank 12). For the 12 students, Table 2.4 displays each student's clinical year grade-point average, his corresponding rank on grade-point average, and his rank according to the oral examination team members. Note that with the grade-point averages the difference between the consecutive ranks 1 and 2 is 0.55 grade points, whereas between consecutive ranks 8 and 9, the difference in averages is only 0.03 grade points. Thus, the ranks neglect distances between students.

Table 2.4. Ranking data: rank of 12 senior medical students according to grade-point average and performance on an oral examination

Student	Grade point average[a]	Rank	Rank on oral examination
a	1.42	1	1
b	1.97	2	5
c	2.12	3	3
d	2.20	4	8
e	2.27	5	11
f	2.33	6	2
g	2.43	7	4
h	2.57	8	7
i	2.60	9	9
j	2.68	10	10
k	2.76	11	6
l	2.87	12	12

[a] The scoring is A = 1 to D = 4.

The obvious goal with these data is to determine the degree of correspondence between the grade-point rank and the rank by the team of oral examiners. Inspection indicates perfect agreement on rank for 5 out of 12 students (ranks 1, 3, 9, 10, 12). For one student, the ranks differed by one; for the remaining 6, the ranks differed by three or more. Thus, there is a suggestion of some correspondence, though it clearly is far from perfect.

Methods for quantification of the degree of correspondence are described in Chapter 7 (p. 223). As before, there is an underlying concept of statistical inference. On the basis of these sample results on 12 students, what conclusion can be drawn regarding the correspondence of these two indicators in a larger population of senior medical students?

Sometimes the results of a ranking are grouped in broader categories. For instance, with medical students, it has been customary to classify their ranking in the upper, middle, or lower third of the class. With the small series of data illustrated in Table 2.4, the top four ranks (1 to 4) constitute the upper third, the next four (5 to 8) the middle third, and the last four (9 to 12) the lower third of the series. One is tempted to equate these broader groupings with the ordered classification scale described before. There is, however, a subtle and important distinction. With the *ranking* of medical students, one *must allocate one-third of all students* to each of the three categories: upper, middle, and lower third. With an ordered classification having the analogous labels "superior," "average," and "fair," one is not forced to allocate the group equally to each of the three categories. At the extremes, one could place the entire class either in the superior category or in the fair category. Thus, ranking within broad groups is a more restrictive form of measurement scale than ordered classifications. Ranking indicates the relative position within the group; ordered classifications imply the use of some external or absolute standard of assessment

Numerical Discrete

Numerical discrete data occur when the observations are integers that correspond with a count of some sort. Some common medical examples are the number of bacteria colonies on a plate, the number of cells within a prescribed area upon microscopic examination, the number of heart beats within a specified time interval, a mother's history of numbers of births (parity) and pregnancies (gravidity), the number of a dental patient's decayed, missing, and

Table 2.5. Numerical discrete data: observed and expected numbers of accidents during a three-year period among 708 Ulster (Northern Ireland) Transport Authority bus drivers

Number of accidents in 3-year period	Number of drivers Observed	Expected
0	117	71.5
1	157	164.0
2	158	187.9
3	115	143.6
4	78	82.3
5	44	37.7
6	21	14.4
7	7	
8	6	
9	1	6.6
10	3	
11	1	
Total	708	708

Data from Cresswell and Froggatt [24].

filled ("DMF") teeth, the number of radioactive particles emitted by a substance within a time interval, and the number of episodes of illness a patient experiences during some time period.

Example 2.5.   Table 2.5 illustrates numerical discrete data from a tabulation of the number of accidents among 708 Ulster (Northern Ireland) Transport Authority bus drivers during a three-year period [24]. Each driver accrued in this period a discrete, integral number of accidents. The results range from 117 drivers who experienced no accidents to one driver who experienced 11.

The expected numbers refer to how the accidents should distribute if they occurred completely at random during the three-year period and if all 708 drivers were at equal risk of an accident. It is equivalent to taking each of the total of 1,623 accidents that occurred and picking a driver at random for that accident.

Comparison of the observed and expected tabulations reveals more than the expected number of drivers with no accidents and with five or more accidents. These data suggest that the accidents did not occur completely at random; in fact, it appears that there is some indication of accident proneness. From this sample, what conclusions are justified concerning the random or nonrandom distribution of bus driver accidents?

Numerical Continuous

Finally, the scale with the greatest degree of quantification is a *numerical continuous scale*. Each observation theoretically falls somewhere along a continuum. One is not restricted, in principle, to particular values such as the integers of the discrete scale. The restricting factor is the degree of accuracy of the measuring instrument. Most clinical measurements, such as blood pressure, serum cholesterol level, height, weight, and age, are on a numerical continuous scale.

Example 2.6.   To illustrate this scale, Table 2.6 presents a summary tabulation of serum uric acid levels among 267 normal males [39]. The raw data of 267 values have been summarized and condensed with the *frequency distribution* of Table 2.6 (the definition of a frequency distribution and some guidelines for its construction appear in the next section).

The reason for collection of these data concerns the genetic mechanism underlying gout. One of the characteristic features of gout is hyperuricemia (excess uric acid in the blood). Although not all individuals with hyperuricemia develop clinical manifestations of gout, it has been long

Table 2.6. Numerical continuous data: serum uric acid levels among 267 normal males

Serum uric acid (mg/ 100 ml)	Number of men[a]
3.0–3.4	2
3.5–3.9	15
4.0–4.4	33
4.5–4.9	40
5.0–5.4	54
5.5–5.9	47
6.0–6.4	38
6.5–6.9	16
7.0–7.4	15
7.5–7.9	3
8.0–8.4	1
8.5–8.9	3
Total	267

[a] Healthy blood donors.
Data from Finn et al. [39].

recognized that the hereditary component of gout is connected with a hereditary tendency toward hyperuricemia. If a simple genetic mechanism controls hereditary hyperuricemia—namely, a single dominant gene—then uric acid levels in the general population should follow a distribution with two peaks (bimodal). If a more complex genetic mechanism determines hyperuricemia—namely, polygenic inheritance—then uric acid levels in the general population would follow a single-peaked distribution (unimodal).

The investigators state that

Recently, attention has been focussed on the frequency distribution curve of uric acid in the general population. The results of these studies have been conflicting. Some authors have found normal* distribution curves, whereas others have found a bimodal distribution of uric acid in the general population.... We have attempted to reexamine the form of the frequency distribution curve of uric acid in the general population....

They conclude that "the frequency distribution curve of uric acid in the general population is shown to be unimodal."

FREQUENCY DISTRIBUTIONS AND OTHER TABLES

Frequency Distributions

With both numerical discrete and continuous observations, a *frequency distribution* (see Tables 2.5 and 2.6) provides the most convenient format for

*The normal distribution is discussed in detail in Chapter 3.

summarizing and presenting the data. In fact, the greater the number of observations, the greater are the economy and clarity achieved with presentation as a frequency distribution. A frequency distribution consists of a series of predetermined classes (such as age intervals) together with counts of the number of observations whose values fall within the interval for each class. There are several simple guidelines for constructing a frequency distribution. These are not hard and fast rules, and they are based mostly on experience and the exercise of common sense.

1. *The number of classes should generally be in the neighborhood of 10 to 20.* Obviously, the use of too many classes differs little from tabulation of the raw data; too few classes may obscure essential information. In practice, it is better to begin with a somewhat larger number of *fine classes.* These fine classes can easily be combined into broader classes. If one starts with broad classes and then wishes a finer tabulation, one must return to the raw data and retabulate the entire series.

2. *The limits for each class must agree with the accuracy of the raw data.* For example, the serum uric acid levels were recorded correct to the nearest tenth of a milligram per 100 ml. The class intervals retain this same accuracy; for example, the first interval is 3.0 to 3.4 mg per 100 ml. It would be inappropriate to employ an interval of 3.00 to 3.49 mg per 100 ml, since the data were not recorded with this degree of accuracy.

3. *Intervals of equal width are convenient and facilitate further computation.* This will be demonstrated in later sections of this chapter. Equal width intervals, however, are not essential.

4. *The class intervals must be mutually exclusive.* For example, in a frequency distribution of age, intervals of 5 to 10 years and 10 to 15 years are not mutually exclusive. With an individual age 10, one would not know whether he falls in the 5 to 10 year or the 10 to 15 year class.

5. *Open-ended intervals should be avoided.* If the last interval in Table 2.6 for serum uric acid levels were "$\geq$ 8.5 mg per 100 ml," one would not know where the observations fell—whether the observations were near 8 or perhaps as high as 10 mg per 100 ml. Although this guideline is commonly neglected, its neglect makes for a certain degree of arbitrariness and difficulty when further manipulations are performed with the frequency distribution. Similarly, graphical depictions of open-ended frequency distributions encounter analogous difficulties.

6. *For further computations from frequency distribution data, determination of the midpoint of each class is essential.* In order to determine the midpoint, it is necessary to distinguish two limits for a class interval: the tabulated limits and the true limits.

The *tabulated* limits of a class refer to the limits that were actually used in tabulating the frequency distribution. Thus, for serum uric acid levels, the tabulated limits for the first class are 3.0 to 3.4 mg per 100 ml.

The *true* limits are what the tabulated limits would correspond with *if* one could measure exactly. Thus, the true limits refer to the underlying continuous scale of measurement, and they are derived from the stated accuracy of the data. For example, if the serum uric acid level data are correct to the nearest tenth of a milligram per 100 ml, then the true limits for the first class are 2.95 to 3.45 mg per 100 ml. This means that any true or hypothetically exact value that was just below 3.45 would, when read as correct to the nearest tenth, be recorded as 3.4 and thus be tabulated in the first class. Any value just above 3.45 would be recorded as 3.5 and be tabulated in the next class.

The midpoint of the class interval consists of the point halfway between its true limits. Thus, with serum uric acid levels, the midpoint of the first interval is $(2.95 + 3.45)/2 = 3.20$.

To illustrate the distinction between tabulated and true limits, several examples are shown in Table 2.7. When the accuracy of a measurement is correct to the nearest unit, the midpoints of the tabulated and true limits are identical. This may be seen in Table 2.7, where serum uric acid is correct to the nearest tenth of a milligram per 100 ml and height is correct to the nearest inch or the nearest eighth of an inch. Age requires special consideration since it is usually recorded correct to the last and not the nearest birthday. Thus, one is age 24 until one's 25th birthday. Hence, for tabulated limits of 20 to 24 years, the true limits are 20 to 25 years, yielding a midpoint of 22.5 years for the interval.

Table 2.7. Examples of tabulated and true limits and their midpoints

Measurement	Accuracy	Tabulated limits	True limits	Midpoint
Serum uric acid level	Nearest 10th of mg/100 ml	3.0–3.4	2.95–3.45	3.2
Height	Nearest inch	50–52	49.5–52.5	51
Height	Nearest eighth of an inch	$50–51\frac{7}{8}$	$49\frac{15}{16}–51\frac{15}{16}$	$50\frac{15}{16}$
Age	Last birthday	20–24	20–25	22.5

It is well to remember the rule that for graphing and for further computations, one employs the true limits and their midpoints.

In tabular presentation of both frequency distributions and other data, some general guidelines are worth mentioning:

1. *Tables should be clearly labeled.* The reader should be able to determine without difficulty precisely what was tabulated.
2. *Totals should be indicated.* These are helpful in summarizing for the reader how much data are in the table and as a means of providing reconciliation with other tables and with textual material.
3. *If percentages are obtained, the base for the percentage should be clearly indicated.* In Tables 2.2 and 2.3, the 100 percent value indicates the percentage base. In a complex table displaying percentages without indication of their base, the reader is uncertain how or which way the percentages add to 100 percent. Such a table can easily be misinter-

preted. A glance at the location of the 100 percent value almost always informs the reader immediately how the percentages in the table were derived.

4. *If units of measurement are involved, they should be clearly indicated.* For example, the serum uric acid levels are in units of milligrams per 100 ml. These units are indicated at the head of the first column of Table 2.6.

5. *Tables can often express results more concisely and clearly than prose.* For example, consider Table 2.1. In prose, these results might be described with the somewhat cumbersome statement: Of 45 patients treated with propranolol, 7 died within the first 28 days after admission while 38 survived this period, giving a survival rate of 84 percent. In contrast, of 46 patients in the control group, 17 died within the first 28 days and 29 survived this period, giving a survival rate of 63 percent.

6. *At the other extreme, exceedingly complex tables are to be avoided.* They can lead to misinterpretation and confusion. Often a certain degree of complexity is necessary to conserve space. However, one should studiously avoid the temptation to compress too much information within a single table.

HISTOGRAMS, FREQUENCY POLYGONS, AND OTHER GRAPHS

Once a frequency distribution has been obtained, it is often helpful to depict it graphically. Two types of graphs of frequency distributions are commonly employed: the *histogram* and the *frequency polygon*.

Histograms

The histogram is the familiar bar-type of diagram. The top half of Figure 2.1 illustrates the histogram for the serum uric acid level frequency distribution. Note that the ordinate begins at zero and that the height of each bar pertains to the number of men in that class; note also that on the abscissa, each bar centers at the midpoint of the class.

With the histogram it is well to remember the key principle that the *area* of the bar depicts the frequency. This point is especially pertinent in considering frequency distributions in which the class intervals are not of equal width. In such a situation, appropriate adjustments are needed so that the area remains in proper proportion.

Example 2.7.   To illustrate this procedure, Table 2.8 gives the age distribution of all deaths in the United States in 1967. The age intervals employed vary in width from 1 (0 to 1 year) to 20 (25 to 44 years). With one year as the narrowest interval in the distribution, all other intervals are scaled to this level. Thus, to retain the proper proportion in area for the histogram, an interval that is 20 times as wide as the smallest interval must, when graphed, have a height 1/20th the

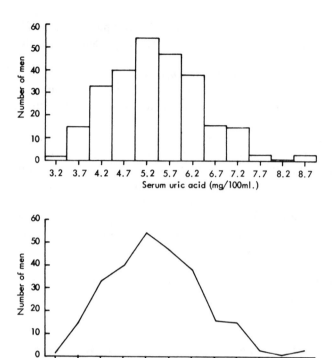

Figure 2.1
Histogram (top) and frequency polygon (bottom) for the depiction of the frequency
distribution of serum uric acid levels among 267 healthy males.

Table 2.8. Age distribution of deaths for total U.S. population, 1967

Age at death (yr)	"True" class limits (yr)	Midpoint of interval (yr)	Width of interval (yr)	Number of deaths	Deaths per year of age[a]
Under 1	0–1	0.5	1	79,028	79,028
1–4	1–5	3	4	13,506	3,377
5–9	5–10	7.5	5	8,809	1,762
10–14	10–15	12.5	5	8,084	1,617
15–24	15–25	20	10	37,706	3,771
25–44	25–45	35	20	108,825	5,441
45–64	45–65	55	20	459,203	22,960
65–74	65–75	70	10	437,919	43,792
75–84	75–85	80	10	469,669	46,967
85+	85–100	92.5	15	227,987	15,199

[a] Deaths per year of age = Number of deaths divided by width of interval.
Data from Public Health Service [90].

frequency of that interval. To achieve the proper heights for histograms, the last column in Table 2.8 indicates the number of deaths per year of age for each interval in the distribution. This column was obtained by dividing the frequencies (number of deaths) by the width of each class. As shown in Figure 2.2 (top), the heights of the bars correspond to the last column of Table 2.8. In this histogram, the area of each bar then appears in proper proportion to the number of deaths.

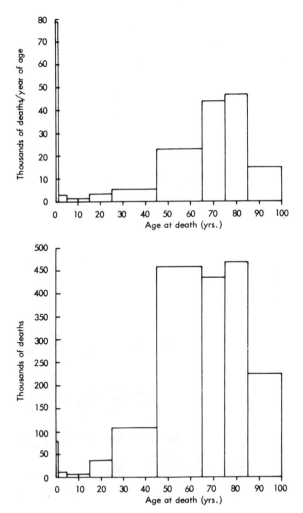

Figure 2.2
Correct (top) and incorrect (bottom) histogram for the depiction of the age distribution of deaths in the United States, 1967.

To illustrate how misleading an incorrect graph can be, the bottom half of Figure 2.2 depicts a histogram in which the height of each bar corresponds directly with the number of deaths. This histogram is entirely inappropriate and one can see how seriously the reader is misled by such a graphical error.

In Table 2.8, it should be noted that the last age interval was open-ended. Thus, for graphing, it was necessary to make an arbitrary decision regarding this class. It was decided to set 100 as the upper class limit.

Frequency Polygons

Though less commonly used than the histogram, the frequency polygon suffices for the depiction of a frequency distribution. For each class of the distribution, one locates a point whose abscissa is the midpoint of the class and whose ordinate or height is the frequency. The series of points, connected by straight lines, gives the frequency polygon that is illustrated in the lower half of Figure 2.1 for the data on serum uric acid levels.

The frequency polygon has an advantage over the histogram when one wishes to plot more than one frequency distribution on the same graph. With the frequency polygon, the same caution that was mentioned above regarding

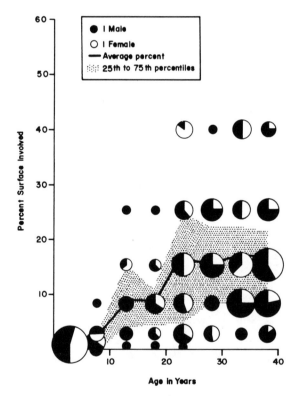

Figure 2.3
Age, sex, and extent of fatty streaks in a study of aortic atherosclerosis among an autopsy series. (From Strong et al. [106].)

histograms prevails with regard to unequal class intervals. For example, with the age distribution of deaths, a frequency polygon would consist of points whose abscissas were the midpoints of the intervals and whose ordinates were determined by the data in the last column (deaths per year of age) of Table 2.8.

Other Graphs

As with frequency distributions and tables, some general comments are in order regarding histograms, frequency polygons, and other graphs.

    1.   *A graph should aid the reader in comprehending the material.*   Often a great deal of ingenuity is employed in designing graphs that contain extensive information. However, the effect on the reader is somewhat dubious.

Example 2.8.   Figure 2.3 was extracted from an article that dealt with atherosclerosis in an autopsy series [106]. The textual description of the graph was:

> The figure depicts graphically the distribution with respect to age, sex and extent of fatty streaks.... The area of each circle is proportional to the number of cases in that category; the black and white areas represent respectively the proportion of males and females; the average extent of fatty streaks at each age and the 25th and 75th percentiles are indicated.

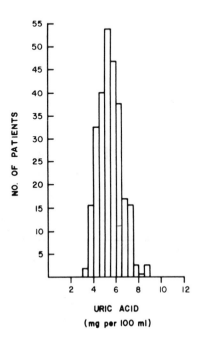

Figure 2.4
Histogram for the depiction of the frequency distribution of serum uric acid levels among 267 healthy males.

2. *Axes should be clearly labeled and units of measurement indicated.* As with tables, it is important for the reader to be able to tell at a glance precisely what is being illustrated and in what units.

3. *Scales are extremely important.* In particular, scales that do not start at zero must be cautiously interpreted. Furthermore, one should be wary of serious distortions of numerical scales.

Example 2.9.   The importance of scale can be gleaned by examining Figure 2.4. This is the depiction of the histogram for the serum uric acid levels of 267 healthy males as presented by the authors in the original paper [39]. Clearly, the impression given by Figure 2.4 differs from that imparted by Figure 2.1. Which is correct?

They both are. The choice of scale in Figure 2.4 is such that, in comparison with Figure 2.1, the abscissa is narrower whereas the ordinate is wider. Both are entirely adequate representations of the frequency distribution.

Example 2.10.   Figure 2.5, taken from an article entitled "Diuretics and hypertension-effect of sodium balance" [61], illustrates a graph that can easily be misinterpreted. A glance at the ordinate indicates that its scale does not start at zero. The use of a histogram to depict mean blood pressure level can be misleading in that the magnitude of the difference is distorted. Recall that the essential feature of a histogram is

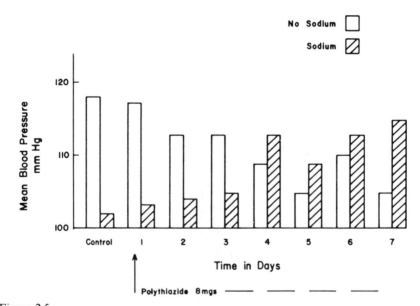

Figure 2.5
Mean blood pressure for a group of subjects before and during daily administration of polythiazide with and without sodium replacement. (From Johnson et al. [61].)

the *area* of the bar. One can envision that if a proper histogram were constructed with an ordinate whose scale started at zero, then the bars would yield quite a different picture for comparison of mean blood pressure levels.

Example 2.11.   Figure 2.6, extracted from an article entitled "Serum lipid patterns in men under 45 years with myocardial infarction" [43], is liable to a different sort of misinterpretation. The chief difficulty is the arbitrary distortion of the scale on the abscissa. The scale clearly is not arithmetical, nor does it correspond to any mathematical rearrangement of scale such as a logarithmic scale. As soon as the bars are connected by lines to indicate the trends over time, the reader can be misled. For example, the last observed values at 24 hours would, if the abscissa were plotted on a proper arithmetical scale, give a somewhat different picture to the time trend of the phenomenon under study. In addition, the built-in lag, with the control values always plotted prior to those for the study group, makes it difficult to compare the two.

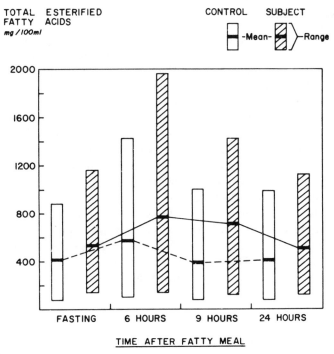

Figure 2.6
Mean and range of total esterified fatty acids at various times after a fatty meal; young adults with myocardial infarction versus controls. (From Freedman and Frajola [43].)

DIFFERENT LOCATION; SAME SPREAD

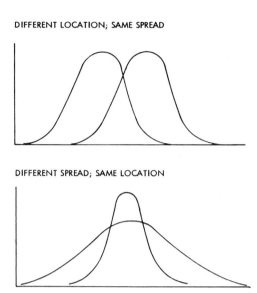

DIFFERENT SPREAD; SAME LOCATION

Figure 2.7
Distributions with different locations but the same spread (top) and with the same location but different spread (bottom).

SUMMARIZATION OF DATA

With a set of data organized into a frequency distribution or with a series of raw, ungrouped observations, interest often focuses on describing the data with one or two summary figures. There are several characteristics that may be examined, the two most common being (1) *location* or *central tendency* and (2) *spread* or *variation*. In Figure 2.7, the top half illustrates two distributions that have the same spread but different locations; the lower half shows two distributions with the same location but with a different spread.

Other characteristics of distributions are occasionally of interest. One such characteristic is the degree of asymmetry or *skewness*. The distributions depicted in Figure 2.7 exhibit symmetry, whereas the distribution of serum uric acid levels (Figure 2.1) indicates some skewness to the right. Another characteristic is the degree of peakedness or *kurtosis* of a distribution. At one extreme are distributions with narrow, sharp peaks (leptokurtic); at the other are those with wide, flat humps (platykurtic). These characteristics are not dealt with in this text. The interested reader will find them discussed in more extensive texts (for example, by Snedecor and Cochran [101]).

Measures of Central Tendency or Location

The three most common measures of location—also called *averages*—are the *mean, median,* and *mode*. Under certain conditions these three measurements are identical; most often, however, they are not. Each has its advantages and disadvantages as a measurement of location.

Mean

The measure familiar to almost everyone is the mean, more appropriately titled the *arithmetic mean*. For a series of ungrouped observations, the mean is defined as the total of the observations divided by the number of observations. If we denote each observation by x, the number of observations by n, and use the summation notation, then the arithmetic mean, which is designated as $\bar{x}$, is

$$\bar{x} = \Sigma x / n$$

The chief advantage of the arithmetic mean is its amenability to mathematical treatment. This advantage, when performing statistical inferences based on the mathematical theory of probability, suffices to explain its extended use throughout this text.

As a purely descriptive measure, however, the mean does have the disadvantage of being seriously affected by extreme values. For example, consider the following data regarding age at death (in years) of five physicians: 34, 64, 68, 70, and 74. Their mean is

$$\bar{x} = \Sigma x / n = 310/5 = 62 \text{ years}$$

Note how the mean is seriously affected by the single aberrant observation of a death at age 34. In fact, four out of the five observations are higher than the mean.

Median

The median is defined as the "middlemost" observation. In other words, the median is that observation which is such that half the observations exceed it and half are below it.

Generally, the median is not as amenable to mathematical treatment as the mean. Although much recent work in theoretical statistics has greatly advanced the statistical manipulations that can be accomplished with the median, these techniques are not widely used by research workers in the medical field. The use of statistical tests involving the median is growing rapidly, but it is unlikely that the mean will be displaced as the prime measurement used in statistical inference.

As a descriptive measure, the median maintains the advantage of being unaffected by extreme observations. For example, with the data on age at death of five physicians, their median is 68. The extreme of a death at age 34, in fact, could have been at any age up to 68 years and the median would remain unchanged at 68 years.

Mode

The mode is the "most popular" or most frequently occurring observation. The mode is even less amenable to mathematical treatment than the median. A particular disadvantage is that, with a small number of observations, there may be no mode. For example, with the data on age at death of five physicians, there is no mode; none of these data occurs more than once. In addition, sometimes there may be more than one mode such as when dealing with a bimodal (two-peak) distribution. The mode is rarely encountered in the scientific literature as a descriptive measure and almost never as the basis for performing statistical inferences.

In unimodal (one-peak) symmetrical distributions, it may be seen that the mean, median, and mode are identical. In unimodal skew distributions, it may be handy to remember that the mean, median, and mode occur in alphabetical order when the longer tail is at the left of the distribution or in reverse alphabetical order when the longer tail is at the right of the distribution.

Which to Use?

As a general guideline, in distributions with some degree of skewness (i.e., distributions that are prone to some tendency toward extreme values), the median is the better descriptive measure than the mean. For purposes of statistical analysis and performing inferences, the mean is more likely to be used. However, when there is considerable skewness, an investigator would do well to consider statistical techniques based on medians or on more specialized methods of analysis.

Other Measures

Clearly, there is a somewhat arbitrary nature to these definitions of measures of central tendency. One might go on almost indefinitely defining ways to manipulate the data so as to obtain measurements of central tendency.

An example of a commonly occurring alternative measure is the geometric mean. The *geometric mean* (GM) is defined as the nth root of the product of the observations. With n observations $x_1, x_2, \ldots, x_n$,

$$\mathrm{GM} = \sqrt[n]{(x_1)(x_2)\cdots(x_n)}$$

The computation is not as formidable as it appears in the above equation. If one takes the logarithm of both sides,

$$\log \mathrm{GM} = \Sigma(\log x)/n$$

In other words, the logarithm of the geometric mean is the arithmetic mean of the logarithms of the individual observations. Thus, for computation, one would obtain the mean of the logarithms and take the antilog of the result to derive the geometric mean.

Another type of mean occasionally encountered is the harmonic mean. The *harmonic mean* (HM) is defined as

$$\mathrm{HM} = n/\Sigma(1/x)$$

Taking reciprocals of both sides gives

$$1/(HM) = \Sigma(1/x)/n$$

In other words, the reciprocal of the harmonic mean is the mean of the reciprocals of the individual observations.

Measures of Spread or Variation

The simplest measure of variation and one that has great intuitive appeal is the *range,* which is defined as the highest minus the lowest value. One disadvantage with the range as a measure of variation is its tendency to increase as the number of observations increases. Clearly, as one accrues more and more observations from a population, one is increasingly likely to obtain values in both tails of the distribution; hence, the range increases. It would be desirable for a measure of variation to remain rather stable, regardless of the sample size. Another disadvantage with the range, despite its great intuitive appeal, is its rather cumbersome nature with regard to the mathematical treatment required in deriving the techniques of statistical inference. Further, on an intuitive basis, the range employs only the two extreme observations and neglects all the information regarding variation that can be obtained from the remaining observations.

As a measure of variation wherein all observations are employed, one might logically consider calculation of deviations from the mean for each observation, $x - \bar{x}$, and then the average of these deviations, namely $\Sigma(x - \bar{x})/n$. This is not helpful, since it can be shown mathematically that $\Sigma(x - \bar{x}) = 0$. In other words, the sum of the deviations about the mean is equal to zero.

One way of avoiding this difficulty would be to add the deviations about the mean and ignore signs; that is, to take the absolute values of the deviations to obtain

$$\Sigma|x - \bar{x}|/n$$

This defines the *mean deviation.* Again, with regard to the goal of statistical inference, the reader may recall from high school and college mathematics that manipulations with absolute values are somewhat difficult. Consequently, the mean deviation is not useful in the mathematical procedures required for performing statistical inferences. The mean deviation is a rarely used measurement.

Another device for disposing of the negative values of deviations from the mean is to square them, since "minus times minus makes plus." Following this line, one can average the squares of the deviations about the mean. This defines the *variance* (V):

$$V(x) = \Sigma(x - \bar{x})^2/(n - 1)$$

Note that in the formula for the variance, $n - 1$ rather than n appears in the denominator. The reason is that in anticipation of the future use of variance in performing statistical inferences, one does better mathematically with $n - 1$ rather than n in the denominator. A proof or rationale for this observation is beyond the scope of this text.

A concept worthy of mention at this point is that of degrees of freedom. For a series of numerical quantities, the *degrees of freedom* (df) refer to the number of independent quantities among the entire series. Alternatively, the degree of freedom may be better conceptualized by defining it as the total number of quantities in the series minus the number of restrictions imposed upon the quantities. In the present consideration of the definition of variance, the quantities involved are deviations about the mean, namely, the series of $x - \bar{x}$ values. There is a total of n such deviations. There is one restriction imposed on these deviations, namely, that their sum is zero, as indicated on p. 32. With n deviations and one restriction, this means $n - 1$ df. In other words, if one were to assign numerical values for a series of n deviations about the mean, then once one had assigned $n - 1$ such numbers, the last number would automatically follow since the sum of all deviations must be zero. Thus, n deviations about the mean contain $n - 1$ df.

A general principle of the mathematical theory underlying statistical inference is that in any form of variance calculations obtained from sample data—be it in the present simple situation or in a more complex form—one does best when one employs the corresponding df in the denominator. Hence, in the present situation, the viewpoint of statistical inference indicates that the variance in a sample be defined as the sum of squares of deviations about the mean divided by their respective df, namely, $n - 1$.

This concept of df arises again later in this text in the uses of t tests for inferences on means (Chapter 4), in the uses of the chi-square test for inferences on proportions (Chapter 5), and with the methods of inference for linear regression and correlation (Chapter 6).

Some textbooks use n in defining the variance of a population and $n - 1$ in defining the variance of a sample. This text employs $n - 1$ almost consistently in an attempt to avoid confusion; the one exception occurs on p. 79. When the sample size or population is large, of course, it matters little which is used.

The variance is quite amenable to mathematical manipulation. Consequently, it is the measure of variation that is used extensively in statistical methods of inference. As a descriptive measure, since it involves squares, it suffers the disadvantage of its units being the square of the units for the original observations. A way of obtaining a measurement of variation in the same units as the original observations is to take the square root of the variance. This defines the *standard deviation* (SD):

$$SD(x) = \sqrt{V(x)} = \sqrt{\Sigma(x - \bar{x})^2/(n - 1)}$$

The standard deviation is the most frequently employed measure of variation in the medical literature.

As with the measures of central tendency, one could go on almost indefinitely defining various measures of variation. There is little purpose in doing so in this text. Knowledge of the meaning of variance and standard deviation suffices for almost all situations the physician is likely to encounter in his reading of the medical literature or in the analysis of his own data.

Because of the importance of the mean, median, and standard deviation in all statistical work, the following section is devoted to the details of their calculation with both ungrouped and grouped observations.

Calculation of Mean, Median, Variance, and Standard Deviation

The formulas for calculating the mean and standard deviation for ungrouped and grouped data are displayed in Table 2.9.

Table 2.9. Formulas for the calculation of the mean and SD with ungrouped and grouped data

	Ungrouped data	Grouped data[a]
Mean	$\Sigma x/n$	$\Sigma fx/\Sigma f$ where f is frequency and x is midpoint of class
SD	$\sqrt{\dfrac{\Sigma(x-\bar{x})^2}{n-1}}$	$\sqrt{\dfrac{\Sigma f(x-\bar{x})^2}{\Sigma f-1}}$
	or their algebraic equivalents, which are computationally simpler:	
	$\sqrt{\dfrac{\Sigma x^2-(\Sigma x)^2/n}{n-1}}$	$\sqrt{\dfrac{\Sigma fx^2-(\Sigma fx)^2/\Sigma f}{\Sigma f-1}}$

[a] The formulas for grouped data result directly from the assumption that all observations within each class of a frequency distribution occur at the midpoint of that class.

For ungrouped data, Table 2.10 illustrates the calculations with a series of 10 pulse rates (in beats per minute) among male first-year medical students. The mean is calculated as 68.7 beats per minute. In the formula for standard deviation, two alternative forms arise from the following algebraic identity for a sum of squares about the mean:

$$\Sigma(x-\bar{x})^2 = \Sigma x^2 - (\Sigma x)^2/n$$

The result can be derived by expanding $(x-\bar{x})^2$, summing terms, and replacing $\bar{x}$ with $\Sigma x/n$. The righthand expression in the equation above is the more convenient computational form. The use of both forms is illustrated in Table 2.10.

In applying the computational form for the sum of squares about the mean, it is well to recognize the distinction between Σx^2 and $(\Sigma x)^2$. The operation Σx^2 means: take each observation, square it, then sum the squares. The operation $(\Sigma x)^2$ means: take the observations, obtain their sum, then square the sum. With any set of numbers, the expression $\Sigma x^2 - (\Sigma x)^2/n$ must be positive. A negative value indicates the presence of a computational error.

With regard to determination of the median, when there is an even number of observations in a series, the median is taken as the value halfway between the $(n/2)$th and $(n/2+1)$th observation. Thus, when the data in Table 2.10 are arrayed in ascending order, the median falls halfway between the fifth (65 beats per minute) and sixth (72 beats per minute) observation. This gives a median of $(65+72)/2 = 68.5$ beats per minute (note the closeness of the median and mean here).

Table 2.10. Calculation of the mean and SD from ungrouped data: pulse rates of 10 male medical students

x Pulse rate (beats/min)	$x-\bar{x}$	$(x-\bar{x})^2$	x^2
59	−9.7	94.09	3,481
72	3.3	10.89	5,184
58	−10.7	114.49	3,364
65	−3.7	13.69	4,225
77	8.3	68.89	5,929
83	14.3	204.49	6,889
72	3.3	10.89	5,184
77	8.3	68.89	5,929
62	−6.7	44.89	3,844
62	−6.7	44.89	3,844
Total 687	0	676.10	47,873

Mean: $\bar{x} = \Sigma x/n = 687/10 = 68.7$ beats per minute

$SD: \sqrt{\Sigma(x-\bar{x})^2/(n-1)} = \sqrt{676.10/9} = \sqrt{75.12} = 8.67$ beats per minute

or

$$\sqrt{\frac{\Sigma x^2 - (\Sigma x)^2/n}{n-1}} = \sqrt{\frac{47,873 - (687)^2/10}{9}} = \sqrt{676.10/9} = \sqrt{75.12}$$

$$= 8.67 \text{ beats per minute}$$

For grouped data, the rationale in calculation of the mean and SD is the assumption that the observations in each class of the frequency distribution are all located at the midpoint of the class. Thus, in calculating a mean for a class with f observations, the value of the midpoint, x, is added f times. In other words, the contribution of that class to the total of the observations is fx. The same reasoning applies to the calculation of the SD. For the SD with grouped data (Table 2.11), there are again two ways of obtaining the sum of squares about the mean, the more convenient computational form being

$$\Sigma fx^2 - (\Sigma fx)^2/(\Sigma f)$$

Table 2.11. Calculation of the mean, SD, and median from grouped data: serum uric acid levels of 267 healthy males

Serum uric acid (mg per 100 ml)	x Mid-point	f Number of men	fx	fx^2	Cumulative number of men
3.0–3.4	3.2	2	6.4	20.48	2
3.5–3.9	3.7	15	55.5	205.35	17
4.0–4.4	4.2	33	138.6	582.12	50
4.5–4.9	4.7	40	188.0	883.60	90
5.0–5.4	5.2	54	280.8	1,460.16	144
5.5–5.9	5.7	47	267.9	1,527.03	191
6.0–6.4	6.2	38	235.6	1,460.72	229
6.5–6.9	6.7	16	107.2	718.24	245
7.0–7.4	7.2	15	108.0	777.60	260
7.5–7.9	7.7	3	23.1	177.87	263
8.0–8.4	8.2	1	8.2	67.24	264
8.5–8.9	8.7	3	26.1	227.07	267
Total		267	1,445.4	8,107.48	

Mean: $\bar{x} = \Sigma fx/\Sigma f = 1,445.4/267 = 5.41$ mg per 100 ml

SD: $\sqrt{\dfrac{\Sigma fx^2 - (\Sigma fx)^2/\Sigma f}{\Sigma f - 1}} = \sqrt{\dfrac{8,107.48 - (1,445.4)^2/267}{266}}$

$$= \sqrt{1.0633} = 1.03 \text{ mg per 100 ml}$$

Median[a]

1. Find uric acid level corresponding to $(267 + 1)/2 = 134$th man;
2. Occurs in class 5.0–5.4 mg per 100 ml;
3. "True" beginning limit of class is 4.95 mg per 100 ml;
4. Estimate value by linear interpolation:
   Median $= 4.95 + [(134 - 90)/54](0.5) = 4.95 + 0.41 = 5.36$ mg per 100 ml

[a] Unlike the calculation of the mean and SD with grouped data, the assumption in calculating the median is that within each class of the frequency distribution, observations are uniformly or evenly distributed over the class interval.

The calculations are illustrated in Table 2.11 for the data on serum uric acid levels. In these calculations, a frequently occurring error concerns the column headed fx^2. Too often, this column is erroneously calculated by squaring the previous column, fx. This yields $(fx)^2 = f^2x^2$, which is not the desired quantity. The correct calculation is obtained by multiplying the fx column values by x, the midpoints indicated in the second column. This then yields the required $(fx)(x) = fx^2$.

Calculation of the median involves a different assumption concerning the distribution of the observations in each class. For the median, it is assumed that observations are uniformly distributed within each class. Thus, determination of the median is analogous to linear interpolation in a mathematical table. The details of the calculation of the median are displayed at the foot of Table 2.11. Here, too, the mean and median for the data employed turn out to be quite similar.

Coded Method for Calculating the Mean and SD with Grouped Data

The calculations in Table 2.11 are rather cumbersome arithmetically. The two-digit numbers for the midpoints x and for the frequencies f yield six-digit numbers in the fx^2 column. In this situation, the computations can be greatly simplified by using the coded method described in this section.

The derivation of this method is as follows. Let x denote the original units in which the data are recorded. Consider a new unit called v, a working unit defined as

$$v = (x - M)/c$$

where M and c are two constants. In mathematical terminology, v is a linear transformation of x. Rewriting the above equation in terms of x gives $x = cv + M$. Now, applying the formula for a mean, it may be seen that $\bar{x} = c\bar{v} + M$. Thus, from calculation of the mean of the v values, the above relation yields the mean of the values of x. Subtracting the equation for $\bar{x}$ from the equation for x gives $x - \bar{x} = (cv + M) - (c\bar{v} + M) = c(v - \bar{v})$. Applying the formula for standard deviation gives SD of $x = c$(SD of v). Hence, from the calculation of the SD of the values of v, the SD of the values of x can be obtained by multiplication by c.

The key is to pick the constants c and M such that the mean and SD of the v values are arithmetically simple. This choice is, of course, completely arbitrary. With unimodal distributions and with equally spaced class intervals, however, the calculations are usually simplified by choosing M to correspond with the midpoint of the class with the highest frequency and c to correspond with the width of the class interval (using true limits). With this choice, the v units become integers, both positive and negative. The calculations using this method for the data on serum uric acid levels are presented in Table 2.12. The simplification in arithmetic is clearly demonstrated upon comparison with Table 2.11.

Table 2.12. Calculation of mean and SD from grouped data using coded method: serum uric acid levels of 267 healthy males

Serum uric acid (mg per 100 ml)	x Mid-point	v Working unit	f Number of men	fv	fv^2
3.0–3.4	3.2	-4	2	-8	32
3.5–3.9	3.7	-3	15	-45	135
4.0–4.4	4.2	-2	33	-66	132
4.5–4.9	4.7	-1	40	-40	40
5.0–5.4	5.2	0	54	0	0
5.5–5.9	5.7	1	47	47	47
6.0–6.4	6.2	2	38	76	152
6.5–6.9	6.7	3	16	48	144
7.0–7.4	7.2	4	15	60	240
7.5–7.9	7.7	5	3	15	75
8.0–8.4	8.2	6	1	6	36
8.5–8.9	8.7	7	3	21	147
Total			267	114	1,180

Mean of v:

$$\bar{v} = \Sigma fv / \Sigma f = 114/267 = 0.427$$

SD of v:

$$SD_v = \sqrt{\frac{\Sigma fv^2 - (\Sigma fv)^2 / \Sigma f}{\Sigma f - 1}} = \sqrt{\frac{1,180 - (114)^2/267}{266}} = \sqrt{4.2531} = 2.062$$

Class interval: $c = 0.5$
Midpoint of interval corresponding with $v = 0$: $M = 5.2$
Mean of x: $\bar{x} = c\bar{v} + M = (0.5)(0.427) + 5.2 = 5.41$ mg per 100 ml
SD of x: $SD_x = cSD_v = (0.5)(2.062) = 1.03$ mg per 100 ml

Other Points Regarding Means and SDs

A common way to present results is "mean $\pm$ 1 SD." Thus, the pulse rate results might appear as "68.7 $\pm$ 8.7 beats per minute," and the serum uric acid results could be reported as "5.41 $\pm$ 1.03 mg per 100 ml."

In addition, in presenting results it is customary to use one more digit for the mean and SD than appears in the raw data.

It should be noted that many investigators employ this same format for presentation of the mean and of another quantity calculated from sample data, the *standard error of the mean* (p. 106). The reader will frequently encounter results expressed as "mean $\pm$ 1 standard error of the mean." Since both forms occur, an author, if he presents his results as "mean $\pm$ some quantity," must clarify to the reader whether the "some quantity" is the standard deviation or the standard error of the mean. Failure to indicate precisely what is the term following the "$\pm$" sign leaves ambiguity and can result in considerable confusion to the reader.

Both the mean and SD are in the same units as the original observations. Thus, to compare the degree of spread of two different clinical quantities, for example, pulse rate and serum uric acid level, it is meaningless to compare the magnitudes of the respective SDs. The pulse rate SD is in beats per minute whereas the serum uric acid SD is in milligrams per 100 milliliters.

The relative spread of distributions can be compared using the *coefficient of variation* (CV), a quantity defined as

$$CV = 100\% \ SD/mean$$

The CV, of course, is a dimensionless quantity. The pulse rate data given above have a CV of 100% (8.7/68.7) = 12.7%, and the serum uric acid levels have a CV of 100% (1.03/5.41) = 19.0%. Thus, the serum uric acid levels are relatively more spread out than pulse rates.

As a means of understanding the use of the standard deviation, it is helpful to remember the following relations among distributions that are unimodal and roughly symmetric:

Mean ± 1 SD encompasses roughly ⅔ of observations

Mean ± 2 SD encompasses roughly 95% of observations

Mean ± 3 SD encompasses virtually all the observations

Finally, with regard to the variability of clinical measurements, it is helpful to add a note concerning the meaning of three commonly misused words *unbiasedness*, *precision*, and *accuracy*. "Unbiasedness" refers to the tendency to arrive at the true or correct value. "Precision" refers to the degree of spread of a series of observations. Thus, medical data may be unbiased but imprecise, and vice versa.

The distinction between unbiasedness and precision is indicated in Figure 2.8. In the top scale of this figure, the observations are unbiased in that, on the average, they tend to the true value. The observations have considerable spread, however, so they lack precision. The bottom scale illustrates little spread among the observations, thus indicating precision, but the observations tend to center at a value displaced from the true value so they are biased.

The term *accuracy* encompasses both unbiasedness and precision. Accurate measurements are *both* unbiased and precise. Inaccurate measurements may be either biased or imprecise or both. Thus, both the top and bottom

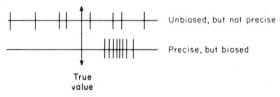

Figure 2.8
Distinction between unbiasedness and precision.

diagrams of Figure 2.8 depict inaccuracy. The top observations are inaccurate because of their imprecision; the bottom observations are inaccurate because of their bias.

VARIATION AND THE STANDARD DEVIATION

Sources of Variation

Since the standard deviation is used to measure variation, it is important to distinguish among various sources of variation in medical observations. This section is concerned with such sources when dealing with a series of quantitative clinical measurements, such as cholesterol levels, blood pressure readings, or serum uric acid determinations.

Generally, these types of clinical determinations are prone to three main sources of variation: *true biological, temporal,* and *measurement error.* "True biological variation" refers to all those factors that tend to make one individual different from another; e.g., age, sex, race, genetic factors, diet, socioeconomic status, and past medical history. "Temporal variation" refers to all those factors that produce variation in observations within an individual from one time to another; e.g., emotional state, activity state, climate, or circadian rhythms. "Measurement error" concerns all the factors that tend to produce differences with different measurements of the same phenomenon; e.g., observers, measuring instruments, technician error, laboratory conditions, or the stability of the reagents used.

To simplify discussion, temporal error will be neglected and attention will be focused on two sources of variation: true biological and measurement error variability. How does one go about segregating these two components? One common technique is replicate (i.e., duplicate, triplicate, and so on) determinations on all or a portion of the material under observation.

An Example of Replicate Determinations

The data in Table 2.13 are triplicate determinations of inulin clearance rates on six dogs.

Table 2.13. Three replicate determinations of inulin clearance rate on six dogs

Dog	First determination	Second determination	Third determination	Total	Means of three determinations
A	75	65	72	212	70.7
B	96	92	76	264	88.0
C	98	109	99	306	102.0
D	91	97	99	287	95.7
E	132	128	126	386	128.7
F	133	136	121	390	130.0
				1,845	615.1
				(Grand total)	(Total)

In describing the variation of these measurements in terms of an SD, there are several SDs that may be calculated. Actually, rather than the SD, its square, the *variance* (V), is calculated. First, the most obvious calculation is to compute the variance of all 18 observations. This gives

$$\frac{\Sigma x^2 - (\Sigma x)^2/n}{n-1} = \frac{75^2 + 65^2 + \cdots + 121^2 - (1{,}845)^2/18}{17} = 509.7$$

This variance, however, is of little value and difficult to interpret. It does not distinguish between observations on the same and on different dogs. It indiscriminately lumps measurement error with true biological variability.

A second possibility is to obtain the mean inulin clearance rate for each dog and then to calculate the variance among these six means. The means of the three determinations are given in the last column of the table. The resulting variance among the six means is

$$\frac{\Sigma x^2 - (\Sigma x)^2/n}{n-1} = \frac{70.7^2 + \cdots + 130.0^2 - (615.1)^2/6}{5} = 542.1$$

This variance deals mainly with *inter*subject variability and is most appropriate for the determination of the true biological variation. This variance does contain a component of measurement error variation, since the basic observations are means of three determinations and each determination is subject to measurement error. With suitable modification, the measurement error component can be eliminated so a pure estimate of true biological variability is obtained. The important point, however, for the present discussion is that the above variance calculation is the basis for estimating the magnitude of true biological variation.

A third variance is obtained as follows. First, for each dog calculate the variance of the three determinations. For dog *A* this gives

$$\frac{\Sigma x^2 - (\Sigma x)^2/n}{n-1} = \frac{75^2 + 65^2 + 72^2 - (212)^2/3}{2} = 26.3$$

For dogs *B, C, D, E,* and *F,* it may be verified that the variances among their three determinations are 112.0, 37.0, 17.3, 9.3, and 63.0, respectively. Next, obtain the mean of these six variances:

$$\text{Mean variance} = \frac{26.3 + 112.0 + 37.0 + 17.3 + 9.3 + 63.0}{6} = 44.2$$

The resulting mean variance deals with *intra*subject variability and is concerned directly with measurement error variation. This estimate of measurement error variance indicates the precision of the technique for measuring inulin clearance rate.

Thus, the two variances above, 542.1 and 44.2, form the basis for segregating true biological and measurement error variation. For any further analysis of the data, one must ask which source of variation is most relevant to the goals of such analysis. For example, further statements regarding the precision of measurement would employ the variance of 44.2. Further analysis regarding subject-to-subject variation—for example, drawing a conclusion regarding a population of dogs for which these data represent a sample of six—would employ the variance of 542.1.

This example illustrates the principles of a very important and frequently employed statistical technique called the *analysis of variance*. The variation among the total of 18 observations has been segregated into two components: inter- (or *between*) subject and intra- (or *within*) subject variation. The reader who proceeds to more advanced texts in statistics (e.g., [2, 12, 29, 101]) will encounter considerable coverage of the analysis of variance. The general principle is the same that is used here, namely, to isolate and assess the contribution of different factors to variation of data. Of course, the subject-matter of analysis of variance ranges from the present simple situation of two components—"between" and "within" variation—to more complex situations in which one may isolate many components of variation within a complex experimental arrangement for data collection.

Assumptions Underlying Variance Calculations

It should be noted that the variance calculations result from a series of assumptions concerning the nature of the data. The three most important assumptions are:

1. *Additivity.* Each observation in Table 2.13 consists of the sum of a true inulin clearance rate for the dog plus a component that is due to measurement error.

2. *Constancy of measurement error variation.* The effect of measurement error is the same, no matter what the level of the inulin clearance rate. In other words, the magnitude of measurement error for the data in Table 2.13 is unrelated to whether the dog's true inulin clearance rate is high, low, or in the middle.

3. *Independence of measurement errors.* The magnitude of measurement error on any one of the total of 18 observations reported in Table 2.13 is unaffected by the magnitude of the measurement error component for any other observation.

Although it is beyond the scope of this text, it is possible to use the data collected to test the validity of these assumptions.

Mishandling of Replicate Data

Often an investigator obtains replicate observations and fails to account for this in his analysis. In addition to incorrect data analysis, the reader is often misled into believing there are many more observations than there actually are. For example, in a study of the distribution of inulin clearance rates in the general population, the claim of a sample size of several hundred observations might actually involve many replicate observations on only a few individuals, say, no more than 25. Data analysis that fails to distinguish between observations on the same individual and observations on different individuals is entirely meaningless. If the goal pertains to the distribution of inulin clearance rates in the general population, the most important item regarding sample size is the number of different individuals and *not* the total number of observations. With such an objective, the data analysis would most profitably be carried out by a determination of the means of the replicate observations on each individual.

Example 2.12.   Consider the following plan for determining the antihypertensive effects of new drugs in ambulant hypertensive patients [45]. The essense of the scheme is that known hypertensive patients would be observed for an extended period of time on a test drug and for the same duration of time on a standard antihypertensive drug in the following way:

> The members of the team who obtain the information are without knowledge of the agent they dispense. They merely give the patient a small pill box bearing a number of 3 or 4 digits. The pill box contains the number of capsules required for the week. The following week the number on the box is different. The contents may be the same or different.

> The patient takes the capsule every day as instructed. He visits the clinic on Monday and Friday for measuring the blood pressure. When 5 readings are made at a visit, every week yields 10 blood pressure readings. Their average represents the blood pressure for the week. If the treatment period is 8 weeks, the average of 80 readings represents the blood pressure during the use of the particular agent. If 10 test-patients are used, the blood pressure value during the use of that agent represents the average of 800 blood pressure readings. . . .

> The averages are based on such a large mass of readings that verification by statistics of any differences which might occur is unnecessary.

Without doubt, the 800 blood pressure readings on a drug do represent a large mass of readings. The readings, however, are not on 800 different patients. Table 2.14 displays a layout for the 800 observations analogous to the inulin clearance data used previously. The key feature of Table 2.14 is the 10 rows corresponding to the 10 subjects.

In assessing the effect of the new agent, the mass of 800 observations is *not* the important feature of the sample size. Obviously, one cannot simply proceed to analyze the 800 observations as if they derived from 800 different patients. The analysis of 800 observations on 800 different subjects must differ from that of 80 observations on 10 subjects, which, in turn, must differ from that of 800 observations on a single subject. The assessment of the drug's effect involves a statistical inference from the sample of 10 to a larger population of hypertensive subjects.

Table 2.14 indicates that the design is well set up for temporal variation. One could quantitate the temporal variation of five repeat measurements over a relatively short time period, the temporal variation from the beginning to the end of a work week, and, finally, the temporal variation from week to week during a period of approximately two months' usage. However, appropriate conclusions regarding the drug's effect rely on subject-to-subject variation, which is essentially the variance among the means of the 80 measurements on each subject. The sample size of 10 is crucial to such analysis.

Table 2.14. Format for 80 blood pressure readings on 10 hypertensive patients during eight-week use of an antihypertensive agent

| | Week 1 | | | Week 8 | |
| | Monday | Friday | | Monday | Friday |
Patient	1 2 3 4 5	1 2 3 4 5	⋯ ⋯	1 2 3 4 5	1 2 3 4 5
1	————	————	⋯ ⋯	————	————
2	————	————	⋯ ⋯	————	————
3	————	————	⋯ ⋯	————	————
4	————	————	⋯ ⋯	————	————
5	————	————	⋯ ⋯	————	————
6	————	————	⋯ ⋯	————	————
7	————	————	⋯ ⋯	————	————
8	————	————	⋯ ⋯	————	————
9	————	————	⋯ ⋯	————	————
10	————	————	⋯ ⋯	————	————

A moral to be derived from this example is that care should be taken to avoid being misled by great masses of observations. Upon close scrutiny, these masses may often vanish. The "great mass" may merely consist of many replicate measurements on a handful of subjects. The following situations involving great masses of data are prone to such mishandling and misinterpretation: episodes, attacks, or exacerbation of a disease, menstrual cycles during use of some contraceptive, or units of blood transfused. The key question is, observations on how many different patients? The further purpose of the investigation must also be clearly stated so that one can determine whether it is true biological variation, measurement error, or temporal variation that is of chief concern.

Variation and the Interpretation of Clinical Measurements

When presented with a clinical or laboratory measurement obtained from a patient, interpretation involves—either explicitly or, more often, implicitly—the following three basic statistical sets of questions:

1. *How reproducible is the observation?* Would repeat determination by the same physician, by another physician, or by the same or a different

laboratory yield a similar result? In other words, what is the effect and magnitude of measurement error variation? If this error is large and the observation is not reproducible, then the observation is of little value.

2. *How does the measurement distribute in normal and abnormal individuals?* What is the "normal range" and what is considered abnormal? In other words, one must have knowledge of the true biological variation if one is to interpret the result properly.

3. *Are there any unusual occurrences or untoward events that might explain the observation?* For example, might the observation be affected by the patient's anxiety state, his degree of physical activity, the time of day, or whatever? Here, the focus is on temporal variation in addition to other possibilities for the explanation of what may appear as an aberrant result.

VITAL STATISTICS

As indicated in Chapter 1, vital statistics constitute the body of techniques used to describe the health status of populations. The goal of this section is to review briefly the techniques of vital statistics that the physician is likely to encounter in his reading of the medical literature. Emphasis naturally falls on those methods regarding vital statistics that deal with mortality.

Mortality Rates

Rates form the essential ingredients of vital statistics methods. For mortality, the numerator of a death rate for some period of time is a count of deaths during that time period as reported to local and, subsequently, to national

Table 2.15. Deaths, midyear population, crude, and age-specific mortality rates for total U.S. population, 1967

Age (yr)	Deaths during year	Midyear population (in thousands)	Age-specific death rates (per 100,000 population)
< 1	79,028	3,539	2,233.1
1–4	13,506	15,652	86.3
5–9	8,809	20,910	42.1
10–14	8,084	19,885	40.7
15–24	37,706	32,265	116.9
25–44	108,825	46,656	233.2
45–64	459,203	40,160	1,143.4
65–74	437,919	11,678	3,749.9
75–84	469,669	5,945	7,900.2
85+	227,987	1,174	19,419.7
Total	1,850,736	197,864	935.4
			(Crude death rate)

Data from Public Health Service [90].

authorities. The denominator is the population at risk during that time period as determined by census, special population enumerations, and the reporting and recording of births.

To illustrate rates commonly employed in summarizing mortality, Table 2.15 displays the deaths and midyear population by age of the United States in 1967. Note that the age distribution of deaths has already been presented in Table 2.8.

The *crude annual death rate* is the simplest of the mortality rates and is defined as the total deaths during the year divided by the total midyear population. To avoid many decimal places, it is customary to multiply death rates by 100,000 and express the results as deaths per 100,000 population. The foot of Table 2.15 indicates that the crude annual death rate for the United States in 1967 was 935.4 deaths per 100,000 population.

One refinement in death rate calculations is to distribute both deaths and population among several categories along the dimension of some crucial variable and then to calculate death rates separately within each category. These are called *specific death rates*. Age, almost invariably, comprises a crucial variable in mortality; thus the reader most often encounters *age-specific death rates*. For the age groups in Table 2.15, the age-specific death rates are shown in the last column. The tremendous variation in these rates underlines the importance of age in relation to mortality. In addition to age, often sex and race relate closely to mortality, and, in many instances, the reader will encounter death rates specific for age, sex, and race simultaneously.

One mortality rate that is of particular interest and is widely employed in the medical literature is the *infant mortality rate*. This is defined as the ratio of the number of deaths during a calendar year among infants under one year of age to the total number of live births during that year. Many experts consider the infant mortality rate as a particularly responsive and sensitive index of the health status of a country or geographical area. No doubt, a number of readers will already be familiar with the controversy that has existed concerning the interpretation of the United States' international ranking according to infant mortality rate (see, for example, Rutstein [95]).

In many circumstances, attention focuses on *cause-specific death rates*. When a death certificate is completed, in addition to vital information regarding the decedent's age, sex, race, and so forth, the attending physician is required to list the underlying cause of death. Completed death certificates are filed with local authorities (usually the town or county) and then are sent to the state office where the causes of death are coded. The number scheme employed for coding deaths is one agreed upon on an international level and is called the *International Classification of Diseases* [119]. This coding scheme is periodically reviewed and updated under the auspices of the World Health Organization. The death certificates filed with state authorities eventually reach the federal government (through the offices of the National Center for Health Statistics in the U.S. Public Health Service), where extensive tabulations on a national level are prepared. Many of these tabulations involve cause-specific death rates. A mortality rate that is specific for cause consists of the number of deaths from that cause during a calendar year in the numerator and the total midyear population, as before, in the denominator. For example, the ingredients for the study that will be described in Chapter 11 (p. 272) consisted of motor vehicle accident mortality rates. Furthermore, the rates employed for this study were age-, sex-, race-, and state-specific as well.

Morbidity Rates

Morbidity rates, which are analogous to the mortality rates described above, report the impact of a disease on a population. The numerator of a morbidity rate is the number of cases of a particular disease; the denominator is the population in risk of the disease. In the analysis of morbidity data, interest often focuses on the determination of morbidity-rates specific for age, sex, race, and so forth.

With morbidity, however, there is one point worth stressing, and this is the distinction between the prevalence and incidence rates of a disease. *Prevalence* refers to the cases of the disease that exist at a specified instant of time or during some period of time. *Incidence* refers to the number of new cases of the disease that develop during some specified time interval. Thus, a prevalence rate (or, more precisely, ratio) is the number of cases divided by the population at that instant of time, or, over a time period, it is the number of existing cases divided by the mid-period population during that period. On the other hand, an incidence rate has as its numerator the number of new cases of the diseases that arise during the specified time interval and, as its denominator, the population in risk but free of the disease at the beginning of the time interval.

Epidemiologists and biostatisticians are quite fussy about the use of the words "incidence" and "prevalence"; the two words mean quite different things. The word "incidence," however, is among the most generally misused terms in the medical literature. One commonly sees it used improperly either when "prevalence rate" is the appropriate term, or, sometimes, when the quantity under consideration is not even a rate but just a raw count of the number of cases (see Example 12.1). One should remember that an incidence rate should *always* be expressed in terms of time; for example, cases per population per year, month, or some other time interval unit.

For chronic diseases, the determination of prevalence is considerably simpler than the determination of incidence. For example, a *prevalence* study of coronary heart disease in a community would consist in identifying all cases of coronary heart disease that existed, say, during a year's time. This would include new cases that developed during the year as well as those cases that had been identified in previous years (provided, of course, the old cases were alive during the year of study). The denominator would consist of the midyear population of the community. A one-year *incidence* study of coronary heart disease in this same community, however, would entail determining the population that is free from coronary heart disease at the beginning of the year. One would need to identify all new cases that develop during the year.

With the number of new cases as the numerator and the population free of the disease at the start of the interval as the denominator, one can determine the incidence rate.

Adjusted Rates

One of the main difficulties in the comparison of crude rates among various geographical areas or over a period of time is that the basic characteristics of the population may also differ substantially, particularly with regard to age. The calculation of specific rates will assist in ensuring a proper comparison, but these may involve a considerable number of figures for comparison. There would be some advantage in determination of a single summary rate figure— be it for mortality or morbidity—that accounts or adjusts for the differences among populations regarding these other variables. The two principal techniques of adjustment of vital statistics rates are referred to as the *direct* and *indirect methods*. The direct method is illustrated first. The data chosen for illustration concern the adjustment for age of cancer mortality rates. Of course, adjustments in rates can be made for any subclassification of the data, such as sex and race. Likewise, adjusted rates apply as well to morbidity as to mortality.

Direct Method

The requirements for the calculation of an age-adjusted rate by the direct method are (1) the availability of age-specific rates in each of the population groups under study and (2) the designation of a standard population age distribution. The illustrative data concern cancer mortality among American females during the period 1929 to 1931. The goal is to compare cancer mortality rates of single and married women, with adjustment being made for differences in the age distribution of the two groups. Table 2.16 displays the cancer deaths (columns 3 and 6), population (columns 2 and 5), and age-specific cancer mortality rates (columns 4 and 7) of single and married women. At the foot of columns 4 and 7 appear the crude death rates: 61.7 per 100,000 for single women and 137.2 per 100,000 for married women, more than a twofold difference. Without doubt, the age distributions of the two groups differ, the married women, of course, being older. Therefore, a good portion of the difference in crude rates may be explained by the greater proportion of older women in the married group who are in high risk of cancer mortality. The purpose in calculating an age-adjusted rate is to remove the effect of age differential so a meaningful comparison of cancer mortality according to marital status would result.

The standard population for the calculation of the age-adjusted death rate was chosen as the total American female population divided according to age in 1930 (i.e., the total of single, married, widowed, and divorced women as shown in column 8 of Table 2.16). The age-adjusted mortality rates are derived by applying the age-specific rates for each of the two groups—single and

Table 2.16. Calculation of age-adjusted rates by the direct method: cancer mortality for single and married females, United States, 1929–31 (adjusted to total U.S. female distribution by age)

	Single women			Married women			
1	2	3	4	5	6	7	8
Age (yr)	Population (× 1,000)	Cancer deaths	Cancer death rate (per 100,000 pop.)	Population (× 1,000)	Cancer deaths	Cancer death rate (per 100,000 pop.)	Pop. distribution for all women (× 1,000)
15–24	6,129.5	226	3.69	2,627.5	141	5.37	8,847.1
25–34	1,485.4	251	16.90	5,923.8	1,335	22.54	7,725.2
35–44	759.0	612	80.63	5,610.3	4,630	82.53	6,924.3
45–54	522.4	1,198	229.33	3,876.4	7,894	203.64	5,189.4
55–64	343.5	1,511	439.88	2,124.3	8,155	383.89	3,454.1
65–74	187.9	1,340	713.15	828.2	5,346	645.50	2,002.0
≥ 75	45.1	707	1,567.63	154.2	1,513	981.19	825.0
Total	9,472.8	5,845	61.70	21,144.7	29,014	137.22	34,967.1

Age-Adjusted Cancer Mortality Rates (Per 100,000 Population):

Single women
$$\frac{(8{,}847.1)\,(3.69) + \ldots + (825.0)\,(1{,}567.63)}{34{,}967.1} = \frac{6{,}152{,}004}{34{,}967.1} = 175.94$$

Married women
$$\frac{(8{,}847.1)\,(5.37) + \ldots + (825.0)\,(981.19)}{34{,}967.1} = \frac{5{,}277{,}634}{34{,}967.1} = 150.93$$

married women (columns 4 and 7)—to the standard population (column 8) and dividing by the total in the standard population (34,967,100; from the foot of column 8). This procedure is outlined at the bottom of Table 2.16, and it yields age-adjusted mortality rates of 175.9 per 100,000 population for single women and 150.9 per 100,000 population for married women. These age-adjusted rates are interpreted as the cancer mortality rates that would apply if both the married and single women's age composition were the same as that for the total female population. Thus, when the effect of age is removed, it may be seen that *single women, compared with married women, have a slightly higher age-adjusted mortality rate from cancer.*

The study from which these data were taken receives more detailed discussion in Chapter 12 (p. 294). The point is that comparison of mortality by marital status requires, at the very least, correction for age differential. Age-adjusted rates calculated by the direct method provide an appropriate correction. The most meaningful comparison of cancer mortality in single and married women is, of course, the detailed age-specific rates of columns 4 and 7. The purpose of calculating an age-adjusted rate is merely to condense this comparison into a single, summary statistic.

It should be noted that with rate adjustment by the "direct" method, the results depend somewhat on the choice of the standard. Different standard populations will lead to different adjusted rates. The point, however, is that one usually encounters adjustment of rates within the context of comparison of two or more groups. As one goes from one standard population to another, the magnitude of the *differences* for the various adjusted rates will not alter materially, provided that the standard populations do not differ radically. In other words, for the example under consideration, the choice of some other standard population would matter little in the magnitude of the difference between single and married women in their age-adjusted cancer mortality rates.

Indirect Method

The requirements for the calculation of an age-adjusted mortality rate by the indirect method are (1) the distributions by age in each of the population groups under study and (2) the choice of a set of age-specific rates for a standard population. The data used before to illustrate the direct method—i.e., cancer mortality among single and married American females during 1929 to 1931—serve to illustrate the indirect method as well.

Table 2.17 demonstrates the procedure. Columns 2 and 3 present the required age distributions for single and married women, respectively. The standard population chosen was the total number of American females in 1929 to 1931, and column 4 presents the requisite age-specific mortality rates in the standard population. The essence of the calculation is the determination in each of the groups under study of the total *expected* deaths. These are the deaths one would expect to occur under the presumption that the age-specific rates of the standard population prevailed in each of the groups under study.

Table 2.17. Calculation of age-adjusted rates by the indirect method: cancer mortality for single and married females, United States, 1929–31 (age-specific cancer mortality for total U.S. females chosen as standard)

1	2	3	4
	Population distribution		Age-specific cancer mortality rates in standard population (total U.S. females, 1929–31) (rates per 100,000 population)
Age (yr)	Single women (× 1,000)	Married women (× 1,000)	
15–24	6,129.5	2,627.5	4.27
25–34	1,485.4	5,923.8	22.03
35–44	759.0	5,610.3	84.88
45–54	522.4	3,876.4	214.40
54–64	343.5	2,124.3	411.40
64–74	187.9	828.2	695.88
≥75	45.1	154.2	1,095.88
Total	9,472.8	21,144.7	160.90 = Crude mortality rate in standard population

	Single women	Married women
Cancer deaths:		
Observed	5,845	29,014
Expected (at rate in standard population)	5,567.9	30,681.7
Standard mortality ratio (100 × Observed ÷ Expected)	105.0	94.6
Adjusted cancer mortality rate (per 100,000 population)	(160.90) (1.050) = 168.9	(160.90) (0.946) = 152.2

Thus, the expected deaths result from application of the age-specific death rates among the standard population (column 4) to the study populations of single women (column 2) and married women (column 3). For single women, the expected deaths are

$$\tfrac{1}{100}[(6,129.5)(4.27) + (1,485.4)(22.03) + \cdots + (45.1)(1,095.88)] = 5,567.9$$

whereas for married women the expected deaths are

$$\tfrac{1}{100}[(2,627.5)(4.27) + (5,923.8)(22.03) + \cdots + (154.2)(1,095.88)] = 30,681.7$$

(Note that the factor of 1/100 comes from the fact that the mortality rates are per 100,000 population but the population figures are in thousands, thus requiring multiplication by 1,000/100,000 = 1/100.)

One now compares the expected cancer deaths with the observed cancer deaths in each group (the observed deaths are 5,845 for single and 29,014 for married women). The ratios of observed to expected deaths (100 times those observed divided by those expected) are 105.0 for married and 94.6 for single women. Many uses of the indirect method end at this stage with the calculation of these ratios, called *standard mortality ratios*. (Had the basic ingredients been morbidity rather than the present mortality rates, the term, of course, would be *standard morbidity ratio*.) At this point the results indicate that, after age adjustment, single women have a 5 percent higher cancer mortality rate than that of all women, whereas married women have a 5 percent lower cancer mortality rate than that of all women.

One could also proceed to calculate the actual age-adjusted rate in each group. These rates derive from multiplication of the crude mortality rate in the standard population (the rate of 160.90 cancer deaths per 100,000 at the foot of column 4) by the respective standard mortality ratios. The age-adjusted rates are shown at the bottom of Table 2.17. Thus, by the indirect method and with the choice of age-specific cancer mortality rates of all American females in 1929 to 1931 as the standard, the age-adjusted cancer mortality rates are 168.9 deaths per 100,000 population for single women and 152.2 deaths per 100,000 population for married women.

The numbers may differ slightly for age-adjustment by the direct method compared with the indirect method, but the conclusion is the same. With adjustment or removal of the effects of age, single women have somewhat higher cancer mortality than married women: their rate is approximately 10 to 15 percent higher than that of married women.

The question of whether to use the direct or indirect method often depends on the data available. If age-specific rates are available in each of the population groups under comparison, one will find investigators more likely to choose to adjust by the direct method. When the age-specific rates by population groups are not available, the investigator has no other choice but to adjust by the indirect method. With vital statistics data for large units such as states or countries, the requisite age-specific rates are usually available, and the reader will most often encounter adjustment by the direct method. With vital statistics for small units—such as counties, towns, or municipalities—and with many epidemiological investigations of morbidity, the age-specific rates for each unit are not available. Here the reader will most frequently encounter the indirect method of adjustment, often with the calculations proceeding no farther than the determination of standard morbidity or mortality ratios.

Population Life Tables

The *population life table* is a convenient format for summarizing the mortality experience of a large community, such as a country or a state. At the outset, it is well to emphasize that the life-table values summarize mortality experience *at a particular time*. As such, they are denoted as "period life tables." The quantities contained in population life tables derive from the age-specific mortality rates in that population at that particular period of time.

Table 2.18. Abridged life tables by race and sex, United States, 1968

WHITE, MALE

Age interval (yr) x to x+n	Proportion of persons alive at beginning of age interval dying during interval nq_x	Number living at beginning of age interval l_x	Number dying during age interval nd_x	Average number of years of life remaining at beginning of age interval $\mathring{e}_x$
0–1	0.0219	100,000	2,186	67.5
1–5	0.0033	97,814	326	68.0
5–10	0.0024	97,488	232	64.3
10–15	0.0025	97,256	239	59.4
15–20	0.0073	97,017	710	54.6
20–25	0.0098	96,307	943	49.9
25–30	0.0083	95,364	794	45.4
30–35	0.0091	94,570	860	40.8
35–40	0.0131	93,710	1,232	36.1
40–45	0.0208	92,478	1,927	31.6
45–50	0.0341	90,551	3,088	27.2
50–55	0.0557	87,463	4,876	23.0
55–60	0.0872	82,587	7,198	19.2
60–65	0.1320	75,389	9,949	15.8
65–70	0.1864	65,440	12,197	12.8

ALL OTHER, MALE

Age interval (yr) x to x+n	Proportion of persons alive at beginning of age interval dying during interval nq_x	Number living at beginning of age interval l_x	Number dying during age interval nd_x	Average number of years of life remaining at beginning of age interval $\mathring{e}_x$
0–1	0.0378	100,000	3,778	60.1
1–5	0.0060	96,222	576	61.4
5–10	0.0034	95,646	322	57.8
10–15	0.0038	95,324	364	53.0
15–20	0.0107	94,960	1,015	48.2
20–25	0.0182	93,945	1,706	43.6
25–30	0.0225	92,239	2,077	39.4
30–35	0.0293	90,162	2,642	35.3
35–40	0.0380	87,520	3,322	31.2
40–45	0.0521	84,198	4,387	27.4
45–50	0.0701	79,811	5,591	23.7
50–55	0.0956	74,220	7,092	20.3
55–60	0.1344	67,128	9,023	17.2
60–65	0.1830	58,105	10,633	14.5
65–70	0.2605	47,472	12,368	12.1

Left table (WHITE, FEMALE)

Age				
70–75	0.2722	53,243	14,494	10.2
75–80	0.3571	38,749	13,835	8.1
80–85	0.4675	24,914	11,646	6.2
85 and over	1.0000	13,268	13,268	4.5

WHITE,
FEMALE

Age				
0–1	0.0164	100,000	1,637	74.9
1–5	0.0027	98,363	270	75.1
5–10	0.0017	98,093	165	71.3
10–15	0.0014	97,928	139	66.4
15–20	0.0029	97,789	281	61.5
20–25	0.0032	97,508	314	56.7
25–30	0.0035	97,194	344	51.9
30–35	0.0048	96,850	465	47.1
35–40	0.0076	96,385	731	42.3
40–45	0.0119	95,654	1,141	37.0
45–50	0.0186	94,513	1,762	33.0
50–55	0.0280	92,751	2,599	28.6
55–60	0.0412	90,152	3,715	24.3
60–65	0.0616	86,437	5,323	20.2
65–70	0.0965	81,114	7,828	16.4
70–75	0.1554	73,286	11,392	12.9
75–80	0.2426	61,894	15,013	9.8
80–85	0.3749	46,881	17,578	7.0
85 and over	1.0000	29,303	29,303	4.8

Right table (ALL OTHER, FEMALE)

Age				
70–75	0.3524	35,104	12,370	10.5
75–80	0.3393	22,734	7,713	9.9
80–85	0.3669	15,021	5,512	8.7
85 and over	1.0000	9,509	9,509	7.4

ALL OTHER,
FEMALE

Age				
0–1	0.0311	100,000	3,114	67.5
1–5	0.0049	96,886	476	68.7
5–10	0.0024	96,410	229	65.0
10–15	0.0021	96,181	202	60.2
15–20	0.0041	95,979	390	55.3
20–25	0.0069	95,589	660	50.5
25–30	0.0100	94,929	948	45.9
30–35	0.0151	93,981	1,417	41.3
35–40	0.0222	92,564	2,055	36.9
40–45	0.0317	90,509	2,866	32.7
45–50	0.0432	87,643	3,790	28.6
50–55	0.0589	83,853	4,935	24.8
55–60	0.0846	78,918	6,675	21.2
60–65	0.1245	72,243	8,996	17.9
65–70	0.1987	63,247	12,569	15.1
70–75	0.2327	50,678	11,794	13.2
75–80	0.2406	38,884	9,354	11.5
80–85	0.3054	29,530	9,020	9.3
85 and over	1.0000	20,510	20,510	7.3

Data from Public Health Service [89].

A population life table refers to a hypothetical population. The key to its interpretation is that it represents the mortality experience of a hypothetical 100,000 infants born alive and who are subjected to the age-specific death rates that prevail in the population at the particular time. Table 2.18 exhibits four life tables for four sex and race categories of the American population in 1968. For example, the life table for white males represents the mortality experience of a hypothetical 100,000 infants born alive and subjected to the age-specific mortality rates of American white males in 1968.

The life tables in Table 2.18 bear the label "abridged" in that they present quantities for age in intervals rather than for single years of age. Life tables for single years of age are calculated and published, but it is the abridged life tables that the medical reader most frequently encounters.

The column headed $_nq_x$ represents essentially the death rates for each age interval. More precisely, $_nq_x$ denotes the proportion of persons alive at the beginning of the age interval who die during that interval. It is shown in Chapter 3 that these values may be interpreted as "conditional probabilities." They represent the chance that an individual dies during a particular age interval, conditional upon his having survived to the beginning of that interval. For example, among white males 20 to 25 years old, the chance is .0098 that a white male who survived to age 20 will die before reaching his 25th birthday (provided, of course, that the 1968 white male mortality rates prevail).

The l_x column represents the cumulative survival to the beginning of each interval. At age 0, there are of course the 100,000 born alive. At age 1, after the death rate during the first year of life has taken its toll, there are 97,814 of the 100,000 who remain alive. At age 25, after successive applications of the appropriate death rates, 95,364 remain alive. At age 65, there remain 65,440 alive. Finally at age 85, there are 13,268 of the original 100,000 left alive, and, since this is the last tabulated interval, beyond age 85 all die.

The l_x values can be used to determine the chance of survival from any one age to some other age. If one is interested in the chance of survival from time of birth, one needs only to divide the l_x figures by 100,000. Thus, the chance is .97814 that a newborn white male survives to his first birthday, .95364 that he survives to his 25th birthday, .65440 that he survives to his 65th birthday, and .13268 that he survives to his 85th birthday. It may be seen for white males that the median survival—i.e., the age at which half the original 100,000 (or 50,000) remain alive—occurs somewhere in the interval of 70 to 75 years. Thus, a white male, exposed throughout his lifetime to the 1968 mortality rates, has better than an even chance of surviving to celebrate his 70th birthday.

To determine the chance of survival from any age other than birth, one has merely to divide by the appropriate l_x values. For example, what is the chance that a 25-year-old white male survives to age 65? Since 95,364 of the hypothetical 100,000 are alive at age 25 and 65,440 are alive at age 65, then the chance that a 25-year-old white male survives to age 65 is 65,440/95,364 = .6863. (This result will be shown in Chapter 3 to involve conditional probabilities and the use of the multiplicative law of probability.)

Attached to the determinations in the above two paragraphs is the condition, "provided that the 1968 mortality rates prevail." A recent white male medical school graduate at age 25 who is contemplating his chances of surviving to a retirement age of 65 surely has better prospects than that indicated above. The calculated chance is based on the American white male population mortality in 1968. One has many reasons to expect a continuation of improved mortality experience over the years, due in part to general social and economic improvements and to medical and technological advances. Thus, the chance of .6863 may be taken as a lower limit to what he might anticipate. Parenthetically, one reason for considering the figure as a lower limit is that numerous studies have demonstrated a more favorable survival rate for physicians as compared with the general population (see, for example, Williams et al. [116]).

Subtraction between the successive l_x values gives, of course, the number of deaths during each age interval, namely, the $_nd_x$ column. For example, the $_nd_x$ value of 2,186 for white males age 0 to 1 is obtained as $100,000 - 97,814 = 2,186$. Alternatively, it may be seen that $_nd_x = (_nq_x)(l_x)$. In other words, the number of deaths is the product of the death rate for the interval and the number of survivors at the beginning of the interval. (Note that in the notation for life-table functions, a subscript n preceding a quantity indicates that the quantity refers to what happens during the interval; no preceding subscript indicates that the quantity refers to the beginning of the interval. Thus, $_nd_x$ and $_nq_x$ represent deaths and death rates during the interval; l_x represents survivors at the beginning of the interval.)

The last column of the life table, $\overset{\circ}{e}_x$, is the most frequently cited of the life-table values. This is the expectation of life. At age 0, it represents the mean lifetime of the 100,000 hypothetical newborn babies who die at the indicated rates. American white males born in 1968 have a life expectancy of 67.5 years. This has nothing to do with the average age at death or the age of the 1968 American white male population. It means only that a group of hypothetical babies who are subject to the 1968 white male death rates would survive, on the average, 67.5 years. Comparison of the $\overset{\circ}{e}_x$ values at age 0 for males and females shows that females outlive males by about seven years for both whites and nonwhites. Furthermore, a comparison of life expectancies at birth for whites and nonwhites reveals whites outlive nonwhites by about seven years for both males and females.

The $\overset{\circ}{e}_x$ values for ages other than birth refer to the average number of years of expected survival among those who have already survived to the beginning of the age interval. These, too, are to be interpreted within the constraints of the 1968 age-specific mortality rates applied to a hypothetical cohort of newborn infants. The recent white male medical graduate at age 25 might note that white males in the general population have, on the average, 45.4 more years of life remaining, provided that they are subject to the 1968 mortality rates. For the reasons mentioned above, however, his own life expectancy would be higher.

Another interesting feature of the average duration-of-life figures is that for each sex-race group, the value is higher at age 1 than at age 0. Thus, those who survive to age 1 have greater life expectancy than newborn infants. This is not an anomaly, but reflects the tremendous impact of infant mortality.

Finally, note that the life expectancy at birth for each sex-race group is lower than the median duration of life (the median is determined by the age group wherein the l_x value is 50,000). For example, white males have a life expectancy of 67.5 years at birth but their median age of survival is between 70 and 75 years. This indicates that the distribution of survival is far from symmetrical. The distribution is skewed to the left because the mean is affected considerably by the deaths at younger ages.

Life tables are also extremely useful in summarizing results obtained in longitudinal investigations. The use of the life table in this format—e.g., to determine the prognosis or outcome in the study of chronic disease—appears in Chapter 9.

EXERCISES

1. A class experiment with 60 first-year male medical students involved their measuring blood pressure on one another. The measurements were to be read to the nearest even number of mm Hg. The results for systolic blood pressure (in mm Hg) are:

142	142	134	110	98	130
136	120	118	130	116	140
118	122	128	128	114	138
104	116	110	100	128	128
124	140	108	146	116	114
152	118	140	128	116	110
138	132	118	120	122	120
108	112	94	130	130	118
120	128	108	120	124	110
124	132	132	130	102	118

A. The measurements were stated to be correct to the nearest even number of mm Hg. On examining these data, is there any evidence that this degree of accuracy was not always achieved? (Hint: What would you expect for the frequencies of the last digits of the above observations?)

B. Obtain a frequency distribution of these 60 observations and draw a histogram.

C. What are the "true" limits and the "true" midpoint for the lowest class of your frequency distribution?

D. State why the use of frequency distribution groups (in mm Hg) of 95 to 99, 100 to 104, 105 to 109, 110 to 114, and so on, is inappropriate.

E. From your frequency distribution in part B, calculate the median, mean, SD, and the coefficient of variation.

F. The variation in blood pressure readings consists of two major components: the "true" biological variation and measurement error variability. From what you know about blood pressure and its usual determination with a sphygmomanometer, list some of the factors that influence the magnitude of these two major components of variation.

G. A handbook of clinical norms states that the normal range for systolic blood pressure in males age 20 to 24 is 105 to 140 mm Hg.
   (1) Are the results of your tabulations generally compatible with this statement?
   (2) Suppose these blood pressure observations were duplicated on a large number of medical students. Giving your reasons, state whether you agree or disagree with the use of these results to establish a clinical norm.

2. An investigator at a university hospital is preparing a report on the natural history of angina pectoris. He searches through all the case records in his hospital during the last 20 years and locates 50 with the diagnosis of angina pectoris. One of his first interests is to determine the average age at first symptoms. He tabulates the age at first symptoms for each of his 50 histories, collects his data, arranges it in a frequency distribution, and constructs the following worksheet for calculating the mean and SD using the coded method:

Age at first symptoms in years	f	Working unit, v	fv	fv^2
20–40	3	− 2	− 6	36
40–50	11	− 1	− 11	121
50–60	20	0	0	0
60–70	13	1	13	169
70–90	3	2	6	36
	50		2	362

A. There are three errors in the above worksheet. What are they?

B. He corrects these errors and finds the mean age at onset of first symptoms is 55.2 years with an SD of 9.9 years. In referring this investigator's findings to all patients with angina pectoris, discuss the sources of selection that would make his sample nonrepresentative.

C.   Discuss the limitations of the measurement "age at first symptoms" in a disease such as angina pectoris.

3.   Fill in the blanks with one or more of the following words: *mean, median, mode.*
   A.   At birth an infant has an equal chance of living longer than the _____ length of life.
   B.   An investigator tabulates the changes in blood pressure following the administration of an antihypertensive agent to a sample of hypertensive patients. He then calculates the mean, median, and mode of the changes in blood pressure.
       (1)   If the sign of the largest change were incorrect, it would be necessary to recalculate the _____.
       (2)   If the magnitude of the largest change were incorrect by one unit, it would be necessary to recalculate the _____.
   C.   By taking the logarithm of the amount of a drug that is required to produce an effect in dogs, a symmetrical frequency distribution is obtained in which, of course, the mean, median, and mode are identical. If the data were *not* transformed into logarithms and the original dosage units were used, the highest measure of location would   be   the   _____,   the   next   highest   the _____, and the lowest the _____.
   D.   A study that began 10 years ago comprised 100 newly diagnosed patients with some disease. During the 10-year span, 70 patients are known to have died, and at present, 30 remain alive. For all 100 patients, one can definitely calculate the _____ survival, one might be able to calculate the _____ survival, but one cannot possibly calculate the _____ survival.
   E.   Among patients dying from a disease, the _____ duration is   equal   to   the   _____   age   at   death   minus   the _____ age at onset.
   F.   The total number of days of hospitalization is derived from multiplying the total number of admissions by the _____ length of stay.
   G.   In citing the average income of people 65 years and older, the proponents of Medicare would likely find the _____ most advantageous,   whereas   the   opponents   would   likely   find   the _____ most advantageous.

4.   The data tabulated on p. 59 give the results of duplicate determinations of the fasting levels of triglycerides in six male subjects:
   A.   Find the variance:
       (1)   Among all 12 observations;
       (2)   Among the means of the six subjects.

B. Verify algebraically that the variance among two observations, denoted as x_1 and x_2, can be expressed as

$$s^2 = (x_1 - x_2)^2/2$$

C. Using the result in part B, obtain the variance among the two duplicate observations for each of the six subjects. Then obtain the mean of these six variances.

	Fasting level of triglyceride (mg percent)			
Subject	Determination 1	Determination 2	Mean	Difference
A	170	186	178	−16
B	193	205	199	−12
C	110	118	114	−8
D	135	123	129	12
E	135	119	127	16
F	115	131	123	−16
		Total	870	
		Mean	145.0	

Total (all 12 observations) = 1,740
Sum of squares (all 12 observations) = 264,920
Also useful: $(1740)^2/12 = 252,300$

D. For each of the following situations, indicate which variance is most appropriate and why:
   (1) Evaluating the precision of a new technique for measuring triglyceride levels.
   (2) Determining whether there are significant changes in triglyceride levels before and after various meals.
E. A new technique for measuring triglyceride levels is proposed. Discuss how you would determine the unbiasedness and precision of this new technique. Assuming the new technique is unbiased and more precise than the previous one, what else would you consider before recommending its adoption?

5. For widows in the United States in the period 1929 to 1931, the following table gives their distribution by age, the distribution by age for all cancer deaths among widows, and the corresponding age-specific cancer mortality rates:
   A. Compute the crude cancer mortality rate for widows and compare this with the crude cancer mortality rates of single and married females (p. 47 and Table 2.16).

B.   Using the population distribution by age for all women (see the last column of Table 2.16) as the standard, compute the age-adjusted cancer mortality rate for widows by the direct method and compare it with the corresponding age-adjusted rates for single and married women (p. 49 and foot of Table 2.16).

C.   Using the 1929–1931 age-specific cancer mortality rates in the total American female population as the standard (see the last column of Table 2.17), compute the age-adjusted cancer mortality rate for widows by the indirect method. Compare the result with the corresponding age-adjusted rates for single and married women (p. 51 and foot of Table 2.17) and with the age-adjusted rate calculated in part B by the direct method.

	U.S. widows 1929–31		
Age (yrs)	Population (× 1,000)	Cancer deaths	Cancer death rate (per 100,000 pop.)
15–24	39.8	7	17.59
25–34	176.8	74	41.86
35–44	423.4	496	117.15
45–54	705.4	1,805	255.88
55–64	945.5	4,324	457.32
65–74	972.4	7,107	730.87
≥ 75	623.1	6,779	1,087.95
Total	3,886.4	20,592	

6.   The following data have been extracted from the Framingham Heart Study [27, 28]. The first column gives the number of subjects undergoing the initial examination according to their age and sex. The second column gives the number of cases of coronary heart disease (CHD) discovered on initial examination. The cohort was reexamined every two years, and the third column indicates, according to age and sex, the number of new cases of CHD that arose during a fourteen-year interval.

A.   Compute and graph the sex- and age-specific prevalence rates of CHD on initial examination.

B.   Compute and graph the sex- and age-specific fourteen-year incidence rates of CHD.

C.   Are there sufficient data to compute the sex- and age-specific prevalence rates of CHD at fourteen years? If so, then compute the rates and compare them with the prevalence rates on initial examination; if not, state what additional data are needed to compute the rates.

| Sex and age (yr) | Initial Examination | | New cases of CHD during fourteen-year interval |
	Number examined	Number with CHD	
Males			
35–44	865	7	86
45–54	731	26	135
55–64	348	18	83
Females			
35–44	1.095	4	15
45–54	883	13	76
55–64	437	11	72

Chapter 3
Probability

It was stated earlier that the mathematical theory of probability underlies the methods for drawing statistical inferences in medicine. The purpose of this chapter is not to develop this theory in detail, but to introduce some of the basic concepts and rules for manipulations of probability. Thus, the intent is to provide an understanding of probability and to set the groundwork for the development of statistical inference that begins in the next chapter.

DEFINITIONS AND BASIC LAWS

Definition of Probability

There is no completely satisfactory definition of probability. Probability is one of those elusive concepts that virtually everyone knows but which is nearly impossible to define entirely adequately. During the past few centuries, much has been written in mathematics and philosophy about probability and its meanings, from its origins in games of chance to its present use in the quantification of personal beliefs regarding degrees of uncertainty. For the purposes of this text, the following definition, called the *frequentist definition*, suffices: *The probability of an event is the event's long-run relative frequency in repeated trials under similar conditions.*

This definition excludes what are called *subjective* or *personal probabilities*. The key phrase that excludes these is "repeated trials under similar conditions." Personal probabilities are used every day and are exemplified by such phrases as "the chance of a particular war terminating within some fixed time period" or "the chance that a particular individual will take some particular action." In the field of medical education, an example comes to mind where a colleague on a medical school promotion board assessed a freshman student in academic difficulty as having a "30 percent chance" of successful graduation. These events do not meet the definition of "repeated trials under similar conditions" and thus are excluded from consideration in this text.

It should be noted that what, in one sense, seems to be a personal probability, can, in another context, satisfy the frequentist definition. For example, consider the chance of the death of the president of the United States during his term of office. This, on one hand, can reflect a subjective probability indicating someone's degree of belief. On the other hand, if one considers the president as one of many American males at a certain age, then the American male mortality experience for that age group during the four-year period would reasonably satisfy the frequentist definition. Likewise, in the instance cited above concerning the student's 30 percent chance of successful graduation, the probability has meaning in the frequentist sense if the statement is based on a backlog of experience. This would mean that this student is one of many in similar circumstances of academic difficulty. Experience would indicate that 30 percent of such students eventually graduate successfully.

Since the frequentist definition of probability employed in this text involves the term "relative frequency," then it is clear that the numerical value of a probability must fall somewhere between 0 and 1. Thus, probabilities are expressed as either decimals, fractions, or percentages.

It also follows from the definition of the probability of an event's occurrence that the probability that the event does *not* occur—the *complementary event*—is obtained by subtraction from unity. Hence, if $Pr(A)$ is the probability that event A occurs, the probability for the complementary event—i.e., that A does not occur—is $1 - Pr(A)$.

Mutually Exclusive Events and the Additive Law

Two events that cannot happen together are defined as *mutually exclusive*. Thus, if events A and B are mutually exclusive, the occurrence of A precludes the occurrence of B, and vice versa. For example, in the toss of a coin, the event A, it lands heads, and event B, it lands tails, are mutually exclusive. In the throw of a pair of dice, the event A, the sum of the faces is 7, and B, the sum of the faces is 11, are mutually exclusive.

The *additive law*, when applied to two mutually exclusive events, states that *the probability of either of the two events occurring is obtained by adding the probabilities of each event*. Thus, if A and B are mutually exclusive events,

$$Pr(A \text{ or } B) = Pr(A) + Pr(B)$$

Example 3.1. In the throwing of a pair of dice, calculations derived below (see next example) indicate that the chance of a 7 is 6/36 and of an 11 is 2/36. Consequently, the chance of a 7 *or* an 11 is $6/36 + 2/36 = 8/36$.

Extension of the additive law to more than two events indicates that if A, B, C, ... are mutually exclusive events,

$$Pr(A \text{ or } B \text{ or } C \text{ or } \cdots = Pr(A) + Pr(B) + Pr(C) + \cdots$$

As a corollary to the additive law, if there is a total of n mutually exclusive and equally likely outcomes for an event and if some subset of these outcomes, n_A, is favorable to a particular event A, then the probability of A is n_A/n. This follows because each of the n mutually exclusive outcomes, if they are equally likely, has the probability $1/n$. If n_A outcomes correspond with event A, then the additive law states that $1/n$ is added n_A times, giving the probability n_A/n.

Example 3.2. The toss of a single die results in $n = 6$ mutually exclusive outcomes, which, if the die is fair, are equally likely. Hence, if one denotes event A as the appearance of an odd number, there are $n_A = 3$ favorable outcomes: 1, 3, and 5. The probability of an odd number is thus $3/6 = .5$.

To determine the probability of a 7 in the toss of a *pair* of dice, one would enumerate the number of possible ways out of the total of 36 in which the sum of the faces is 7. There are six ways (1+6, 2+5, 3+4, 4+3, 5+2, 6+1), giving a probability of $6/36$. Likewise, for an 11, there are two ways (6+5 and 5+6), giving a probability of $2/36$.

The above condition—n_A favorable out of n mutually exclusive and equally likely events—is employed in many statistics texts in the definition of probability. As with the frequentist definition used here, it serves the purpose entirely well. It has been pointed out, however, that such a definition is somewhat circular since it contains the phrase "equally likely events," which itself involves the notion of probability.

Many texts and courses delve into more complex probability situations by developing the rules and methods for counting the number of favorable outcomes out of the total number of mutually exclusive and equally likely outcomes. These calculations involve the concepts of permutation and combination of items, a subject which should be familiar from high school and college mathematics. For example, to determine the chance of a particular hand in poker (say, a straight flush), one enumerates the number of favorable outcomes (compatible with occurrence of a straight flush) out of the total possible five-card hands that can be dealt from a deck of 52 cards. The underlying premise is that all of the possible five-card hands that can be dealt (there are 2,598,960 of them!) are mutually exclusive and equally likely outcomes. The interested reader is referred to elementary texts on probability for an introduction to such methods of enumeration (for example, [79]). These enumeration methods are used to a limited extent later only insofar as they are necessary to develop the needed methods of statistical inference.

A common pitfall in dealing with mutually exclusive outcomes is the often erroneous additional assumption of "equally likely outcomes" when this is clearly not appropriate. The point is that only under special conditions are mutually exclusive outcomes equally likely as well. Perhaps because in many games of chance the mutually exclusive outcomes are also equally likely, there is a tendency to assume erroneously that the two phrases always go together. This can lead to serious errors in probability determinations.

Example 3.3.   Consider the toss of a fair coin. Knowledge of the physical situation and the specification "fair" indicate that the two mutually exclusive outcomes—heads and tails—are also equally likely, each with probability ½. If, however, one tosses a thumbtack, it cannot be assumed that the two mutually exclusive outcomes—sideways (➚) or upside down (⬇)—are also equally likely. Some experiments in tack-tossing will clearly illustrate how erroneous it is to state that the probability a tack lands sideways is ½.

Example 3.4.   In the toss of a single fair die, the physical situation indicates that the six mutually exclusive outcomes are also equally likely, so each outcome has the chance 1/6. However, if one considers throwing a pair of dice, then for the sum of the two faces there are 11 mutually exclusive outcomes, corresponding with the numbers 2 to 12. These are clearly not equally likely outcomes, as any experienced crap-shooter can confirm. It may be shown that there are 36 mutually exclusive and equally likely outcomes corresponding with each possible pair that can be formed among the numbers 1 to 6. The correct probability calculation is to determine how many such pairs correspond with the sum 2, how many with the sum 3, and so on. The point, however, is that the mutually exclusive outcomes *for the sum* are not equally likely.

Example 3.5.   This author recalls an instance involving some material distributed to medical students concerning radioactive decay. The notes stated that during some very small unit or instant of time, an atom either emits or does not emit a particle. It was further stated that, as a consequence, the probability of an atom's emitting a particle is ½. This is erroneous. Emission and nonemission of a particle are mutually exclusive events, but they are not necessarily equally likely. For some particular substance the chance could be ½, but this is clearly not the general situation. In general, the chances of atomic particle emission or nonemission are undoubtedly unequal. The proper model for radioactive decay is that the chance of atomic particle emission during some small time interval is proportional to the length of the interval; surely, this probability cannot be assumed to be ½.

In the classic coin-tossing, dice-throwing, and card-playing illustrations of probability, knowledge of the physical situation and the specifications of *fair* coins and dice and *well-shuffled, thoroughly mixed* cards permit the "equally likely" restriction to be attached.

Conditional Probabilities and the Multiplicative Law

Sometimes the chance a particular event happens depends on the outcome of some other event. This applies obviously with many events that are spread out in time. For example, in card playing, when several cards have already been played, the chance of a particular card on the next draw depends on the cards already played. An ideal medical example concerns survival (see Chapter 9). The chance a patient with some disease survives the next year depends, of course, on his having survived to the present time. Such probabilities are called *conditional*. The notation is

$$Pr(B|A),$$

which is read as "the probability event B occurs given that event A has already occurred."

Example 3.6.   Consider the successive drawing of two cards from a deck of 52 and the following events

Notation	Event
A	First card is a spade
$B|A$	Second card is a spade given that the first card was a spade

Each card from a deck of 52 is equally likely to be drawn, and since there are 13 spades, $Pr(A) = 13/52$. Now in drawing the second card, the $52 - 1 = 51$ remaining cards are also, of course, equally likely. If event A occurred and the first card was a spade, there are $13 - 1 = 12$ spades remaining. Hence, $Pr(B|A) = (13 - 1)/(52 - 1) = 12/51$.

Example 3.7.   Extracting data from the survival curve illustration used later in the text (Table 9.3), consider the events corresponding with the patient surviving each year in the two years subsequent to diagnosis. The following notation may be used:

Notation	Event	Probability
A	Survive first year following diagnosis	.8131
$B|A$	Survive second year given that the patient has survived first year	.8378

Survival for the second year depends, of course, on having survived the first. The life-table calculations that provide the probabilities of A and $B|A$ are described later, and there is no need now for concern with how they were derived. The above probabilities are used below to illustrate the multiplicative law of probability.

The *multiplicative law* of probability states that *the chance that two events* A *and* B *both* *happen is*

$$\Pr(A \text{ and } B) = \Pr(B|A)\Pr(A)$$

Example 3.8.   It may be seen from the example of drawing two cards that the probability of both the first and second cards being spades is

$$\Pr(A \text{ and } B) = (12/51)(13/52) = 156/2652 = .0588$$

Example 3.9.   For the survival study, the probability that a patient survives both the first and second years following diagnosis is

$$\Pr(A \text{ and } B) = (.8378)(.8131) = .6812$$

This determines the two-year survival rate.

One should note that the multiplicative law is also sometimes used to determine a conditional probability from knowledge of $\Pr(A \text{ and } B)$ and $\Pr(A)$:

$$\Pr(B|A) = \Pr(A \text{ and } B)/\Pr(A)$$

This can be considered as an alternative form of the multiplicative law.

Example 3.10.   A population life table provides a good illustration (see Table 2.18). In the 1968 population life table for American white males, the chance that an infant lives to age 25 is .95364, whereas the chance that he lives to age 65 is .65440. For the latter, it is understood that to survive to age 65 means to survive both from birth to age 25 *and* from age 25 to 65. Now, what is the chance that a white male 25 years of age survives to age 65? Consider the following notation:

Notation	Event	Probability
A	Survive birth to age 25	.95364
A and B	Survive both birth to age 25 and age 25 to 65	.65440
$B|A$	Survive age 25 to 65 given survival to age 25	?

Then

$$\Pr(B|A) = .65440/.95364 = .68621$$

That is, a white male, age 25, has a 68.6 percent chance of living to age 65, according to the 1968 U.S. life tables.

Independent Events

Often there are two events such that the occurrence or nonoccurrence of one does not in any way affect the occurrence or nonoccurrence of the other. This defines *independent events*. Thus, if events A and B are independent, this means $Pr(B|A) = Pr(B)$.

Example 3.11.   A classic example is n tosses of a coin and the chances that on each toss it lands heads. These are independent events. The chance of heads on any one toss is independent of the number of previous heads. No matter how many heads have already been observed, the chance of heads on the next toss is ½.

Example 3.12.   A similar situation prevails with the sex of offspring. The chance of a male is approximately ½. Regardless of the sexes of previous offspring, the chance the next child is a male is still ½. These are *independent* events.

Often, what is referred to as the "law of averages" is invoked to justify predicting that after a run of, say, three female children, a couple is more likely to have a male for their fourth. Similarly, if five successive tosses of a coin yield heads, some might be willing to give better than even odds that the sixth toss will be tails. This argument is fallacious. A useful explanation of the law of averages is that it operates by long-run *swamping* and not by short-run *compensation* [79]. In the long run, after very many tosses, the ratio of heads to tails will stabilize at nearly 1 to 1. Likewise, if a couple were to continue to produce offspring indefinitely (should nature and physical stamina permit), the ratio of males to females would stabilize at approximately 1 to 1.

With independent events, the multiplicative law becomes

$$Pr(A \text{ and } B) = Pr(A)Pr(B)$$

Example 3.13.   Consider the drawing of two cards from a deck of 52. This time, however, the first card is replaced and the deck is thoroughly shuffled before the second is drawn. What is the probability that both will be spades? Event A, the first card is a spade, has the probability $13/52 = 1/4$, as before. Since the first card, however, is replaced and the deck is remixed, then event B, the second card is a spade, is independent of event A. Clearly, $Pr(B) = 13/52 = 1/4$. Hence, the chance both are spades is

$$Pr(A \text{ and } B) = (1/4)(1/4) = 1/16 = .0625$$

Note that with the replacement of the first card, the probability that both cards are spades is slightly higher than the probability for the previous situation without replacement.

In an analogous manner, the chance that n tosses of a coin are all heads or the chance that n offspring are all females is $\frac{1}{2}^n$, i.e., the multiplication of the probability $\frac{1}{2}$ on each occasion for all n occasions.

Summary of Basic Laws

The two basic manipulative rules of probability necessary for the development of methods of statistical inference are the additive and multiplicative laws. To aid in distinguishing between them, the following outline may be useful:

Type of Events	Law Usually Implied	Operation
Mutually exclusive	Additive	$Pr(A \text{ or } B) = Pr(A) + Pr(B)$
Independent	Multiplicative	$Pr(A \text{ and } B) = Pr(A)Pr(B)$

A Misapplication of the Laws of Probability

One particular instance where the incorrect law is likely to be applied is in situations requiring determination of the "probability of at least one."

Example 3.14.   With each administration of a drug to a particular patient, there is a 10 percent chance of his having a toxic reaction. The patient requires five consecutive drug administrations. What is his chance of having a toxic reaction?

In essence, with five consecutive administrations of the drug, the patient will exhibit a toxic reaction if he does so on at least one administration. In other words, the patient exhibits the toxic reaction whether he does so on only one, or on two, or on as many as all five administrations. The question asks what is the probability of *at least one* administration resulting in a toxic reaction?

The faulty line of reasoning to which many people succumb is as follows: Since there is a 10 percent chance on each administration, then the chance on five administrations is $5 \times 10\% = 50\%$. This approach easily can be seen to be erroneous by considering the case of 11 administrations. Following the suggested line of reasoning, the chance of at least one of the 11 administrations producing a toxic reaction becomes $11 \times 10\% = 110\%$. Obtaining an impossible answer of a probability in excess of 100 percent shows that something must be wrong.

What is wrong is that the additive rather than the multiplicative law was applied. The computation, $5 \times 10\%$, derives from *addition* of the 10 percent probabilities on each of the five occasions. However, the events of toxic reaction on each of the five occasions are *independent*, not mutually exclusive. Hence the appropriate law is the *multiplicative*, not the additive law.

The simplest method for obtaining the correct answer is to make use of the complementary relationship

$$\text{Pr(at least one)} = 1 - \text{Pr(none)}$$

Then Pr(none) can be computed directly using the multiplicative law. Since the chance of the complementary event of no toxic reaction on each administration is $1 - .1 = .9$, the chance of no toxic reaction on all five administrations is

$$\text{Pr(no toxic reaction on all 5)} = .9^5$$

Hence

$$\text{Pr(at least one toxic reaction)} = 1 - .9^5 = 1 - .59 = .41 \text{ or } 41\%$$

If there had been eleven administrations,

$$\text{Pr(at least one toxic reaction)} = 1 - .9^{11}$$

which yields a number under unity.

BAYES' THEOREM

The additive and multiplicative laws and the notion of conditional probabilities can be used to derive Bayes' theorem, which is of interest to many physicians as well as to many theoretical statisticians. For physicians, Bayes' theorem plays a key role in recent developments in automated and computer-assisted diagnosis; it pertains directly to the logic system underlying the process of performing a medical diagnosis. For theoretical statisticians, Bayes' theorem forms the cornerstone for a new structure of statistical inference aptly labeled *neo-Bayesian*. This structure differs considerably from that considered in this book. Many prominent theoreticians subscribe to the Bayesian viewpoint. However, it will be a long time before the Bayesian methods supplant the methods of statistical inference currently pervading the scientific literature.

This section develops the principle of Bayes' theorem by means of a numerical example and then proceeds to indicate how Bayes' theorem is used in a computer approach to medical diagnosis.

An Example to Develop Bayes' Theorem

This example concerns pregnancy, bacteriuria, and pyelonephritis. Suppose it is known that roughly 6 percent of pregnant women attending a prenatal clinic at a large urban hospital have bacteriuria (bacteria in the urine). Consider the two events: A_1, a pregnant woman has bacteriuria, and A_2, she does not have bacteriuria. Clearly A_1 and A_2 are mutually exclusive and complementary, so $Pr(A_1) = .06$ and $Pr(A_2) = 1 - .06 = .94$. Suppose it is further known that 30 percent of bacteriuric and 1 percent of nonbacteriuric pregnant women proceed to develop pyelonephritis. Using B to denote the occurrence of pyelonephritis, then

Notation	Event	Probability
$B\|A_1$	Pyelonephritis given that the pregnant woman was bacteriuric	.30
$B\|A_2$	Pyelonephritis given that the pregnant woman was nonbacteriuric	.01

1. With these definitions consider the following probability questions:
    A. What is the chance a pregnant woman will have both bacteriuria and pyelonephritis?
        Answer: Use multiplicative law:

$$Pr(A_1 \text{ and } B) = Pr(B|A_1)\,Pr(A_1) = (.30)(.06) = .0180$$

B. What is the chance a pregnant woman will *not* have bacteriuria but will have pyelonephritis?
    Answer: Use multiplicative law:

$$Pr(A_2 \text{ and } B) = Pr(B|A_2)Pr(A_2) = (.01)(.94) = .0094$$

2. What is the chance of pyelonephritis?
    Answer: In this particular example, pyelonephritis can happen in two mutually exclusive ways, with or without bacteriuria. Hence, application of the additive law to the probabilities determined in 1A and 1B gives

$$Pr(\text{pyelonephritis}) = Pr(B)$$
$$= Pr(A_1 \text{ and } B) + Pr(A_2 \text{ and } B)$$
$$= .0180 + .0094 = .0274$$

3. Finally, with the knowledge that a pregnant woman has developed pyelonephritis, what is the chance she had been bacteriuric?
    Answer: Using the notation developed, the question asks for the probability of $A_1|B$, i.e., the presence of bacteriuria given that the pregnant woman has pyelonephritis. From the alternative form for the multiplicative law of the preceding section (p. 68) and the answers to 1A and 2 above,

$$Pr(A_1|B) = Pr(A_1 \text{ and } B)/Pr(B) = .0180/.0274 = .6569$$

In other words, if a pregnant woman has developed pyelonephritis, there is a 65.7 percent chance that she had been bacteriuric.

This now completes the illustration of Bayes' theorem. Knowledge of the chances of pyelonephritis when bacteriuria is present and when it is absent along with knowledge of the relative frequency of bacteriuria among pregnant women has permitted the determination of a conditional probability, namely, the chance that the pregnant woman had been bacteriuric, given that she has developed pyelonephritis.

Substituting letters for numbers and working backward from the expression in the answer to Question 3, it may be seen that

$$P(A_1|B) = \frac{\Pr(A_1 \text{ and } B)}{\Pr(B)} = \frac{\Pr(A_1 \text{ and } B)}{\Pr(A_1 \text{ and } B) + \Pr(A_2 \text{ and } B)}$$

$$= \frac{\Pr(B|A_1)\Pr(A_1)}{\Pr(B|A_1)\Pr(A_1) + \Pr(B|A_2)\Pr(A_2)}$$

This last expression is the usual formulation of Bayes' theorem.

If instead of only the two mutually exclusive and exhaustive outcomes A_1 and A_2, one now had several, say k, outcomes $A_1, A_2, \ldots, A_k$, it may be shown that Bayes' theorem becomes

$$\Pr(A_1|B) = \frac{\Pr(B|A_1)\Pr(A_1)}{\Sigma\Pr(B|A_i)\Pr(A_i)}$$

where i is the index of summation. If one wanted to determine $\Pr(A_2|B)$, one would replace each subscript 1 in the above expression with 2, and so on for other A subscripts.

Application to Computer Diagnosis

In the theory of computer diagnosis, the events $A_1, A_2, \ldots, A_k$ correspond with mutually exclusive possible diagnoses, and the event B corresponds with a particular complex of symptoms, signs, and laboratory results [15, 50, 67]. Then the left-hand side of the equation defining Bayes' theorem, $\Pr(A_i|B)$, is the chance of the occurrence of the ith diagnosis, given that the patient presents with the symptom constellation B. The probabilities necessary to derive this chance appear on the right side and are

1. $\Pr(B|A_i)$: The chance that the patient exhibits symptom constellation B given that he has the ith diagnosis. (These conditional probabilities must be known for each of the k mutually exclusive diagnoses.)
2. $\Pr(A_i)$: The proportion of patients with the ith diagnosis. (These proportions must be known for each of the k diagnoses and their total must, of course, be unity.)

In other words, knowledge of the frequency of a particular symptom constellation in each of k possible diseases, coupled with knowledge of the relative frequency of each of the k diagnoses in the population at hand, permits one to determine, with the use of Bayes' theorem, the likelihood of a diagnosis if a patient presents with the symptom complex. In this way, given the symptoms, the most probable diagnosis—i.e., the A_i whose $\Pr(A_i|B)$ is largest—can be determined.

THE CHANCE OF x SUCCESSES IN n INDEPENDENT TRIALS WITH CHANCE π OF SUCCESS ON EACH TRIAL

This section illustrates the application of the additive and multiplicative laws of probability to obtain the probability of a compound event. The results are important and are employed again in Chapter 5.

The explanation begins by considering a simple event for which there are two mutually exclusive outcomes: success (S) or failure (F). The probability of success is denoted by π, and of failure, by $1 - \pi$. There are n independent trials in which, for each trial, there is a constant probability π of success and $1 - \pi$ of failure. What is the probability of exactly x successes in n trials?

Some examples where this situation applies are the chance of x heads in n tosses of a coin, the chance of x boys in a family with n children, the chance of x deaths among n patients with a certain disease, and the chance of x remissions as a result of treating n patients with some drug.

The process of determining the chance of x successes in n trials consists of listing all the possible mutually exclusive outcomes, calculating the probability of each outcome using the multiplicative law, and then combining the probability of all those outcomes that are compatible with the desired result by use of the additive law.

Consider two trials ($n = 2$). The four mutually exclusive outcomes of two trials are listed below. For each outcome—since the trials are *independent*—the application of the multiplicative law yields the probabilities shown. (Since all possible outcomes are considered, the probabilities total unity.)

Outcome			
First trial	Second trial	Probability	Number of successes
F	F	$(1-\pi)(1-\pi) = (1-\pi)^2$	0
F	S	$(1-\pi)(\pi) = \pi(1-\pi)$	1
S	F	$(\pi)(1-\pi) = \pi(1-\pi)$	
S	S	$(\pi)(\pi) = \pi^2$	2

Total probability: $(1-\pi)^2 + 2\pi(1-\pi) + \pi^2 = [(1-\pi) + \pi]^2 = 1$

Note that the event of one success in two trials corresponds with the two mutually exclusive outcomes, FS and SF, each with probability $\pi(1 - \pi)$. Hence, by the additive law, the probability of one success in two trials is $2\pi(1 - \pi)$.

The same process applies for three trials, in which there are eight mutually exclusive outcomes:

First trial	Second trial	Third trial	Probability	Number of successes
	Outcome			
F	F	F	$(1-\pi)(1-\pi)(1-\pi) = (1-\pi)^3$	0
F	F	S	$(1-\pi)(1-\pi)(\pi) = \pi(1-\pi)^2$	
F	S	F	$(1-\pi)(\pi)(1-\pi) = \pi(1-\pi)^2$	1
S	F	F	$(\pi)(1-\pi)(1-\pi) = \pi(1-\pi)^2$	
F	S	S	$(1-\pi)(\pi)(\pi) = \pi^2(1-\pi)$	
S	F	S	$(\pi)(1-\pi)(\pi) = \pi^2(1-\pi)$	2
S	S	F	$(\pi)(\pi)(1-\pi) = \pi^2(1-\pi)$	
S	S	S	$(\pi)(\pi)(\pi) = \pi^3$	3

Total probability $(1-\pi)^3 + 3\pi(1-\pi)^2 + 3\pi^2(1-\pi) + \pi^3 = [(1-\pi) + \pi]^3 = 1$

Since the three trials are *independent*, the *multiplicative* law produces the probabilities shown for each outcome. Since the event "one success in three trials" pertains to three *mutually exclusive* outcomes above, each with probability $\pi(1-\pi)^2$, the *additive* law yields a probability of $3\pi(1-\pi)^2$. The probability of two successes in three trials, by an analogous argument, becomes $3\pi^2(1-\pi)$. Again, since all possible outcomes are considered, the probabilities total unity.

The mathematically inclined reader may recall the binomial theorem of college algebra and will note that with two trials the probabilities of 0, 1, and 2 successes correspond to the terms in the binomial expansion of $[(1-\pi) + \pi]^2$. With three trials, the probabilities of 0, 1, 2, and 3 successes correspond to the terms in the binomial expansion of $[(1-\pi) + \pi]^3$. In general, then, it appears that with n trials, the probabilities of 0, 1, 2, ..., n successes should correspond with the terms in the binomial expansion of $[(1-\pi) + \pi]^n$. They do, as can be proved by mathematical induction for those who wish a proof of this result.

In the expansion of the binomial $[(1-\pi) + \pi]^n$, the xth term, corresponding with exactly x successes in n trials, will involve the expression $\pi^x(1-\pi)^{n-x}$ preceded by some numerical coefficient. This coefficient is denoted by ^nC_x, which, for those familiar with permutations and combinations, is called the *combination of* n *objects taken* x *at a time.* The term is defined as

$$^nC_x = \frac{n!}{x!\,(n-x)!} = \frac{n(n-1)\cdots 1}{[x(x-1)\cdots 1][(n-x)(n-x-1)\cdots 1]}$$

$$= \frac{n(n-1)(n-2)\cdots(n-x+1)}{1\cdot 2\cdot 3\cdot\cdots\cdot x}$$

Thus, with n trials, the probabilities of 0, 1, 2, ..., x, ..., $n - 1$, n successes are:

Number of successes in n trials	Probability
0	$^nC_0\pi^0(1 - \pi)^{n-0} = (1 - \pi)^n$
1	$^nC_1\pi^1(1 - \pi)^{n-1} = \dfrac{n}{1}\pi(1 - \pi)^{n-1}$
2 ⋮	$^nC_2\pi^2(1 - \pi)^{n-2} = \dfrac{n(n - 1)}{1 \cdot 2}\pi^2(1 - \pi)^{n-2}$
x ⋮	$^nC_x\pi^x(1 - \pi)^{n-x} = \dfrac{n(n - 1) \ldots (n - x + 1)}{1 \cdot 2 \ldots x}\pi^x(1 - \pi)^{n-x}$
$n - 1$	$^nC_{n-1}\pi^{n-1}(1 - \pi)^{n-(n-1)} = n\pi^{n-1}(1 - \pi)$
n	$^nC_n\pi^n(1 - \pi)^{n-n}\pi^n = \pi^n$

The boxed relation gives the result required, the probability of exactly x successes in n independent trials with chance π of success on each trial.

RANDOM VARIABLES AND PROBABILITY DISTRIBUTIONS

Discrete Case

Often numbers can be associated with the mutually exclusive outcomes of a simple or compound event. For example, in the preceding section, the integers 0, 1, ..., n correspond to the number of successes among n independent trials. In such a situation, one generates a *probability distribution*. If the numbers are denoted by x, then the probability distribution of x is denoted as $f(x)$. In other words, presented with an integer x, there is a mathematical function or formula that indicates the appropriate probability for that particular x. One could also draw a graph with x as the abscissa and the probability, or $f(x)$, as the ordinate (Fig. 3.1). Generally, in situations where a number x corresponds with a probability $f(x)$, x is called a *random variable* having the *probability distribution* $f(x)$.

Example 3.15. The random variable x denotes the number of successes among n independent trials with probability π of success on each trial. Therefore, the probability distribution of the random variable x is, from the boxed-in formula in the preceding section,

$$f(x) = {}^nC_x\pi^x(1 - \pi)^{n-x} \text{ for } x = 0, 1, \ldots, n$$

This particular probability distribution is called the *binomial distribution* since it is generated by the terms in the binomial

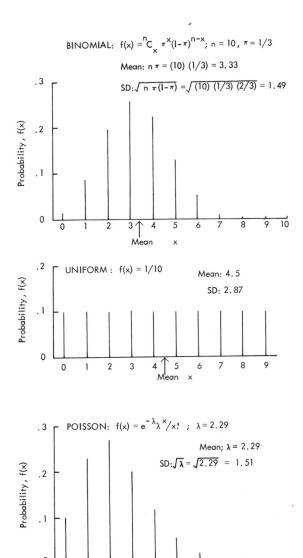

Figure 3.1
Theoretical probability distributions: binomial, uniform, and Poisson.

expansion $[(1 - \pi) + \pi]^n$. In the binomial distribution, the integer values of x can range from 0 to n.

Example 3.16. Each of the numbers 0, 1, ..., 9 is equally likely to occur as the last digit of a series of clinical measurements. For example, if the serum uric acid levels in Table 2.6 were determined correct to the nearest 10th of a milligram per 100 ml, then each reading is equally likely to end with the digits 0, 1, ..., 9 (the digit after the decimal point). Letting x denote the digit, the fact that each occurs with equal chance indicates that $f(x) = 1/10$ for $x = 0, 1, ..., 9$. Here x is a random variable having a *uniform probability distribution* since the probabilities for the occurrence of each x are equal or uniform.

Example 3.17.   A thoroughly mixed large volume of bacterial suspension contains λ bacteria per unit volume. Samples of one unit volume each are obtained, and the number of bacteria in each sample is counted. Let x denote the number of bacteria in each sample. If the bacteria are randomly distributed in the suspension, then x is a random variable whose probability distribution is

$$f(x) = e^{-\lambda}\lambda^x/x! \quad \text{for } x = 0, 1, ...$$

This is called the *Poisson probability distribution*. Its formula will not be derived here, but it can be deduced mathematically from the specification that the bacteria are randomly distributed in the suspension. The x values can theoretically range from zero to infinity.

Example 3.18.   In a similar manner, one can distribute a large number of accidents at random among a group of bus drivers. Let x denote the number of accidents for a bus driver. With random distribution of accidents, x is a random variable with a Poisson probability distribution. For example, if there are 1,623 accidents distributed at random among 708 bus drivers, the overall accident rate is $1623/708 = 2.29$ per driver. The probability that a driver has x accidents is then

$$f(x) = e^{-2.29}2.29^x/x!$$

This probability distribution is shown in Figure 3.1, and the results of multiplication of the probabilities by 708 is depicted in the "Expected" column in Table 2.5.

Properties of Probability Distributions

A probability distribution, $f(x)$, is a theoretical percentage distribution of x. Hence, the percentages must total 100 percent or the probabilities must total unity. Mathematically,

$$\sum_{\text{all } x} f(x) = 1$$

Examples
   1.   Binomial:

$$\sum_{x=0}^{n} {}^nC_x\pi^x(1 - \pi)^{n-x} = [(1 - \pi) + \pi]^n = 1$$

2. Uniform:

$$\sum_{x=0}^{9} 1/10 = 10(1/10) = 1$$

3. Poisson:

$$\sum_{x=0}^{\infty} e^{-\lambda}\lambda^{x}/x! = e^{-\lambda} \sum_{x=0}^{\infty} \lambda^{x}/x! = e^{-\lambda}e^{\lambda} = 1$$

The previous chapter dealt with empirical distributions (e.g., serum uric acid levels) wherein the mean and SD were calculated. The theoretical probability distributions now under consideration also have means and SDs. If one takes the probability values $f(x)$ and multiplies each by a constant n, the resulting $nf(x)$ values are analogous to the frequencies of an empirical frequency distribution. One may then substitute the $nf(x)$ values for the f values in the formulas given in Table 2.9 for the mean and SD of an empirical distribution. This gives as the mean of a theoretical probability distribution:

$$\bar{x} = \frac{\Sigma fx}{\Sigma f} = \frac{\Sigma[nf(x)]x}{\Sigma nf(x)} = \frac{n\Sigma xf(x)}{n\Sigma f(x)} = \Sigma xf(x)$$

The last step follows by canceling the ns and using $\Sigma f(x) = 1$ from the above equation.

In the formula for SDs, since the goal is not inference and since theoretical distributions are now of concern, it is better to use $\Sigma f = n$ instead of $\Sigma f - 1 = n - 1$ in the denominator. Substitution then yields the SDs of a theoretical probability distribution:

$$SD = \sqrt{\frac{\Sigma f(x - \bar{x})^2}{\Sigma f}} = \sqrt{\frac{\Sigma[nf(x)](x - \bar{x})^2}{\Sigma nf(x)}}$$

$$= \sqrt{\frac{n\Sigma(x - \bar{x})^2 f(x)}{n\Sigma f(x)}} = \sqrt{\Sigma(x - \bar{x})^2 f(x)}$$

Using the alternative formula for SDs, an equivalent form is

$$SD = \sqrt{\frac{\Sigma fx^2 - [(\Sigma fx)^2/(\Sigma f)]}{\Sigma f}} = \sqrt{\Sigma x^2 f(x) - [\Sigma xf(x)]^2}$$

The following summarizes the application of the above formulas to the binomial, uniform, and Poisson probability distributions:

Distributions	Range of x	$f(x)$	Mean	SD
Binomial	0 to n	$^nC_x\pi^x(1 - \pi)^{n-x}$	$n\pi$	$\sqrt{n\pi(1 - \pi)}$
Uniform	0 to 9	$1/10$	4.5	2.87
Poisson	0 to ∞	$e^{-\lambda}\lambda^x/x!$	λ	$\sqrt{\lambda}$

The means and SDs for these distributions are also displayed in Figure 3.1.

Continuous Case

There is no necessity that the numbers associated with probabilities be integers. In the previous examples, x was an integer; hence, these were labeled as *discrete cases*. The values of x might include intermediate values between integers. This situation defines *continuous* probability distributions. Graphically, when plotting $f(x)$ against x, a continuous, smooth curve replaces the preceding discrete lines or bars. The previous requirement that the total probability in the distributions of x be unity becomes the requirement that the area under the smooth curve be unity. With use of the integral calculus, this is simply the statement

$$\int_{-\infty}^{\infty} f(x)\,dx = 1$$

There are corresponding changes in the definition of the mean and SD for continuous distributions. Integration ($\int$) replaces the previous summation (Σ). Hence, for continuous probability distributions,

$$\text{Mean} = \bar{x} = \int_{-\infty}^{\infty} xf(x)\,dx$$

$$\text{SD} = \int_{-\infty}^{\infty} (x - \bar{x})^2 f(x)\,dx = \int_{-\infty}^{\infty} x^2 f(x)\,dx - \left[\int_{-\infty}^{\infty} xf(x)\,dx\right]^2$$

Example 3.19. The *exponential* is a continuous probability distribution. Its equation is

$$f(x) = \theta e^{-\theta x} \text{ for } 0 < x < \infty$$

This distribution corresponds with the time intervals between successive occurrences of random events. For instance, in radioactive decay each particle in a mass has a constant chance of disintegration over time. Disintegrations occur completely at random and at a constant rate. In consequence, the times elapsed between successive disintegrations follow the exponential distribution.

Research on the theory of component reliability uses the exponential distributions extensively. The classic illustration of the exponential is in the life-testing of light bulbs.

Correspondingly, in the medical field the length of life of patients following the onset of disease often closely approximates the exponential distribution. Other aspects of medicine where the exponential distribution is relevant include elapsed times between arrivals at an emergency ward, between outbreaks of epidemics, between occurrences of disastrous accidents, and so forth.

Application of integral calculus to the exponential distribution reveals that the total area under the curve is unity, i.e.,

$$1 = \int_{-\infty}^{\infty} f(x)\,dx = \int_{0}^{\infty} \theta e^{-\theta x}\,dx$$

Likewise, the mean, is $1/\theta$, and the SD is $1/\theta$.

Example 3.20.   The most important theoretical probability distribution in statistics is the *normal* or *Gaussian* distribution. Empirically,

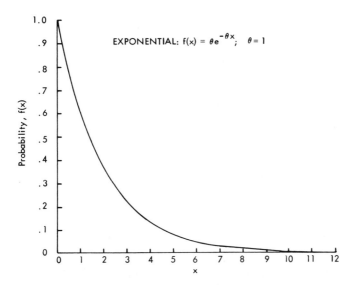

EXPONENTIAL: $f(x) = \theta e^{-\theta x}$; $\theta = 1$

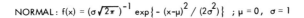

NORMAL: $f(x) = (\sigma\sqrt{2\pi})^{-1} \exp\{-(x-\mu)^2 / (2\sigma^2)\}$; $\mu = 0$, $\sigma = 1$

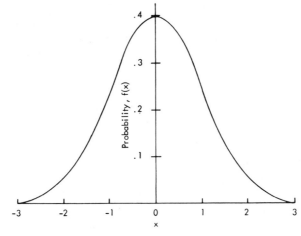

Figure 3.2
Theoretical probability distributions: exponential and normal.

this continuous distribution corresponds quite well with the distribution of quantitative variables in many populations. Its more important use, however, is in the procedures for performing a statistical inference, which form the main focus of this text. Hence, because of the central role of the normal distribution, the next section is devoted solely to describing it and illustrating its use.

Example 3.21.   There are many other continuous theoretical probability distributions that the statistician employs in his pursuit of procedures for performing statistical inferences. Examples are the *t* and *chi-square distributions*, whose uses are discussed later. Each of these is a continuous distribution in that, for a specified *x*, there is a mathematical relation or formula that gives a probability, $f(x)$. The interest of this text is not in the definition or theory of these distributions but in their proper use for making appropriate inferences in the analysis of data. Hence, since these distributions are all well tabulated, there is no need to indicate the mathematical formulas that define them.

To illustrate continuous probability distributions, the exponential and normal distributions are depicted in Figure 3.2.

NORMAL DISTRIBUTION

The ubiquitous normal distribution is the most important one in statistical work. "Normal" is perhaps not the most appropriate label for this distribution, since the statistical meaning of the term differs from the medical meaning of "normal." Some authors prefer to call it the "Gaussian distribution" in order to avoid confusion. However, since "normal" is its more common designation in the medical literature, this text uses the expression *normal distribution*. When so used, the reference is solely to the theoretical probability distribution discussed in this section and not to the medical or any other meaning of normal.

Why Use It?

The normal distribution is important because, empirically, the distribution of many medical measurements in populations approximate the normal in shape (e.g., serum uric acid levels, cholesterol levels, blood pressure, height, and weight). More important, in the techniques of performing statistical inference, the normal distribution occupies a central role.

As will be shown in the following chapter, even if one is sampling from a population whose shape departs severely from a normal distribution, the normal distribution, under certain general conditions, still forms the basis for performing statistical inferences. Some investigators have the misconception that the methods of statistical analysis hinge on the fact that one is sampling from a normal population. This is not entirely so. Lack of normality in the underlying population does not preclude meaningful statistical analysis and inference.

What is true, however, is that one is in a more secure position if one is fortunate enough to be dealing with an underlying normal population. There are fewer restrictions in the application of statistical methods. Hence, it is often extremely advantageous to make some adjustment of the raw data, if possible, in order to yield derived data that are more nearly normally distributed. Knowledge of when to make such adjustments depends on the cumulation of a backlog of empirical evidence in the field.

One common adjustment with raw data is a *log transformation*, i.e., taking the logarithm of each observation and then working the analysis entirely in log units. Pharmacology affords a good illustration. Often, in dealing with the minimal dose of a drug required to produce a particular effect on an animal, it turns out empirically that, from animal to animal, the logarithms of the just-effective dosages are more nearly normally distributed than are the raw doses. A classic example is the assay of digitalis. One of the earlier methods for this assay involved infusion of digitalis into the bloodstream of a cat until the heart stopped beating. The just-effective dose for each cat was determined. Empirical observations on many cats revealed that the log doses, not the original doses, more closely adhered to the normal distribution. Hence, for these and other reasons, analysis is performed in "log dose" units.

Another example of the logarithmic transformation occurs in epidemiology with the distribution of incubation periods (defined as time between exposure and onset of clinical disease) of communicable diseases. Sartwell collected data on the distribution of incubation periods for many communicable diseases ranging from onset within hours to onset within months [96]. The typical pattern of these data revealed that the logarithm of the incubation period tended to be normally distributed. Hence, in further analysis of data on incubation periods of communicable diseases, the "log incubation period" is the appropriate scale for analysis.

Description

1. The normal distribution is a theoretical, continuous probability distribution whose equation is

$$f(x) = \frac{1}{\sqrt{2\pi}\,\sigma} e^{-\frac{1}{2}\frac{(x-\mu)^2}{\sigma^2}} \quad \text{for } -\infty < x < \infty$$

Of course, it follows that the area under the entire curve is unity, a fact that can be verified mathematically.

2. The normal distribution is determined by two quantities: its mean (μ) and SD (σ). Recall that the equation of a straight line, $f(x) = a + bx$, is also determined by two quantities, its slope b and intercept a. In this same sense,

μ and σ are the two quantities (or, in mathematical terms, the two *parameters*) that define a normal curve. Changing μ alone shifts the entire normal curve along the abscissa. Changing σ alone changes the degree to which the distribution is spread out.

3. The normal distribution is unimodal, bell-shaped, and symmetrical about $x = \mu$.

4. Extensive tables of the normal distribution are available. Hence, there is no need to employ the above mathematical expression. The chief concern is how to use the tables properly.

For purposes of statistical inference, one must ascertain areas in the normal curve corresponding to various points on the abscissa. For example, for a given point on the abscissa, how much of the area of the normal curve is above that point or below that point? How much of the area lies between two given points on the abscissa? The answers to each of these questions involve the integration of the above equation defining the normal curve. For example, the area between two points c and d on the abscissa is

$$\int_{c}^{d} \frac{1}{\sqrt{2\pi}\,\sigma} e^{-\frac{1}{2}\frac{(x-\mu)^2}{\sigma^2}}\, dx$$

This form cannot be integrated analytically. However, tables of areas under the normal curve are available and the following paragraphs describe their use.

Use of Tables of Areas in the Normal Curve

The tabulated normal curve is that for which $\mu = 0$ and $\sigma = 1$ and is called the *standardized normal curve*. For points on the abscissa, denoted by z, the body of Appendix Table A1 indicates the area in the standardized normal curve above z (i.e., the area in one tail).

Example 3.22. What is the area in the standardized normal curve
  A. above 1.00?
  B. below -1.00?
  C. between -1.00 and 1.00?
  D. between -1.28 and 1.65?
  Answers:
  A. Finding $z = 1.00$ in Appendix Table A1, a direct reading gives 0.159 as the required area.
  B. The symmetry of the normal curve indicates that the area above any positive z value is the same as the area below that same negative z value. Thus, the area below -1.00 is the same as that above 1.00, namely, 0.159.
  C. Since the total area under the curve is unity, the area between ± 1.00 is obtained by subtracting the area above 1.00 and the area below -1.00 from unity, namely, $1 - 0.159 - 0.159 = 0.682$.
  D. In a similar manner, the area between -1.28 and 1.65

obtains by subtracting the areas above 1.65 and below −1.28 from unity, namely, 1 −0.100 − 0.049 = 0.851.

Appendix Table A1 can, of course, be used in reverse to determine the appropriate z value from the specification of an area.

Example 3.23.   In the standardized normal curve, what z value cuts off
    A.   10 percent in the upper tail?
    B.   5 percent in the lower tail?
    Answers:
    A.   The area 0.100 in Appendix Table A1 corresponds with $z = 1.28$.
    B.   The area 0.050 in Appendix Table A1 corresponds with 1.65. Since the question asks about the lower tail, $z = -1.65$.

The two-tailed table (Appendix Table A2) gives, for a specified z value, the combined area above $+z$ and below $-z$. Thus, on the basis of symmetry, the entries in the body of the two-tailed table, apart from rounding-off errors, are double the entries in the body of the one-tailed table.

Example 3.24.   In the standardized normal curve,
    A.   What is the area above 2.58 and below −2.58?
    B.   What is the area between ± 1.00?
    C.   What z values encompass 95 percent of the distribution?
    Answers:
    A.   From Appendix Table A2, the combined area above 2.58 and below −2.58 is obtained directly as 0.010.
    B.   Since the total area is unity, the area between ± 1.00 is $1 - 0.317 = 0.683$, the same result as in Example 3.22 (apart from rounding error).
    C.   If 95 percent is encompassed in the central portion of the distribution, 5 percent must be in the combination of two tails. Finding 0.050 in body of Appendix Table A2 will show that $z = \pm 1.96$.

For any other normal distribution, the relation

$$z = \frac{x - \mu}{\sigma}$$

permits the use of the tables of the standardized normal distribution. The quantity $(x - \mu)/\sigma$ above is termed the *critical ratio, relative deviate, standardized value,* or *normal deviate* (the last being an appropriate statistical labeling, although a rather anomalous word pair in medical terminology).

Example 3.25.   Assume that among diabetics the fasting blood level of glucose is approximately normally distributed with a mean of 105 mg per 100 ml and an SD of 9 mg per 100 ml.

A. What proportion of diabetics have levels between 90 and 125 mg per 100 ml?

B. What level cuts off the lower 10 percent of diabetics?

C. What levels encompass 95 percent of diabetics?

Answers: In each situation, the relation $z = (x - \mu)/\sigma$ is used to convert from standardized to actual scale, or vice versa. For each question, there is a diagram illustrating both the original and z scales.

A. Convert the "mg per 100 ml" scale to a standard z scale:

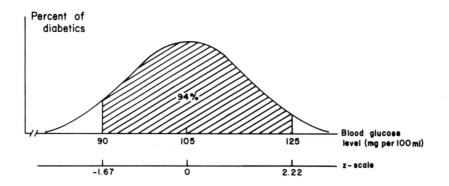

(1) $z = (90 - 105)/9 = -1.67$;
$z = (125 - 105)/9 = 2.22$.

(2) From Appendix Table A1, the area in the standard normal curve between -1.67 and 2.22 is $1 - 0.013 - 0.049 = 0.938$ or 93.8 percent.

B. Use a standard one-tailed table, then convert the z scale to mg per 100 ml:

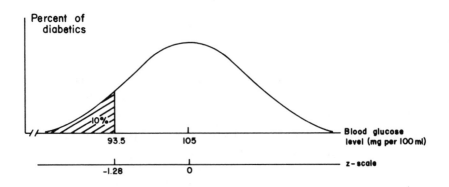

(1) From Appendix Table A1, -1.28 cuts off the lower 10 percent of the standard normal curve.

(2) Set $-1.28 = (x - 105)/9$.

(3) Solve for x: $x = (-1.28)(9) + 105 = 93.5$ mg per 100 ml.

C. Use a standard two-tailed table, then convert to mg per 100 ml:

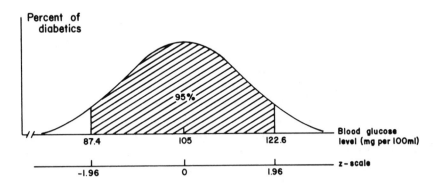

(1) From Appendix Table A2, ± 1.96 cuts off 5 percent in both tails.

(2) Set $\pm 1.96 = (x - 105)/9$.

(3) Solve for x: $x = (\pm 1.96)(9) + 105 = 87.4$ and 122.6 mg per 100 ml.

It was stated previously that for unimodal distributions which are not too skew,

Mean $\pm$ 1 SD encompasses approximately ⅔ of observations

Mean $\pm$ 2 SD encompasses approximately 95% of observations

Mean $\pm$ 3 SD encompasses virtually all the observations

These guidelines are derived from the properties of the theoretical normal distribution. From the two-tailed table (Appendix Table A2), it may be seen that, corresponding to $z = 1, 2,$ and 3, the areas in the standard normal curve are 68.3, 95, and 99.7 percent.

An Application of the Normal Distribution to the Screening of Blood Donors

Prince and Gershon describe the use of serum enzyme determinations as a means of screening hospital blood-bank donors for possible anicteric hepatitis [88]. One of the serious risks of blood transfusion is the possibility of transmission of hepatitis virus. If there were a way to screen the donors' blood and reject the blood from donors likely to harbor hepatitis virus, then the risk of transmitting the virus to the patient needing the blood would be subsequently reduced. The authors state:

A considerable body of literature provides evidence that serum énzymes, particularly the transaminases, may be elevated considerably before, and also after, the clinical course of icteric viral hepatitis; as well as during the course of anicteric viral hepatitis. . . . The above findings would appear to suggest the feasibility of detection of anicteric and preicteric cases of viral hepatitis by chemical screening procedures. Indeed these findings would offer hope that it may be possible to detect anicteric serum hepatitis carriers by routine serum enzyme determinations carried out on bloods prior to transfusion.

The enzyme determination under consideration is serum glutamic pyruvic transaminase (SGPT). It is not necessary in this text to define this measurement, to indicate the causes for its possible elevation during hepatitis, nor to provide any further background or review of hepatitis. Suffice it to say that hepatitis is an untoward consequence of blood transfusion, that a reduction of its risk is desirable, and that in this particular investigation the determination of SGPT and the establishment of a screening procedure offer the possibility of achieving some reduction in risk. The purpose of this example is primarily to illustrate the use of the normal distribution and secondarily to elucidate several of the basic principles of mass screening programs.

As a background for establishing the screen, the authors refer to the empirical results of extensive surveys that indicated that the logarithm (to base 10) of the SGPT determination was approximately normally distributed both among healthy individuals (i.e., known to be free from hepatocellular damage) and diseased individuals (i.e., known to have definite hepatocellular damage). In the healthy population, the log SGPT was found to have a mean of 1.25 and an SD of 0.12 (these are log SGPT units), whereas in the diseased population, the mean log SGPT was 1.55 with an SD of 0.13. Note that this is a particular instance in which conversion to logarithms achieves the desired normality of distribution. The theoretical percentage distributions for the healthy and diseased groups are illustrated in Figure 3.3.

The intent of the proposed screening procedure is to establish a cut-off log SGPT value. The blood of a potential donor whose log SGPT exceeds this cut-off value would be rejected by the blood bank; if his log SGPT falls below the cut-off value, his blood is accepted. Suppose it is specified that the cut-off point be located such that the screening procedure will accept 95 percent of the blood of healthy individuals. What is the cut-off value? Using the normal curve on the left in Figure 3.3, one determines the log SGPT value that cuts off the upper 5 percent of the distribution:

1. From Appendix Table A1, 1.65 cuts off the upper 5 percent in standard one-tailed normal distribution.
2. $1.65 = (x - 1.25)/0.12; x = 1.448.$

Hence, a log SGPT cut-off of 1.448 achieves the specification of accepting 95 percent of healthy blood.

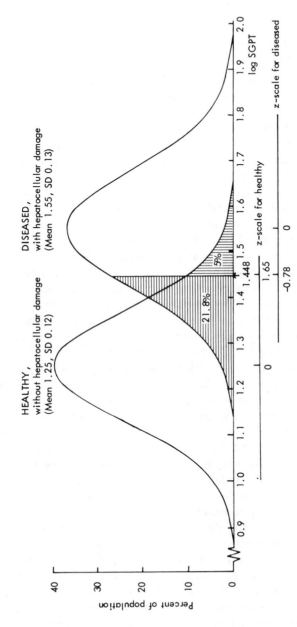

Figure 3.3
Theoretical percentage distributions of log SGPT among healthy blood donors and blood donors with hepatocellular damage.

Now, the following question arises: What percentage of diseased blood will be accepted by the screen? With the cut-off at 1.448 and using the normal curve on the right in Figure 3.3, one must find the proportion of the curve that is below 1.448. Converting to the standard z scale for this curve,

1. $z = (1.448 - 1.55)/0.13 = -0.78$.
2. The standard one-tailed table (Appendix Table A1) indicates that the area below -0.78 is 21.8 percent.

Hence, the 1.448 cut-off point results in the screening procedure's accepting 21.8 percent of blood from diseased donors.

Both determinations above deal with errors. First, if the blood bank accepts 95 percent of the blood from healthy individuals, it obviously must be rejecting 5 percent of the blood of healthy individuals. In other words, the blood of healthy donors whose log SGPT exceeded 1.448 would be mislabeled in the screen as being suspect of disease and thereby not accepted for the blood bank. This form of error is called a *false positive*; in this example, a healthy subject would be falsely labeled as positive or suspect for the disease under study. In this instance, the cut-off point for the screen was devised in order to set the rate of false positive errors at 5 percent.

The second determination above yielded the frequency with which blood from diseased donors will pass the screen and be accepted by the blood bank. This form of error is called a *false negative*, namely, a diseased individual who is falsely labeled as healthy. In this instance, the false negative rate was found to be 21.8 percent. It is the false positive and false negative rates that form the inherent ingredients of any screening program, be it one of testing blood for hepatitis, of testing blood for syphilis, or of reading the results of a tyne test for tuberculosis. In Figure 3.3, the false positive rate corresponds with the upper tail of the curve on the left; the false negative rate corresponds with the lower tail of the curve on the right.

Suppose now that the investigator decided that a false negative rate of 21.8 percent was too high to tolerate and he wished to reduce it. Inspection of Figure 3.3 indicates that the area of 0.218 in the lower tail of the "diseased" curve can be reduced only by lowering the cut-off below 1.448. However, as the cut-off is lowered, the area in the upper tail of the "healthy" curve increases. In other words, a smaller false negative error is achieved only by increasing the false positive error, and vice versa. In essence, it is the degree of overlap between the healthy and diseased populations that dictates the false positive and false negative error interrelationship.

In the determination of what levels are appropriate for false positive and false negative errors, one would want to consider more carefully the consequences of each type of error and then attempt to strike a satisfactory compromise. The magnitude of the errors depends on the degree of overlap of the healthy and diseased groups. The overlap may be sufficiently great so as to negate the feasibility of establishing a screen. In such a case, the best course of action may be "to go back to the drawing board" to attempt to devise some measurement or combination of measurements that will minimize the overlap between the healthy and diseased groups.

There is one major factor in the above analysis that has so far been neglected. Note in Figure 3.3 that the curves are *percent* distributions for the healthy and diseased groups. Hence, the important missing feature is the relative magnitude of the diseased and healthy groups.

To illustrate the consequences of the size of the respective groups, suppose that 12 percent of the population have the disease. (Of course, only the 12 percent rate is known; one cannot identify the specific individuals in the population who are diseased and healthy.) To simplify the arithmetic, suppose further that the screen is applied to a population of 1,000. Thus, among the population there are 880 healthy and 120 diseased individuals.

Considering the 880 healthy individuals, 95 percent of their blood is accepted and 5 percent is rejected. This gives (880)(0.95) = 836 healthy units accepted by the blood bank; correspondingly, (880) (0.05) = 44 healthy units are rejected by the blood bank.

Considering the 120 diseased individuals, 21.8 percent of their blood is accepted, so 100% − 21.8% = 78.2% of their blood is rejected. This gives (120)(0.218) = 26 diseased units accepted, and (120)(0.782) = 94 diseased units rejected.

These results are summarized as follows:

	Blood accepted	Blood rejected	Total
Healthy	836	44	880
Diseased	26	94	120
Total	862	138	1,000

The effectiveness of the screen may be seen in that among the 862 units accepted, only 26 (or 3 percent) are diseased. Thus, from a relative frequency of 12 percent diseased in the unscreened population, the relative frequency of disease among the accepted units has been reduced to 3 percent.

The cost of the screen may be seen with the figure of 138, or 13.8 percent, of the donated blood being discarded. Furthermore, of this discarded blood, 44 of 138 units, or 32 percent, are perfectly good. This may be too high a price to pay for the screen.

It may be worthwhile to indicate that the above calculations can be framed as a direct application of Bayes' theorem. For example, with the accepted blood the following notation is appropriate:

Notation	Event	Probability
A_1	Diseased	.12
A_2	Healthy	.88
$B\|A_1$	Blood is accepted given that individual is diseased	.218
$B\|A_2$	Blood is accepted given that individual is healthy	.95

The direct application of Bayes' theorem gives $Pr(A_1|B) = .03$, namely, the chance that the blood came from a diseased individual given that it was accepted by the screen. For disease rates in the population other than 12 percent, the above calculations would, of course, yield different results.

A systems analyst or operations research expert, if presented with this problem of establishing a screen, would no doubt consider a cost-benefit form of analysis. This would involve quantification of all costs involved (including financial costs, such as that of establishing the screen, and nonfinancial costs, such as that resulting from the discarding of blood from healthy individuals) and of the benefits to be derived. Then he would seek, by a scheme of trade-offs, an optimal screening strategy that strikes a proper balance between cost and benefit.

EXERCISES

1. Each time an individual receives pooled blood products, there is a 2 percent chance of his developing serum hepatitis. An individual receives pooled blood products on 45 occasions. What is his chance of developing serum hepatitis? (Note that the chance is *not* $45 \times .02 = .90$.)

2. Associated with three diseases A, B, and C, there are the respective chances .20, .30, and .50 of being hospitalized. If an individual has all three diseases (A, B, and C) and if these exert their influences independently, what is the chance of his being hospitalized?

3. A clinical trial to evaluate the effect on mortality of a treatment for some disease consists of pairs of subject patients: one member of each pair receives the new treatment, and the other receives a suitably designated control regimen. At the conclusion of the trial's observation period, there are four mutually exclusive outcomes for each pair as follows: both die, both survive, the treatment member survives while the control member dies, or the control member survives while the treatment member dies. Let π_T and π_C represent the respective mortality rates for the treatment and control subjects.
   A. What are the probabilities of each of the four mutually exclusive outcomes for a treatment-control pair?
   B. Pairs where one member survives while the other dies are called "untied." What proportion of the pairs will be untied?

C. Among the untied pairs, what proportion will consist of the treatment member surviving and the control member dying?

D. Show that when the mortality rates for treatment and control patients are equal (i.e., when $\pi_T = \pi_C$), then the proportion of the untied pairs with the treatment member surviving and the control member dying is ½.

E. If the control mortality rate is 40 percent and the treatment mortality rate is 20 percent, show that 44 percent of the treatment-control pairs will be untied and that, among the untied pairs, approximately 70 percent will consist of the treatment member surviving and the control member dying.

4. For screening drugs that may produce remission of some of the symptoms of a chronic disease, an investigator proposes the following program:

Test any drug on six patients. If none of the patients shows remission, reject the drug. Under this program, a drug which produces remissions in 20 percent of a large population of patients has about 3 chances in 4 of passing the screen, while one with a 30 percent remission rate has nearly nine chances in ten of passing the screen.

Verify this claim.

5. A. Table 2.18 shows that at age 65 the probability of surviving for the next 5 years is $1 - .1864 = .8136$ for a white male and $1 - .0965 = .9035$ for a white female. For a married couple who are both white and both age 65, show that the probability that the wife is a living widow five years later is 2.15 times the probability that the husband is a living widower.

B. Using Table 2.18, what are the respective chances that a white male and a white female, each age 65, will survive to age 75? What is the chance that a white married couple who are both age 65 and celebrating their 40th wedding anniversary will celebrate together their 50th wedding anniversary (presuming they will not divorce or separate)?

6. An investigator develops a screening test for cancer. He uses this screening test on known cancer patients and known noncancer patients, and he finds the test has a 5 percent false positive rate (i.e., positive test results for noncancer patients) and a 20 percent false negative rate (i.e., negative test results for cancer patients). He is now going to apply this test to a population in which he knows 2 percent have undetected cancer. Using Bayes' theorem, find the chance that someone with a positive test actually has cancer; also, find the chance that someone with a negative test actually has cancer. In considering the use of this test, what other (nonstatistical) issues are relevant?

7. Among a large series of patients referred for endocrine consultation because of suspected Cushing's syndrome, it was ultimately found that for every three who actually had the disease, there was one who did not. Furthermore, 65 percent of those ultimately diagnosed as having the disease exhibited osteoporosis on initial examination. In comparison, only 3 percent of those ultimately found to be free of the disease had displayed osteoporosis on initial examination.

   A.   What is the chance that a patient who presents with osteoporosis on initial examination will ultimately be found to have Cushing's syndrome?

   B.   If osteoporosis is used as a screening test for Cushing's syndrome, what are the "false positive" and "false negative" rates?

   C.   Assuming that patients present themselves in an approximately random order, what proportion of patients will be found

   (1)   with initial osteoporosis and actually having the disease?

   (2)   without initial osteoporosis and actually free of the disease?

   D.   The two events in question C correspond to the screen's result being "concordant" with the disease status. Otherwise, the screen's result and the disease status are "discrepant." A random sample of n patients is selected. Denoting the respective probabilities in C as π_1 and π_2, give an expression in terms of n, π_1, and π_2 for the chance that there will be at least one discrepant result among the sample of n.

8. It is found that 25 percent of children exposed to a particular infectious agent become ill with the particular disease. Among a playgroup of four children with equal exposure to the infectious agent,

   A.   Show that the probabilities that 0, 1, 2, 3, and 4 children become ill are 81/256, 108/256, 54/256, 12/256, and 1/256, respectively.

   B.   What is the probability that at least one child becomes ill? What is the probability that there will be at least one ill and one healthy child in the playgroup?

   C.   From part A, compute the mean and SD of the distribution of the number of ill children and verify that

$$\text{Mean} = n\pi = 4(\tfrac{1}{4}) = 1$$

$$\text{SD} = \sqrt{n\pi(1 - \pi)} = \sqrt{4(\tfrac{1}{4})(\tfrac{3}{4})} = 0.87$$

9. A drug manufacturer claims that a particular drug provides relief from the symptoms of angina pectoris among 80 percent of patients. You prescribe this drug to five of your patients with angina and find that only two experience relief of symptoms. Assuming the manufacturer's claim is true, what is the chance you would obtain results as bad as or worse than you have observed?

10. In the National Board Examinations, the scores are scaled so that among all medical students taking the exam nationwide, the scores are approximately normally distributed with a mean of 500 and a standard deviation of 100.
    A. What percentage of the students will have scores exceeding 700?
    B. What score is exceeded by 10 percent of the students?
    C. What percentage of students score between 400 and 700?
    D. Previously the scores were scaled so that the normally distributed nationwide scores had a mean of 80 with an SD of 5. Which is the better score, 670 in the present system or 89 in the old system?

11. Among a large group of coronary patients, it is found that their serum cholesterol levels approximate a normal distribution. It was found that 10 percent of the group had cholesterol levels below 182.3 mg per 100 ml whereas 5 percent had values above 359.0 mg per 100 ml. What is the mean and SD of the distribution?

12. The amount of a rectal general anesthetizing agent required to cause surgical anesthesia in patients was found to be approximately normally distributed from patient to patient, with a mean of 50 mg and an SD of 10 mg. The mean lethal dose was 110 mg with an SD of 20 mg, and this was also normally distributed. If a dose were used that brings 90 percent of patients to surgical anesthesia, what percentage of patients would be killed by this dose?

13. From the data in Tables 2.6 and 2.11 and in Figure 2.1, presume that serum uric acid levels in normal males are approximately normally distributed with a mean of 5.4 mg per 100 ml and an SD of 1.0 mg per 100 ml.
    A. What is the chance that a healthy male selected at random will have a serum uric acid level outside the range of 4.0 to 7.0 mg per 100 ml?
    B. What is the chance that among 4 healthy males selected at random there is at least one whose serum uric acid level is outside the range of 4.0 to 7.0 mg per 100 ml?
    C. How many healthy males must be selected so that there is a 95 percent or better chance of at least one having a serum uric acid level outside the range of 4.0 to 7.0 mg per 100 ml?

14. Serum cholesterol levels were determined for a large number of healthy males in the general population. These males were all followed for two years and were subdivided into two groups: those who had a definite coronary event in the two-year period and those who did not. The initial cholesterol levels of each of these two groups were found to be normally

distributed with the following means and SDs (in units of mg per 100 ml serum):

	With coronary	Without coronary
Mean	260	240
SD	60	50

A.   Suppose that an initial cholesterol level of 280 is used as a criterion for predicting a coronary event in the next two years, i.e., that for a value above 280, a coronary event is predicted. What is the probability of predicting a coronary event for a man who will not have one (false positive)? What is the probability of failing to predict a coronary event for a man who will have one (false negative)?

B.   From these data, how useful is the serum cholesterol level in the prediction of coronary events?

C.   If one raises the critical cholesterol level from 280 to 300, which of the following statements about the probabilities of false positives and false negatives are correct? (Calculations are not necessary.)
   (1)   They remain the same.
   (2)   They both increase.
   (3)   They both decrease.
   (4)   False positives increase; false negatives decrease.
   (5)   False positives decrease; false negatives increase.

PART II
STATISTICAL INFERENCE

Chapter 4
Inference on Means

Statistical inference is the process by which one draws conclusions regarding a population from the results observed in a sample. The concern in the following pages is with quantitative data and inferences regarding *population means*. First, a single mean will be considered and then the comparison of two means.

To set the stage, consider the following example cited by Armitage [2]. This concerns a trial of a new drug for the treatment of cancer at some particular site. Previous experience and record analysis indicate that patients with cancer at this site survive (from first diagnosis to death) an average of 38.3 months, with a standard deviation of 43.3 months. One hopes the new drug will prolong survival. An investigator tests this drug by administering it to a sample of 100 newly diagnosed cancer patients. These patients are followed until all die, and the investigator determines their mean survival as 46.9 months.

What can he conclude regarding the drug's ability to prolong survival in this type of cancer? If this drug were adapted for the treatment of all patients with this cancer, do the results on the sample of 100 provide sufficient evidence that drug treatment, on the average, will prolong survival beyond the known mean of 38.3 months without drug use? In essence, the investigator wants to draw an inference from a *sample* of 100 drug-treated cancer patients to the mean survival in a *population* of drug-treated patients. In particular, he wants to compare this mean survival with a known level of 38.3 months mean survival without drug treatment in order to determine whether treatment with the drug does or does not bring about improvement.

In making this inference, it seems reasonable to expect the strength of the inference to be related to:

1. *The sample size.* The larger the sample size, the stronger the inference. In other words, the fact that the sample consists of 100 patients should be accounted for when making the inference; also, a given result in 100 patients should provide a more reliable inference than that same result in, say, 10 patients.
2. *The variability of the response under study.* The less the variability, the stronger the inference. A small variation in survival from one patient to another indicates a consistent, reproducible response. Hence, the smaller the variation, the more certainty one would have regarding the sample observations. The variability of survival time is indicated by the SD of 43.3 months based on previous experience, and, intuitively, this SD should somehow enter into the process of drawing the inference.

Therefore, in making the inference, both the underlying variability, σ, and the sample size, n, are relevant.

In order to answer the question regarding the effect of this anticancer agent, one must first consider the sampling distribution of means.

SAMPLING DISTRIBUTION OF MEANS

Definitions

In statistics there are two kinds of distributions: *population distributions* and *sampling distributions*. The former term refers to the distributions of characteristics in defined populations; e.g., serum uric acid levels among males or survival times of drug-treated cancer patients. The latter term refers to distributions that are derived from population distributions as described below. One rarely encounters sampling distributions empirically, but it is necessary to study them and to know their properties in order to draw a statistical inference. In fact, sampling distributions form the very basis for statistical inference.

One may generate the sampling distribution of means as follows:

1. Obtain a sample of n observations selected completely at random from a large population. Determine their mean and then replace the observations in the population.
2. Obtain another random sample of n observations from the population, determine their mean, and again replace the observations.
3. Repeat the sampling procedure indefinitely, calculating the mean of the random sample of n each time and subsequently replacing the observations in the population.
4. The result is a series of means of samples of size n. If each mean in the series is now treated as an individual observation and arrayed in a frequency distribution, one determines the *sampling distribution of means of samples of size* n.

Example 4.1.   If one obtains repeat samples of 25 from a large population of males, determines the mean serum uric acid level in each sample, replaces the 25 observations each time, and then arrays the means into a distribution, then one generates the sampling distribution of mean serum uric acid levels of samples of size 25.

Example 4.2.   From a large population of drug-treated cancer patients, one obtains repeat samples of 100 patients. For each sample, one calculates the mean survival and then replaces the patients in the population before taking another sample of 100. One arrays the means into a frequency distribution and obtains the sampling distribution of means of size 100 for survival of cancer patients undergoing drug therapy.

Clearly, there appears to be no rationale for taking repeated samples of size *n*. There is certainly no apparent reason for repeat samples of 25 serum uric acid levels, and the repeat samples of 100 survival times among drug-treated cancer patients are obviously a conceptual device. However, the knowledge of the properties of these sampling distributions of means—*if* one hypothetically obtained these repeated samples—permits one to draw a conclusion based upon *one* sample of 25 serum uric acid levels and *one* sample of 100 survival times among drug-treated cancer patients.

Properties

The general notation in this text is to use Greek letters to denote population values and Latin letters to denote sample values. Hence, μ and σ, respectively, denote the mean and SD of an underlying population, whereas, $\bar{x}$ and s, respectively, denote the mean and SD in a single sample of size *n*. From a population with a mean, μ, and an SD, σ, the sampling distribution of repeat sample means of size *n* (that is, repeat $\bar{x}$s) has three extremely important properties:

1. The mean of the sampling distribution of means is the same as the population mean, μ.
2. The SD of the sampling distribution of means is $\sigma / \sqrt{n}$.
3. The shape of the sampling distribution of means is approximately a normal curve, regardless of the shape of the population distribution and provided *n* is large enough.

Each of these three properties can be derived mathematically. The first is what one might expect intuitively: the mean of the means of a large series of repeat random samples is the same as the population mean. The second property might not be easily guessed, but it is roughly consistent with intuition: the variability among means of repeat samples should depend directly upon the variability of the observations in the underlying population. Furthermore, it should have an inverse relation to the size of sample, since larger sample sizes reproduce a greater proportion of the population in each sample. Consequently, the variability between means of repeated samples should decrease with increased sample size. Note especially that this is *not* a simple inverse relation, but is inversely proportional to the *square root of sample size*. Hence, a 100-fold increase in sample size produces a 10-fold reduction in the variability of the sampling distribution of means. The third property of the sampling distribution of means may be somewhat surprising and is quite important. Even though one might start with a population distribution that is distinctly "nonnormal" in shape, the sampling distribution of means of samples of size *n* (if *n* is sufficiently large) will be normal. One can then use the tables of the normal distribution to draw the statistical inference. That is one reason why the manipulation of the normal distribution was stressed in the preceding chapter. The proof of this third property, termed the *central limit theorem*, is fairly complex mathematically. Empirical verification of these three properties is provided by generating sampling distributions from some known populations.

Example 4.3.   Suppose one begins with a population which itself is normally distributed. In particular, consider the standardized

Population - Normal distribution

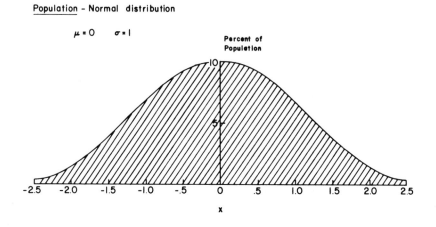

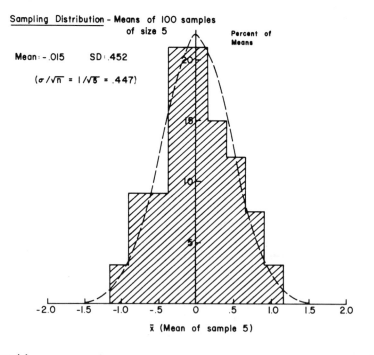

Figure 4.1
Standardized normal population (top) and empirical sampling distribution of means for 100 samples of size 5 (bottom).

normal distribution, i.e., a normal population distribution whose mean is zero and standard deviation is unity, as is illustrated in the top half of Figure 4.1. A series of 100 random samples of five observations each was selected, and the mean for each sample of five was calculated. The mean of the 100 means is -0.015, which is in agreement with the mean of zero that the first property listed above indicates. The SD of the 100 means is 0.452, agreeing with the $\sigma/\sqrt{n} = 1/\sqrt{5} = 0.447$ of Property 2. Finally, in the bottom half of Figure 4.1, the sampling distribution of means is approximately bell-shaped, as is indicated by Property 3. Of course, by continuing beyond 100 samples, the empirical results would more closely approach the theoretical results described by the three properties.

Example 4.4. The population distribution is the uniform distribution, which is clearly not normal in shape (see the top half of Figure 4.2). The uniform distribution is a theoretical popu-

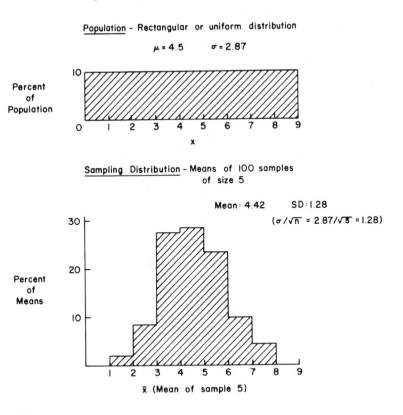

Figure 4.2
Uniform population (top) and empirical sampling distribution of means for 100 samples of size 5 (bottom).

lation distribution in which each of the digits 0, 1, ..., 9 appears with equal frequency. An example to which it applies is a clinical measurement, such as serum uric acid level, that can be read correctly to the nearest tenth of a milligram per 100 ml. Among a large series of serum uric acid level readings, the percentage of readings tabulated by the last digit would theoretically follow the uniform distribution. The uniform probability distribution has a mean of 4.5 and an SD of 2.87 (see Chapter 3, p. 77).

From this population, 100 random samples of five observations were selected and their means determined. The mean of the 100 means is 4.42 compared with the 4.5 predicted by theory (Property 1), the SD is 1.28 compared with the $\sigma/\sqrt{n} = 2.87/\sqrt{5} = 1.28$ of theory (Property 2), and the shape of the distribution of these 100 means (see the bottom half of Figure 4.2) compares well with the normal distribution that theory dictates (Property 3). This last property holds even though the population distribution was definitely nonnormal in shape.

Example 4.5.   The top half of Figure 4.3 displays an empirical population distribution: the age at onset for all cases of poliomyelitis in Massachusetts in 1949. The mean of this distribution is 13.9 years with an SD of 10.3 years. This population distribution is clearly not normal in shape.

From this population, 100 random samples of 10 were selected. The mean of the 100 means is 13.8 years and the SD of the means is 3.5 years. The distribution of the 100 means is illustrated in the bottom half of Figure 4.3. This agrees well with Property 1 (the population mean is 13.9), Property 2 (SD $= \sigma/\sqrt{n} = 10.3/\sqrt{10} = 3.3$), and Property 3 (the shape is approximately normal) of the sampling distribution of means.

It is the tendency toward normality (Property 3) of the sampling distribution of means that permits calculation of critical ratios and use of the standardized normal distribution. The critical ratio was previously defined (Chapter 3) as

$$z = \frac{x - \mu}{\sigma}$$

For the normally shaped sampling distribution of means, the observations are *means*, and the mean and SD of the distribution are those of Properties 1 and 2. Hence, the appropriate critical ratio becomes

$$z = \frac{\bar{x} - \mu}{\sigma/\sqrt{n}}$$

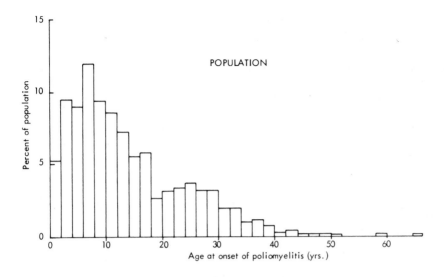

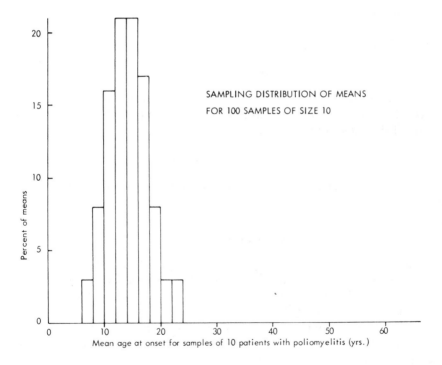

Figure 4.3
Percentage distribution by age of the reported cases of poliomyelitis in Massachusetts in 1949 (top) and empirical sampling distribution of means for 100 samples of size 10 (bottom).

Table 4.1 summarizes the contrast between the population distribution and the sampling distribution of means.

Table 4.1. Summary of properties of the sampling distribution of means compared with the underlying population distribution

Distribution	Mean	SD	Shape	Critical ratio
Population	μ	σ	Any	$z = \dfrac{x - \mu^{a}}{\sigma}$
Sampling distribution of means of samples of size n	μ	$\sigma/\sqrt{n}$	Approximately normal regardless of shape of population distribution[b]	$z = \dfrac{\bar{x} - \mu}{\sigma/\sqrt{n}}$

[a] Valid only if shape of population is approximately normal.
[b] Provided n is large enough.

Sampling distributions involve a special vocabulary. The SD of the sampling distribution of means is called the *standard error of the mean* and is denoted as $SE(\bar{x})$ or $SE_{\bar{x}}$. Hence,

$$\text{Standard error of the mean} = SE(\bar{x}) = \sigma/\sqrt{n}$$

Correspondingly, the variance of the sampling distribution of means is called the *variance of the mean* and is denoted by $V(\bar{x})$. The variance is the square of the standard error, i.e.,

$$\text{Variance of the mean} = V(\bar{x}) = [SE(\bar{x})]^2 = \sigma^2/n$$

Finally, this variability in the sampling distribution of means is referred to as *sampling variation*.

The Condition for Approximate Normality

The one problem in claiming an approximately normal shape for the sampling distribution of means (Property 3) has been the somewhat vague proviso that n be large enough. The reader may well wonder how large is "large enough." Unfortunately, there is no clear-cut answer.

First, if one is sampling from an underlying population that itself is normally distributed, there is no cause for concern. Any n is large enough; i.e., the sampling distribution of means is normal no matter what the value of n, even if $n = 1$.

Second, it is clear that when sampling from nonnormal populations, $n = 1$ is never large enough, since the sampling distribution of means of samples of size 1 merely reproduces the population distribution.

In general, the n at which the sampling distribution of means tends to be approximately normal in shape depends on the extent to which the underlying population distribution departs from a normal shape.

As an example of investigating a "large enough n," consider the uniform population distribution (see the top half of Figure 4.2). The sampling distributions of means of samples of size 2, 3, and 4 from this population are shown in Figure 4.4. By inspection, the sampling distribution of means for

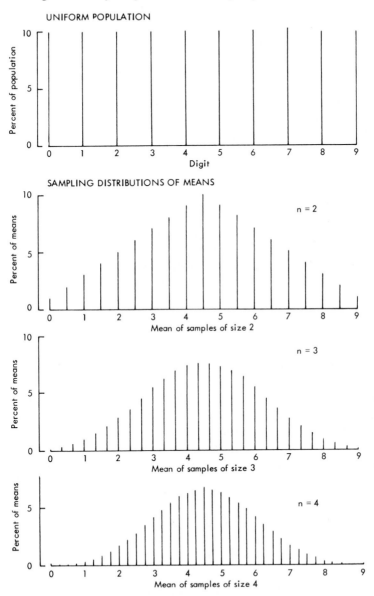

Figure 4.4
Uniform population and theoretical sampling distributions of means for samples of sizes 2, 3, and 4.

$n = 3$ appears sufficiently close to normal, and, even for $n = 2$, the shape does not appear to be very far from normal. In this case, then, $n = 3$ appears to be "large enough."

In cases in which the theoretical form of the underlying population distribution is known—e.g., if it is binomial, Poisson, or exponential (see Chapter 3)—guidelines have been established for "large enough n" to ensure a sampling distribution of means that is sufficiently normal in shape. The guidelines for the binomial distribution are discussed later (p. 153).

There is no cause for concern when the underlying population is normal, and this is clearly an advantageous situation, especially if a small sample size is contemplated. Basically, one hasn't a choice; one samples from the population defined and has no say about its shape. Sometimes, however, some manipulation can produce a situation more analogous to that of sampling from an underlying normally distributed population. Often a simple transformation—such as taking the logarithm of each observation or the square root of each observation—will produce this situation. Knowledge of when to apply such transformations depends on the backlog of experience accumulated in the particular area, or in similar areas, of investigation.

As mentioned in Chapter 3 (p. 83), for example, in pharmacological work it has been established with many drugs that the distribution of the amount of drug required to produce some response in a subject is not normally distributed from one subject to another, but the logarithms of these doses are. Hence, one employs a logarithmic transformation, i.e., one obtains the logarithm of each observed dose, and, with a sample, one works with the mean, SD, and so forth in "log dose" units.

Other Sampling Distributions

So far the discussion has focused on the sampling distribution of *means*. However, the principle for generating the sampling distribution of means can be applied to any other value that may be calculated in a sample. Hence, one can talk about the sampling distribution of the standard deviation, the range, the median, and so on. These sampling distributions derive from calculating the standard deviations, ranges, medians, or whatever in repeat samples of size n from a population. Figure 4.5 shows an empirically determined sampling distribution of the standard deviation: the result of calculating the sample standard deviation in 100 repeat samples of size 10 from the population of age at onset of poliomyelitis (see Figure 4.3).

Note that the three properties for the sampling distribution of means do not necessarily apply to sampling distributions of other quantities.

In the usual nomenclature, the standard deviation of the sampling distribution of any quantity is referred to as the *standard error* of that quantity; hence, one can talk about the standard error of the standard deviation, the standard error of the range, the standard error of the median, and so forth. Furthermore, any quantity determined in a sample is called a *sample statistic*.

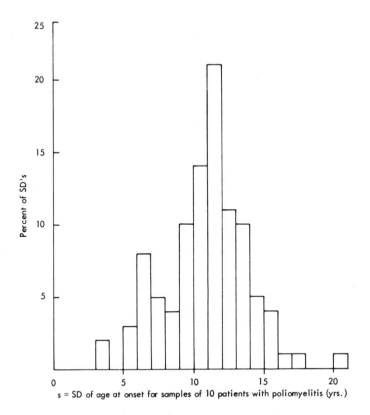

Figure 4.5
Empirical sampling distribution of the SD for 100 samples of size 10 from the population of reported cases of poliomyelitis by age in Massachusetts in 1949.

The mean, SD, range, or median is each a sample statistic. Every sample statistic has a *sampling distribution*, and the standard deviation in the resulting sampling distribution is therefore termed the *standard error of the statistic*. Hence, if u denotes any statistic calculated in a sample, $SE(u)$ denotes the standard error or sampling variation of that statistic. A great deal of the theory of statistics is concerned with the derivation of the mathematical forms for the sampling distributions of various statistics based on the assumption of a particular mathematical form for the underlying population distribution.

Manipulation of the Sampling Distribution of Means

This section concerns the use of the critical ratio to relate the sampling distribution of means to the standardized normal distribution, i.e., the use of

$$z = \frac{\bar{x} - \mu}{\sigma/\sqrt{n}}$$

Such manipulation permits the answers to the following three questions:

1. With a prescribed sample size, what proportion of the sampling distribution of means is above some specified value?
2. With a prescribed sample size, what mean value corresponds to cutting off a specified portion of the sampling distribution of means?
3. What sample size is required so that in the resulting sampling distribution of means a specified proportion of the means will depart by a specified amount from the population mean?

Example 4.6.   The underlying population is the serum uric acid levels of males that was considered in Chapter 2 (Example 2.5). The mean is $\mu = 5.4$ mg per 100 ml, and the SD is $\sigma = 1.0$ mg per 100 ml.

A. Among repeat samples of size 25 from this population, what proportion of samples have means of 5.9 mg per 100 ml or more?

Answer: This is the same as asking what proportion of the normally shaped sampling distribution of means of size 25 is above 5.9 mg per 100 ml. The critical ratio gives

$$z = \frac{5.9 - 5.4}{1.0/\sqrt{25}} = \frac{0.5}{0.2} = 2.50$$

The one-tailed normal curve table (Appendix Table A1) gives 0.6 percent as the required area.

B. What value cuts off the upper 5 percent of the sampling distribution of means of size 25?

Answer: This is equivalent to asking what corresponds to the upper 5 percent point of the normally shaped sampling distribution of means of size 25. Appendix Table A1 gives 1.65 for the upper 5 percent point. Hence, set

$$1.65 = \frac{\bar{x} - 5.4}{1.0/\sqrt{25}} = \frac{\bar{x} - 5.4}{0.2}$$

so that $x = 5.4 + (1.65)(0.2) = 5.73$ mg per 100 ml.

C. How large a sample size is required so that 5 percent of the means of samples of this size will exceed the population mean by 0.2 mg per 100 ml or more?

Answer: Determine n so that the upper 5 percent point of the sampling distribution of means is $x = \mu + 0.2$ (or $x - \mu = 0.2$). Appendix Table A1 indicates 1.65 as the cut-off point for 5 percent of the curve. Hence, set

$$1.65 = \frac{0.2}{1.0/\sqrt{n}}$$

so that

$$n = [(1.65)(1.0)/0.2]^2 = 8.25^2 = 68.06$$

The required sample size, then, is 69 men.

Example 4.7. The population consists of cancer patients with a mean survival $\mu = 38.3$ months and an SD of $\sigma = 43.3$ months. Note that in this population the survival time is not normally distributed, since the mean minus 1 SD gives a negative value. The sample size of 100 or more under consideration, however, is assuredly large enough to ensure that the sampling distribution of means is normal.

A. Among samples of size 100 from this population, what proportion will have mean survival of either 46.9 months and more or 29.7 months and less? (This asks about deviations in *both* directions from the mean.)
Answer: Calculate critical ratios corresponding to these two values:

$$z = \frac{46.9 - 38.3}{43.3/\sqrt{100}} = \frac{8.6}{4.33} = 1.99$$

$$z = \frac{29.7 - 38.3}{43.3/\sqrt{100}} = \frac{-8.6}{4.33} = -1.99$$

Appendix Table A2 yields 4.7 percent as the area cut-off.

B. What limits embrace 95 percent of the means of samples of size 100 from this population?
Answer: Appendix Table A2 indicates that ± 1.96 embrace 95 percent of the standardized normal curve. Hence, using the critical ratio,

$$\pm 1.96 = \frac{\bar{x} - 38.3}{43.3/\sqrt{100}} = \frac{\bar{x} - 38.3}{4.33}$$

$$\bar{x} = 38.3 \pm (1.96)(4.33) = 38.3 \pm 8.5$$

$$= 29.8 \text{ to } 46.8 \text{ months}$$

Therefore, 95 percent of means of samples of size 100 will be between 29.8 and 46.8 months.

C. How large a sample of cancer patients is needed so that 95 percent of the means of samples of this size will be within ± 6 months of the population mean?

Answer: The two-tailed normal curve table (Appendix Table A2) gives ± 1.96 as embracing 95 percent of the standard normal curve, and the question indicates that $\bar{x} - \mu = \pm 6$. Hence, one obtains

$$1.96 = \frac{6}{43.3/\sqrt{n}}$$

$$n = [(1.96)(43.3)/6]^2 = (14.14)^2 = 200 \text{ patients}$$

A STATISTICAL TEST OF SIGNIFICANCE ON A MEAN

The preceding discussion provides the necessary equipment for conducting a test of significance on the mean. In fact, the arithmetic for such a test has already been performed. This section describes the logical basis for the statistical testing of hypotheses, shows how this relates to what has already been calculated, discusses the conclusion to be drawn from this analysis, and then proceeds with further implications and considerations of statistical tests of significance.

Description

One begins with a statement that claims a particular value for the unknown population mean. For example, with drug-treated cancer patients, one might claim that mean survival in this population is 38.3 months; or one might state with a population of male patients with some disease, say, diabetes mellitus, that their mean serum uric acid level is 5.4 mg per 100 ml. In general, μ_0 denotes the particular value of the population mean in this statement.

The statistical inference consists of drawing one of the following two conclusions regarding this statement:

1. Reject the claim about the population mean because there is sufficient evidence to doubt its validity, and conclude that μ_0 is not the population mean.
2. Do not reject the claim about the population mean, because there is not sufficient evidence to doubt its validity. One then concludes that, as far as one can tell, μ_0 may very well be the population mean.

One arrives at one of these two conclusions by the analysis of a random sample of n observations from the population, in particular, by examining the mean, $\bar{x}$, of this random sample and comparing it with μ_0. The following reasoning provides the basis for arriving at either of these conclusions: Suppose the claim is true and the population mean is μ_0. What, then, is the chance that random sampling from such a population would produce a sample mean as deviant as or more deviant than the $\bar{x}$ observed? If this chance *is* sufficiently small, then one reasons that the observed sample mean is not a plausible outcome. Therefore, the basic premise must be faulty. Hence, μ_0 is *not* the mean of the population, i.e., one reaches the first conclusion. If, on the other hand, this chance *is not* sufficiently small, then the observed sample mean is a plausible outcome, and one has not contradicted the basic premise that μ_0 is the population mean. Thus, one reaches the second conclusion.

It is necessary to be specific and define what a "sufficiently small" chance means. This is accomplished by arbitrarily picking a probability value and defining it as sufficiently small; in most medical situations, one picks either 5 percent or 1 percent. A choice of 5 percent indicates that a chance as small as .05 (1 in 20) provides sufficient evidence to contradict the statement that μ_0 is the population mean. A choice of 1 percent (1 in 100) is, of course, a more conservative value.

Now one must implement this strategy. The analysis consists of determining the chance of observing a mean as deviant as or more deviant than the sample mean, under the assumption that the sample came from a population whose mean is μ_0. One then compares this chance with the predetermined "sufficiently small" chance. Substituting "relative frequency" for "chance" and rewording terms, it becomes a matter of determining the relative frequency with which means of samples of size n are as deviant as or more deviant than the observed $\bar{x}$ when μ_0 is the population mean. This is essentially a question about areas in the tails of the sampling distribution of means. As before, one calculates the critical ratio

$$z = \frac{\bar{x} - \mu_0}{\sigma/\sqrt{n}}$$

One then uses tables of the normal distribution (if n is large enough) and compares the result with the predetermined "sufficiently small" chance.

The inference does not involve generating a sampling distribution of means. One uses what is known of this sampling distribution to relate the observation of a *single* sample mean to a population mean.

Before working some examples, another point must be made. The determination of the chance of a sample mean as deviant as or more deviant than that observed requires the specification of whether interest is in deviation in only one or in both directions from μ_0. This dictates whether the one-tailed or two-tailed normal curve table (Appendix Table A1 or A2) is to be used. The majority of medical applications specify *both* directions from the mean and therefore indicate the use of Appendix Table A2. The experimental situation and the aims of the study, however, determine the distinction between one and both directions. A more complete discussion of this point appears later (p. 124).

In summary, a test of significance on a mean requires specification of:

1. A statement that the population mean is some particular value, μ_0.
2. A probability level that is sufficiently small to provide reasonable evidence against μ_0. In general, this probability is denoted as α.
3. Whether concern is with deviations in one or both directions from μ_0.

Example 4.8.   The population consists of serum uric acid levels of male patients with diabetes mellitus.
Specifications:
1.   The serum uric acid level in the population is 5.4 mg per 100 ml serum.
2.   A probability of 5 percent is sufficiently small.
3.   Concern is with deviations in only one direction (above the population mean).
Observation:
In a sample of 25 diabetics, the mean serum uric acid level is 5.9 mg per 100 ml.
Analysis:
The arithmetic for this analysis has been previously performed (see Example 4.6), giving a critical ratio of 2.50. From Appendix Table A1, the chance of a mean this large or larger is 0.6 percent, which is less than 5 percent.
Conclusion:
Reject the statement that the mean serum uric acid level in the population of male diabetics is 5.4 mg per 100 ml. The sample provides reasonable evidence that the diabetics' serum uric acid levels have a population mean above 5.4 mg per 100 ml.

Example 4.9.   The population consists of survival times of cancer patients who have been treated with a new drug.
Specifications:
1.   The mean survival time in the population is 38.3 months.
2.   A probability of 5 percent is sufficiently small.
3.   The concern is with deviations in both directions from the population mean.
Observation:
A sample of 100 drug-treated cancer patients has a mean survival figure of 46.9 months.
Analysis:
The arithmetic for this analysis has also been previously performed (see Example 4.7), giving a critical ratio of 1.99. Appendix Table A2 gives 4.7 percent as the chance that a mean of a sample of 100 would be as deviant as or more deviant than what was observed. This is just below 5 percent.
Conclusion:
Reject the statement that the mean survival of drug-treated cancer patients is 38.3 months. There is sufficient evidence that mean survival in the population of drug-treated cancer patients is longer than 38.3 months.

It is, of course, important to consider the implication of these conclusions. Before doing so, it may be helpful to provide some nomenclature for the statistical tests of significance just performed.

Nomenclature

The initial claim regarding the population mean defines the *null hypothesis*. Thus, the preceding section involved a test of significance of the null hypothesis that the population mean is μ_0. If H_0 denotes the null hypothesis, then in algebraic terms the test was of $H_0 : \mu = \mu_0$.

The specification of a sufficiently small chance, which is denoted by α, determines the *significance level*. Conventionally, one chooses $\alpha = .05$ or $\alpha = .01$.

Specification of interest in deviations in one or in both directions corresponds with determination of a *one-sided* or *two-sided test*.

The conclusion that rejects the statement about the population mean then *rejects the null hypothesis*; the other conclusion *does not reject the null hypothesis* (it is wise to refrain from the expression "accept the null hypothesis" for reasons that will be discussed later—see p. 117). These two conclusions are equivalent, respectively, to claiming *statistically significant* and *not statistically significant* results.

Hence, to perform a statistical significance test on the mean, one must specify a null hypothesis population mean, μ_0, a significance level, α, and whether the concern is with a one-sided or two-sided test. Test results are either statistically significant or not statistically significant.

For the serum uric acid levels of diabetics (Example 4.8), the result of a one-sided test of the null hypothesis—i.e., that the population mean is 5.4 mg per 100 ml serum—was statistically significant at the 5 percent level. Hence, the null hypothesis was rejected.

For the drug-treated cancer patients, the result of a two-sided test of the null hypothesis—i.e., that the population mean survival is 38.3 months—was statistically significant at the 5 percent level. Hence, the null hypothesis that drug-treated cancer patients have a mean survival of 38.3 months was likewise rejected.

Interpretation

It is important to remember that a test of significance *always* refers to a null hypothesis. The concern here is with an unknown population mean, and the null hypothesis states that it is some particular value: 5.4 mg per 100 ml for the serum uric acid levels of diabetics or 38.3 months for the survival time of cancer patients. With any statistical test of significance, the null hypothesis must be either explicitly stated or clearly implied.

The test of significance answers the question: Is chance or sampling variation a likely explanation of the discrepancy between a sample result and the corresponding null hypothesis population value? A "yes" answer—a discrepancy that is likely to occur by chance variation—indicates the sample result is compatible with the claim that the sampling is from a population in which the null hypothesis prevails. This is the meaning of "not statistically significant." A "no" answer—a discrepancy that is *unlikely* to occur by chance variation—indicates that the sample result is *not* compatible with the claim that sampling is from a population in which the null hypothesis prevails. This is the meaning of "statistically significant."

Hence, the following terms can be used interchangeably:

Statistically significant	= Reject null hypothesis	= Sample value not compatible with null hypothesis value	= Sampling variation is an unlikely explanation of discrepancy between null hypothesis and sample values
Not statistically significant	= Do not reject null hypothesis	= Sample value compatible with null hypothesis value	= Sampling variation is a likely explanation of discrepancy between null hypothesis and sample values

The level of significance selected, be it 5 percent, 1 percent, or otherwise, must be clearly indicated. A statement that the results were "statistically significant" without giving further details is worthless.

Consider now the implications of the choice of a significance level, say, the 5 percent level. By specifying this level, an investigator states that he is willing to risk a 5 percent chance of erroneously rejecting his null hypothesis when, in fact, the null hypothesis is true. Alternatively, this means that with many repeated statistical tests of significance, each performed at the 5 percent significance level, on the average 5 percent (or 1 in 20) will erroneously reject true null hypotheses; 95 percent (or 19 in 20) will correctly not reject true null hypotheses. (Of course, only some omnipotent being could identify which of the 1 in 20 are wrong and which of the 19 in 20 are correct.)

It has already been indicated that a 1 percent significance level (i.e., a one in 100 chance of erroneously rejecting the null hypothesis) is, of course, less risky. As with other aspects of life, however, one does not get something for nothing, and one must pay a price for being more conservative. The price will be evident in the discussion of the β or type II error (p. 120).

It is common for investigators to indicate their conclusion and their significance level simultaneously with the format: "statistically significant ($P < .05$)" or "not statistically significant ($P > .05$)."*

Since a result that is significant at some predetermined level is clearly significant for all higher significance levels (e.g., a result significant at the 0.1 percent level is significant at the 1, 5, and 10 percent levels), some investigators customarily state the smallest level at which the sample results are significant, or they merely indicate the probability value determined from the critical ratio. For example, with the serum uric acid levels of diabetics, the result might appear as "a test of the null hypothesis that the population mean is 5.4 mg per 100 ml was found to be statistically significant ($P < .01$)" or "... $P = .006$."

---

* Whereas "Pr" stands for the probability of the occurrence of an event, the notation "P" is used for probability in the sense of statistical significance.

The statement "$P < .01$" indicates that the discrepancy between the sample mean and the null hypothesis mean is significant even if such a conservative significance level as 1 percent is adopted. The statement "$P = .006$" indicates that the result is significant at any level up to 0.6 percent. It must be emphasized that one must not interpret these statements as indicating the probability of the truth of the null hypothesis.

A further caution in the interpretation of significance tests is that "not statistically significant" does not prove the null hypothesis true. The most that can be said with results that are not statistically significant is that the data fail to provide sufficient evidence to doubt the validity of the null hypothesis. The null hypothesis might actually not be valid, but the sample was just too small to reach this conclusion at the predetermined significance level. Hence, "not significant" is like "not proved" or "inconclusive." It indicates that one has to live with the null hypothesis value until other evidence is obtained. In this discussion, the phrase "accept the null hypothesis" as a synonym for "not statistically significant" has been particularly avoided because it connotes there is proof that the null hypothesis is valid. Those well versed in statistical methods often do use the phrase, but with the clear understanding that it does *not* imply proof. If the reader finds an occasional "accept the null hypothesis" later in this text, the interpretation is strictly within the context of "not enough evidence to contradict."

Another warning deals with the confusion between the technical statistical meaning and the everyday meaning of the word "significant." One must not equate "statistically significant" with "medically important." A result may be highly statistically significant, yet medically it may be quite unimportant. An editorial in the *New England Journal of Medicine* entitled "Significance of significant" has most eloquently clarified the confusion [36]:

SIGNIFICANCE, being one of those words that mean everything or nothing, is too convenient for the medical writer. In its refined statistical sense, significance embodies mathematical precision. In its vulgar usage, unrelated to statistical manipulations, it comfortably serves ambiguity. It permits an author to describe his clinical findings as significant, or his patients as prospering significantly, and so to impute importance to his efforts without requiring him to use an acceptable measure of that importance. It affords him, moreover, with a mobile hedge against criticism. With the label of significance, he may circumvent the more direct immodesty of claiming importance, and he can safely insist that a given event is undeniably significant to him. . . . In this, its conventional usage, significant has become a word devoid of significance.

In contrast, the medical writer who uses significance to express a statistical analysis is being rigorously exact. . . . Significance used to summarize a statistical operation is fabulously useful for the clinical investigator. Few other words serve precision so well.

To have one popular word serve the extremes of both exactness and inexactness hardly furthers clarity in medical writing. The *Journal* therefore proposes to discourage the use of significance and its corresponding adjective and adverb in its scientific articles, except when the term is warranted by statistical backing. Writers and other editors, it is hoped, will be persuaded to do likewise.

One must be wary. This goal regarding the usage of significance in medical writing is still far from being achieved.

Returning to the previous example of the serum uric acid levels of diabetics, the following discussion pertains to why the particular null hypothesis mean was selected and what the results of the significance test imply. Recall that the test of significance yielded statistically significant results at the 5 percent level.

For the serum uric acid levels of diabetics, the null hypothesis was a population mean of 5.4 mg per 100 ml. This is based on information from a study of males in the general population in which the mean serum uric acid level was found to be 5.4 mg per 100 ml with an SD of 1.0 mg per 100 ml (see Chapter 2). The null hypothesis is equivalent to stating that mean serum uric acid levels in the population of male diabetics is the same as that of males in the general population. The initial question was: "Do diabetics have a higher mean serum uric acid level than other males?" The null hypothesis of equal means for diabetic and general population males was established with the intent of obtaining evidence that may refute it, i.e., to be able to answer, "Yes, diabetics do have higher serum uric acid levels." This statistical reasoning is analogous to the *reductio ad absurdum* used in many proofs in geometry. One proposes a premise, follows a logical scheme, and shows that the acceptance of this premise leads to a contradiction or, in the present example, improbability. If this is demonstrable, one rejects the premise and turns to an alternative premise. With the sample of serum uric acid levels among diabetics, the analysis led to the conclusion that diabetics have a statistically significantly higher mean serum uric acid level than other males. A result that had not been statistically significant in this case would not have proved that the means were the same. All that could have been said was that the evidence was insufficient to indicate a difference in mean serum uric acid levels between diabetic and general population males.

It is important to note that the test of significance presupposes *random* sampling from the population under scrutiny. Actually, strict random sampling in medical studies is rare. One should always examine how the sample observations were selected, ask how large is the departure from strict random sampling, and determine in what ways the sample may be biased and nonrepresentative of the target population. This is related to the discussion in Chapter 1 on target and sample populations and to the discussion in Chapter 11.

For the comparison of two groups considered in Chapter 10, this assumption of random sampling from an underlying population may be relaxed. A rather different assumption is involved (p. 262). Random assignment to groups (p. 257) in this situation ensures that the assumption holds and permits application of tests of significance with impunity.

In assessing the results of a test of significance, the reader should have, as an immediate question, whether the design of the investigation was such that the author had the right to conduct a test of significance. An editorial, "Statistics in medical research," in the *New England Journal of Medicine* commented [98]:

Unfortunately, the arithmetic computational part of statistical methods can be applied to any set of numbers no matter how derived. The validity of the method is dependent, however, on how the data are collected. Inappropriate data will yield a numerical solution as readily as appropriate data. The temptation to use these methods regardless of the appropriateness of the data is obviously very great, as one may judge from current literature. In interpreting such literature it therefore becomes necessary to ask first not what the test of significance shows—but what justification there is for calculating it.

Considering the example of the drug treatment of cancer patients, the null hypothesis was that the mean survival is 38.3 months. This null hypothesis arose with the statement that cancer patients *without* drug therapy were known to survive a mean of 38.3 months, with an SD of 43.3 months. Hence, the null hypothesis claims that the drug-treated population has the same mean survival as that in the population previously without drug treatment. The investigator, particularly if he were the discoverer of the drug, would hope that the sample results would provide evidence to refute this null hypothesis and would permit him to conclude that drug-treated patients live significantly longer. One might then recommend this drug as the preferred treatment with this type of cancer. Adopting the 5 percent significance level, one can see from the results that drug-treated cancer patients live significantly longer than the previously established mean survival of 38.3 months without drug therapy, so there seems to be a basis for recommending this drug.

Is this recommendation justified? In this author's opinion, the answer is definitely "no." There are reasonable arguments that this investigation fails to provide sufficient evidence to attribute any statistically significant increase in longevity to the drug. The statistical analysis is correct; the investigation is deficient. In simplest terms, this investigation lacks adequate controls. *Historical controls* are used, i.e., present patients receiving the drug are compared with past patients without drug treatment. The test of significance merely indicates that the mean survival of the present drug-treated sample is not compatible with the population mean survival of past patients without drug therapy. The argument is that there are factors other than use of the drug that offer a reasonable explanation for the statistically significant results. What are these factors?

1. *The present cancer patients may be very different from those of the past.* First, present patients may be diagnosed at an earlier stage of their disease. If the methods of diagnosis have improved and it is possible to identify cases earlier, then the present mean survival will, of course, be greater than that of past experience, quite apart from any effect of the drug. Second, the natural history of the disease may have changed over time. It is well known that there are secular trends in diseases, apart from diagnostic advances and fads in diagnosis. Some diseases become more virulent over time, others less so. Perhaps the latter may have occurred with this type of cancer, producing the longer survival. Third, there may be other factors that are closely related to survival which, when scrutinized in the sample under study, could explain the favorable results. For example, age and sex are important prognostic factors with almost any disease. If the best prognosis is for young females, then, if there are proportionately more young females in the drug-treated sample as compared with the controls of past experience, the drug-treated group would achieve longer survival.

2. *The medical management and supervision of present patients may be different from that of the past.* First, the 100 patients, because they are in a trial, are likely to receive closer and stricter medical supervision than past patients. Perhaps this increased medical attention contributes to prolonged survival. Second, there may be some unsuspected aspect of present supportive therapy, not previously applied, that contributes to increased longevity. Third, even a psychological effect is conceivable. The sample of 100 patients may have been told that they were being treated with some new "wonder drug" that represented a present-day miracle. The effect of this on the patients' morale and the subsequent influence on survival is a factor that cannot be discounted.

Only when one can establish beyond reasonable doubt that such factors as the above do not influence the comparison of drug treatment and no drug treatment, can one justify a claim regarding the effect of the drug. The case argued above applies in some respects to almost any therapeutic or clinical study that uses historical controls. Historical controls simply do not provide a valid basis for drawing inferences regarding the effects of new drugs or medical procedures.

What, then, does provide a basis? The obvious answer is *concurrent controls*, i.e., a sample series of observations using the new drug that are obtained simultaneously with a control sample series using no drug or using an established standard drug. The goal is then to compare the mean survival in these two groups. An appropriately designed controlled clinical trial (see Chapter 10) will account for these other factors beyond reasonable doubt. Then the results of a statistical analysis comparing mean survival can be attributed directly to the effect of the drug.

Hence, with concurrent controls the goal is to compare two sample means: treatment versus control. The appropriate statistical analysis of this comparison, as well as its interpretation, constitutes the subject of the latter portion of this chapter.

Two Errors of Hypothesis Testing

The significance level has already been referred to as the risk of erroneously rejecting a null hypothesis that is really true. This error is called the α *error*, *type I error*, or *error of the first kind*. This terminology implies that there is a β *error*, *type II error*, or *error of the second kind*.

A β *error* is defined as the chance of erroneously failing to reject a null hypothesis that is, in fact, false. For example, with the serum uric acid levels of diabetics, suppose the true population mean were really 6.0 mg per 100 ml. In this circumstance, one would prefer that a test of significance of the null hypothesis mean of 5.4 mg per 100 ml yield a "statistically significant" conclusion. It is possible, however, that one will reach the conclusion "not statistically significant." The β error is the chance of reaching this erroneous conclusion.

Example 4.10.   What is the β error for the study of diabetics' serum uric acid levels? Recall that a one-sided test at the 5 percent level

SAMPLING DISTRIBUTIONS OF MEANS OF SAMPLES OF SIZE 25

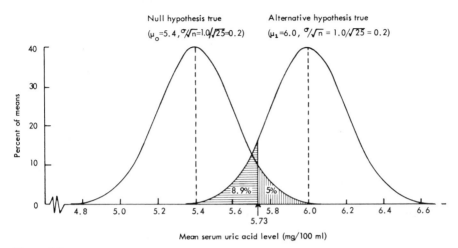

Figure 4.6
Type I and II errors for a test of significance on the mean serum uric acid level in a sample of 25 men.

was performed with a sample size of 25. The determination of the type II error is illustrated in Figure 4.6. First, one determines what mean value for a sample of size 25 would fail to reject the null hypothesis when it is true. This indicates the cut-off point corresponding to the upper 5 percent of the sampling distribution of means, assuming the null hypothesis is true. This question was answered with the manipulation of the sampling distribution of means (Example 4.6) wherein a value of 5.73 mg per 100 ml was obtained. Hence, any mean of a sample of size 25 that is above 5.73 mg per 100 ml will provide evidence to reject the null hypothesis that the mean is 5.4 mg per 100 ml; any mean below this value will not provide a basis for rejecting this null hypothesis. This point is illustrated by the left-hand curve in Figure 4.6.

The β or type II error can now be defined as the chance of not rejecting the null hypothesis when the alternative population mean prevails. In this case, the alternative is 6.0 mg per 100 ml. Again the concern is with a sampling distribution of means of samples of size 25 but now with one whose mean is 6.0 mg per 100 ml, namely, the right-hand curve in Figure 4.6. Since a sample mean below 5.73 mg per 100 ml fails to supply evidence to reject the null hypothesis, the question is: What portion of this right-hand curve falls below 5.73 mg per 100 ml? The critical ratio is

$$z = \frac{5.73 - 6.0}{1.0/\sqrt{25}} = \frac{-0.27}{0.2} = -1.35$$

The one-tailed normal curve table (Appendix Table A1) gives 0.089 as the required area for this value of z. Hence, the β error is 8.9 percent when the population mean is actually 6.0 mg per 100 ml.

The consequence of reducing the significance level, which leads to an α or *type I error*, can be easily seen in Figure 4.6. To cut off less than 5 percent in the upper tail of the left-hand curve, the cut-off point must move above 5.73 mg per 100 ml. This, of course, increases the area in the lower tail of the right-hand curve. Hence, a decrease in type I error increases the type II or β error. Likewise, the type II or β error can be decreased only at the risk of increasing the type I or α error.

The distinction between the two types of error is summarized below:

	Reality	
Conclusion of test of significance	Population mean is μ_0 (null hypothesis is true)	Population mean is not μ_0 but μ_1 (null hypothesis is not true)
Not statistically significant (Do not reject NH)	Correct conclusion	Type II or β error
Statistically significant (Reject NH)	Type I or α error	Correct conclusion

Note that the type II error corresponds with a particular alternative population mean that is denoted by μ_1. One could determine a series of β values for a series of values of μ_1. For example, with the diabetics' serum uric acid levels, one could determine β for $\mu_1 = 5.5$ mg per 100 ml, $\mu_1 = 5.6$ mg per 100 ml, and so on. In fact, one can construct a graph with the series of alternative population means (μ_1) forming the abscissa and the corresponding β values forming the ordinate. This graph yields what is called the *operating characteristic* (OC) of the test. The operating characteristic for the study of diabetics' serum uric acid levels is shown in Figure 4.7.

The complement of the type II error, denoted as $1 - \beta$, is called the *power of the test* at μ_1. If one plots the power of the test (ordinate) against μ (abscissa), the result is called the *power function curve*. In other words, the power function curve is the complement of the operating characteristic curve. These curves are important when one wants to compare several alternative procedures for performing tests of significance. Examination of the power function curve aids in choosing from among these several alternatives.

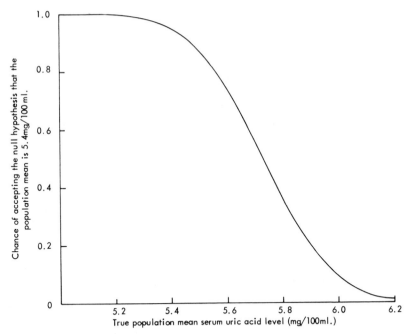

Figure 4.7
Operating characteristic (OC) function for a one-sided test of significance with a sample of 25 men of the null hypothesis that the mean population serum uric acid level is 5.4 mg per 100 ml.

Another point regarding the two types of error is that the magnitude of type II error for a prescribed type I error depends on the degree of overlap of the curves in Figure 4.6. The less the overlap, the better is the situation with respect to type II error. What, then, can be done to decrease overlap?

Aside from sliding the entire right-hand curve to the right, one can reduce overlap by reducing the spread of the two curves. Both curves are sampling distributions of means having SD $= \sigma/\sqrt{n}$. Although one can do nothing with regard to σ (the inherent subject-to-subject variability in the population), one *can* increase n. This reduces $\sigma/\sqrt{n}$ and, therefore, the overlap. Hence, for a prescribed type I error, the type II error decreases when the sample size increases.

This now covers the three essential elements of significance testing: the significance level or α error associated with the null hypothesis mean μ_0, the β error associated with the alternative hypothesis mean μ_1, and the sample size, n. With the specification of n and an α associated with a particular μ_0, the β for a particular μ_1 was determined. Alternatively, one might specify α with a particular μ_0, β with a particular μ_1, and then determine the required n. This is one way that the statistician answers the perennial question: How large a sample is needed? This is discussed in detail later in this chapter (p. 142).

One-sided versus Two-sided Tests

One- and two-sided tests differ with respect to the interpretation of a statistically significant conclusion. With a statistically significant one-sided test result (upper tail), the inference is that the true population value is *above* that specified by the null hypothesis; with a two-sided test, the inference is that the true population value is *either above or below* the null hypothesis value.

Logically, an investigator chooses between a one- and two-sided test *before* he obtains his sample result, i.e., the choice is not influenced by the sample outcome. The investigator asks: Is it important to be able to detect alternatives only above the null hypothesis mean, or is it important to be able to detect alternatives that may be either above or below this mean? His answer, of course, depends on the particular circumstances of the investigation.

With the serum uric acid levels of diabetics, a one-sided test was performed using the upper tail. This means the concern is only with the alternative that diabetics' serum uric acid levels may be above 5.4 mg per 100 ml. The true population mean might actually be below 5.4 mg per 100 ml, but choice of a one-tailed test indicates that this possibility is of no concern.

What is the rationale for a one-sided test? If a population mean above μ_0 has some importance, whereas one below μ_0 has none, then a one-tailed test is justified. For example, suppose one samples drinking water and performs bacterial counts to detect contamination. There is, then, cause for concern only when the population mean count is above some null hypothesis standard that corresponds with a safe level. A population mean count below this standard, i.e., water more pure than the standard, causes no concern. Hence, the statistical testing clearly calls for a one-sided test. The one-tailed test with diabetics' serum uric acid levels has a similar rationale. In the perspective of the entire investigation, a one-tailed test was chosen because the concern was only with the possibility that diabetics' mean serum uric acid level may be higher than that of general population males. There was no interest in a possible conclusion that their mean level is lower.

A one-tailed test is also justified when the investigator can state at the outset that it is entirely inconceivable that the true population mean is below that of the null hypothesis. To defend this position, there must be solid and convincing supporting evidence. In medical applications, this is an uncommon situation.

The two-tailed test is the more conservative. In fact, if there is any doubt, one should perform a two-tailed test. Choice of a two-tailed test indicates that there is equal concern with the possibilities that the true mean is above or below μ_0. This is, by far, the more common situation in medical applications. It certainly is true in most clinical investigations for testing new drugs or new procedures. Although there may be good reason to expect the new drug or procedure to give results as good as or better than those of the control group (in fact, the experiment wouldn't be undertaken if this were not so), the very fact that it is "new" indicates that some contingency must be made for the possibility that the results may be worse. Hence, the two-tailed test is appropriate.

This is the rationale for the use of the two-tailed test in the example of the cancer drug. Certainly there is every reason to expect the drug-treated patients to survive as long as or longer than patients without the drug. However, one cannot discount the possibility, although remote, that the drug may actually be deleterious, and thus survival may be shorter. If this were the case, one would certainly wish to be able to reach this conclusion with the statistical analysis. The two-tailed test, then, is appropriate.

In summary, the contrast between a one- and two-sided test on a population mean is indicated below:

Conclusion	One-sided test		Two-sided test
	Upper tail	Lower tail	
Not significant	$\mu = \mu_0$	$\mu = \mu_0$	$\mu = \mu_0$
Significant	$\mu > \mu_0$	$\mu < \mu_0$	$\mu > \mu_0$ or $\mu < \mu_0$

CONFIDENCE LIMITS ON A POPULATION MEAN

In some situations it is not important to reach one of the conclusions of the test of significance. It may be desirable to use the sample to pinpoint or estimate the unknown population quantity. This occurs often in medical surveys. For example, one might take a random sample of the population of a community (the community might be defined as large as the entire United States) and determine the number of times each sampled member visited his doctor during the past year, the number of disability days during the past year, systolic blood pressure, the levels of various constituents in specimens of blood or urine, or perhaps opinions regarding the quality of the medical care in the community. One might sample the records of all individuals who had been admitted to a hospital during the past year, determine the length of hospital stay, the diagnosis, and the total bill. In each of these situations, the aim of the inference is not to reject or to fail to reject some specific null hypothesis mean, but to arrive at an estimate as to where the population mean lies.

In such situations, the calculation of *confidence limits* is appropriate. The underlying principle for calculating confidence limits is the same as that for tests of significance; i.e., it is based upon properties of the sampling distribution of means. A confidence limit statement is merely an alternative way of drawing an inference about a population quantity based upon observations in a sample. In fact, as shall be demonstrated, confidence limits calculated from a sample must be compatible with any test of significance using the same sample data.

Derivation

Consider the standard normal distribution and the statement

$$\Pr\{-1.96 \leq z \leq 1.96\} = .95$$

This is merely a shorthand algebraic statement that 95 percent of the standard normal curve lies between $+1.96$ and -1.96 on the abscissa. For any other normal curve, one can, of course, substitute the critical ratio for z. If, in particular, one chooses the sampling distribution of means (a normal curve with mean μ and standard deviation $\sigma/\sqrt{n}$), then

$$\Pr\left\{-1.96 \leq \frac{\bar{x} - \mu}{\sigma/\sqrt{n}} \leq 1.96\right\} = .95$$

The expressions within the braces involve inequalities that can be manipulated without altering the probability value of 95 percent. Multiplication of the inequalities by $\sigma/\sqrt{n}$, subtraction of $\bar{x}$ from each side, and then multiplication by -1 (recalling that multiplication of an inequality by a negative number reverses the sign of the inequality) gives

$$\Pr\{\bar{x} - 1.96\sigma/\sqrt{n} \leq \mu \leq \bar{x} + 1.96\sigma/\sqrt{n}\} = .95$$

The quantities $\bar{x} - 1.96\sigma/\sqrt{n}$ and $\bar{x} + 1.96\sigma/\sqrt{n}$ are called *95 percent confidence limits on the population mean* μ. This means that when one claims $\bar{x} \pm 1.96\sigma/\sqrt{n}$ as the limits on μ, there is a 95 percent chance that the statement is correct; i.e., 19 times out of 20 the true unknown population mean will actually be contained within the calculated limits, and 1 time in 20 it will not.

If more than 95 percent certainty regarding the population mean—say, a 99 percent confidence interval—were desired, the only change needed is to use $\pm$ 2.58 (the point enclosing 99 percent of the standard normal curve), which gives

$$\bar{x} \pm 2.58\sigma/\sqrt{n}$$

Example 4.11.   For the survival time of the drug-treated cancer patients, the 95 percent confidence limits on the population mean are

$$46.9 \pm (1.96)(43.3/\sqrt{100}) = 46.9 \pm 8.5$$

$$= 38.4 \text{ to } 55.4 \text{ months}$$

Hence, there is 95 percent certainty that these limits embrace the mean survival in the population from which this sample arose. As before, it is important to define precisely the population sampled, since statistical inference using confidence limits also presumes random sampling from the target population.

The compatibility of confidence limits with a test of significance is exemplified by noting that the null hypothesis mean of 38.3 months, which was just significant with a two-tailed test at the 5 percent level, lies just outside the 95 percent confidence limits. With 95 percent confidence limits, any μ_0 that is included within $\bar{x} \pm 1.96\sigma/\sqrt{n}$ would not be statistically significant for a two-tailed test at the 5 percent level. Any μ_0 outside the confidence limits would be statistically significant at that level.

Interpretation

The confidence limit statement, like the significance test, can be interpreted by considering what happens in the long run. If, whenever one draws a sample, one establishes 95 percent confidence limits on the population mean, then, in the long run, the relative frequency with which the true population mean actually lies within these limits is 95 percent. In other words, 19 out of 20 of a large series of such confidence limits actually contain the population mean; 1 out of 20 does not.

It is important to stress that the concern is with confidence limits on a population mean. Unfortunately, there is a tendency among those unfamiliar with statistical methods to treat confidence limits inappropriately as bounds that enclose a proportion of the population. This is a grave error. For example, it is erroneous, in the case of the survival times of the drug-treated cancer patients, to interpret the 95 percent confidence limits of 38.4 to 55.4 months as indicating that 95 percent of the survival times are within these bounds. The limits concern only the *mean* of the population from which the sample of 100 was selected. The limits that embrace 95 percent of survival times are quite another matter; their determination involves knowledge of the *population distribution* of survival times.

THE *t* DISTRIBUTION

So far the test of significance and confidence limits on a population mean have involved σ, which is the population SD that is assumed to be known.

What does one do, however, in the more frequently occurring situation when σ is not known?

The analysis is similar. It does involve a new theoretical probability distribution called the *t distribution*.

Rationale

It seems logical that if σ is unknown, one should substitute a "reasonable guess" for σ wherever it appeared previously when one is performing a test of significance or obtaining confidence limits. Clearly s, the sample standard deviation, is an estimate of σ and appears to be a logical substitute.

This substitution, however, necessitates an alteration in the underlying theory, an alteration that is especially important when the sample size, n, is small. This is because in addition to the sampling variation of the mean, provision must now be made for the sampling variation of the standard deviation. In other words, to make the inference on a population mean, one must now consider the reliability both of $\bar{x}$ as an estimate of μ and of s as an estimate of σ.

Obviously, as n increases, s is an increasingly reliable estimate of σ. In fact, if n is very large, s is sufficiently reliable so that its substitution for σ is, for all practical purposes, equivalent to σ being known. However, for small samples, it is exceedingly important to give proper attention to the reliability of s, and so what is described in this section is referred to as a *small sample method*.

Thus, when σ is unknown, to perform a test of significance of the null hypothesis that the population mean is μ_0, one would calculate the critical ratio

$$t_{n-1} = \frac{\bar{x} - \mu_0}{s/\sqrt{n}}$$

where

$$s = \sqrt{\frac{\Sigma(x - \bar{x})^2}{n - 1}}$$

The mathematical modification is that this critical ratio does not follow the standardized normal distribution, but what is called *the* t *distribution with* n $-$ 1 *degrees of freedom* (*df*). Hence, the tables of the normal distribution no longer apply. One must now use tables of the *t* distribution with $n - 1$ df. The subscript $n - 1$ is a reminder to refer to $n - 1$ df (see p. 32).

Description and Use

The *t* distribution is a theoretical probability distribution (i.e., its total area is 100 percent) and is defined by a mathematical function. Since it is a well tabulated function, there is no necessity for indicating its equation.* The distribution is symmetrical, bell-shaped, and similar to the normal but more spread out. The *t* distribution involves an additional factor, the degrees of freedom (df), and there is a different *t* distribution for each df.

* The interested reader will find the equation in any introductory mathematical statistics text.

For very large df, the t distribution is indistinguishable from the normal. As the df decrease, the t distribution becomes increasingly spread out compared with the normal.

It is quite cumbersome to provide tables of areas in the tails of the t distribution analogous to the normal curve tables; this would require a page for each df. Since most uses of the t distribution involve tests of significance (one- or two-tailed) or confidence limit statements at the conventional 5 percent and 1 percent levels, a condensed table giving points corresponding to 5, 2.5, 1, and 0.5 percent in the upper tail is sufficient. Appendix Table A3 gives these points for df from 1 to 30.

A feel for the spread of the t distribution with decreasing degrees of freedom can be obtained by glancing up one of the columns of Appendix Table A3. The values of the cut-off points increase at an increasing rate. Note that the bottom line of the table, giving the cut-off point for t with infinite df, corresponds with the normal distribution (see p. 82). Mathematically, this means that the limit of the t distribution as the df increase indefinitely is the normal distribution. In fact, with more than 30 df, the t and normal distributions are sufficiently close so that one can use the normal for most practical purposes. In special situations where it is necessary to use t with more than 30 df or to obtain percentage points for t other than those given in Appendix Table A3, more detailed tables may be used [86].

Example 4.12.   Recall the data in Chapter 2 on the pulse rates for a sample of 10 first-year male medical students (Table 2.10). The sample of 10 was found to have a mean of 68.7 and an SD (or s) of 8.67 beats per minute.

Now, a handbook of clinical norms indicates that the mean pulse rate for young males is 72 beats per minute. Are these data on the 10 medical students compatible with this handbook norm? Is this sample mean likely to arise from a population whose mean is 72 beats per minute? One can now perform a test of significance, namely a t test.

Specifications:
Null hypothesis is $\mu_0 = 72$ beats per minute; test is performed at the 5 percent level; interest is in the two-tailed test.

Observation:

$$\text{Sample size: } n = 10$$

$$\text{Sample mean: } \bar{x} = 68.7 \text{ beats per minute}$$

$$\text{Sample SD: } s = 8.67 \text{ beats per minute}$$

Analysis:
Calculate the critical ratio for t:

$$t_{n-1} = \frac{\bar{x} - \mu_0}{s/\sqrt{n}} = \frac{68.7 - 72}{8.67/\sqrt{10}} = \frac{-3.3}{2.74} = -1.20$$

Refer now to Appendix Table A3 with $n - 1 = 9$ df. Having specified a two-tailed test at the 5 percent level, the table indicates 2.262 as the appropriate cut-off point with 9 df. The critical ratio calculated (-1.20) is less than 2.262. Hence, the calculated t cuts off more than 5 percent in two-tails.

Conclusion:

The result is not statistically significant ($P > .05$). The sample results are compatible with the handbook's statement, i.e., the difference can be explained by chance or sampling variation.

If, instead, one had wanted 95 percent confidence limits on the population mean from which this sample came, one calculates

$$\bar{x} \pm t_{n-1, .05} s/\sqrt{n}$$

This follows from before, with s replacing σ and $t_{n-1, .05}$ replacing the 1.96 of the normal curve. The notation $t_{n-1, .05}$ is used to indicate that one must choose from the table of the t distribution the value corresponding to 5 percent in both tails and with $n - 1$ df.

In the example, 95 percent confidence limits are

$$68.7 \pm (2.262)(8.67)/\sqrt{10}$$

$$= 68.7 \pm (2.262)(2.74)$$

$$= 68.7 \pm 6.20$$

$$= 62.5 \text{ to } 74.9 \text{ beats per minute}$$

In other words, there is 95 percent certainty that the mean pulse rate in the population from which the sample was drawn lies somewhere within these limits.

It is interesting to note that with confidence limits based on the t distribution, an increase in sample size has a twofold effect on the narrowing of the width of the confidence interval. Not only does $s/\sqrt{n}$ decrease as n increases, but $t_{n-1, .05}$ likewise decreases (the latter is evident by glancing down the two-tailed 5 percent column in the t table).

Summary

Table 4.2 summarizes the test of significance and confidence limits on a single mean when the population SD is known (use of normal distribution) and unknown (use of t distribution).

Table 4.2. Summary of inference on a single mean

Situation	Relevant tables	Test of significance	95 percent confidence limits
Population SD known	Normal	$z = \dfrac{\bar{x} - \mu_0}{\sigma/\sqrt{n}}$	$\bar{x} \pm 1.96\,\sigma/\sqrt{n}$
Population SD unknown (Use sample SD as estimate)	t with $n-1$ df	$t_{n-1} = \dfrac{\bar{x} - \mu_0}{s/\sqrt{n}}$	$\bar{x} \pm t_{n-1,.05}\,s/\sqrt{n}$

COMPARISON OF MEANS

The purpose of this section is to extend the arguments of the preceding section to the comparison of *two* sample means. Since much of medicine is, by nature, comparative, this is a rather widespread situation, more common than that of the single means of the preceding section.

In general, there are two samples of observations from two underlying populations (often treatment and control groups) whose means are denoted by μ_T and μ_C and whose standard deviations are denoted by σ_T and σ_C. Recalling that a test of significance involves a null hypothesis that specifies values for population quantities, the relevant null hypothesis is that the means are identical, i.e.,

$$H_o: \mu_T = \mu_C \text{ or } \mu_T - \mu_C = 0$$

The rationale for the test of significance is as before. Assuming the null hypothesis is true (i.e., that there is no difference in the population means), one determines the chance of obtaining differences in sample means as discrepant as or more discrepant than that observed. If this chance is sufficiently small, there is reasonable evidence to doubt the validity of the null hypothesis; hence, one concludes there *is* a difference between the means of the two populations (i.e., one rejects the null hypothesis). As before, it is necessary to specify a sufficiently small chance (i.e., to choose a significance level) and whether interest is in discrepancies in one or in both directions from the null hypothesis statement (i.e., one- or two-tailed test).

The analysis for comparison of two sample means depends on how the observations were obtained, in particular, whether the observations are from *paired* or *independent* samples. It is important to be able to distinguish the two, and the following discussion attempts to clarify their distinction.

Paired Samples

The characteristic feature of paired samples is that each observation in one sample has one and only one mate or matching observation in the other sample. These are the ways in which paired data occur in medicine:

1. The simplest situation is *self-pairing*, in which the subject serves as his own control.

Example 4.13. Therapeutic trials in which each subject receives both of the drugs or procedures under study on two different occasions involve *self-pairing* samples. In assessing the effect of an antihypertensive agent, each member of a group of hypertensive subjects may receive a test drug on one occasion and a standard or "control" drug on another occasion (see p. 42 and p. 134).

Before-and-after comparisons are almost always self-pairing. A set of measurements before performing some procedure on a group of patients (or animals, or cells) is compared with similar measurements obtained afterward.

Humans and animals have pairs of arms, legs, eyes, and ears. The application of one procedure or treatment to one arm, leg, eye, or ear of a patient, while another procedure is applied to the other arm, leg, eye, or ear, defines a self-pairing situation.

2. Next in order are *naturally paired* observations.

Example 4.14. Many laboratory experiments involve litter-mate controls. For example, two mice of the same sex are selected from a litter, and one member of the pair is assigned to one treatment, while the other pair member is assigned to some alternative treatment.

With humans, several clinical investigations select, for each identified patient with a disease, a sibling control of the same sex who is closest in age to the patient and is without the disease. There have been studies of coronary heart disease where, for each member of a sample of immigrants to the United States, a sibling is selected who did *not* emigrate but remained in the old country. These are examples of natural pairing by birth. Many studies on twins are obviously paired.

Natural pairing need not be by birth, of course. As an illustration, a study may identify index cases of school children with a disease and then choose as controls children without the disease from the same schoolroom. An investigator may identify the site and time of day of an automobile accident, then return to the site at the same time on the following day and pick as a control a vehicle not involved in an accident. Many hospital record studies involve identification of the admission date of a patient with the disease of interest. This is followed by the selection, as a control, of the next occurring hospital admission without the disease and in the same sex, race, and age bracket as the index case.

3.   Last is *artificial pairing* created by the investigator. The goal is to match subjects on important characteristics so that members of a pair are as alike as possible with regard to these characteristics. *Important* characteristics refer to those that are related to the outcome under study.

Example 4.15.   A study of prematurity is concerned with birth weight as the principal outcome. It is known that mother's age, race, weight, blood pressure, parity (number of children), gravidity (number of pregnancies), and smoking status are related to birth weight. An investigator who plans to test the effect of a new procedure, perhaps a new drug or diet, on prematurity might choose to pair women on several or perhaps all of these characteristics. For each such pair, he might randomly assign one member to the new drug under test and the matching member to the control.

There are two difficulties with artificial pairing. The first is that a prior knowledge of the characteristics relevant to the outcome under study is required. These characteristics may be clear and well-delineated in some situations, whereas in others they may be completely unknown. Second, when the characteristics are known and there are several, as with prematurity, it is exceedingly difficult to pair with respect to all factors simultaneously. For example, if the first expectant mother is a 25-year-old black, weighs 130 pounds, is hypertensive, has no previous children or pregnancies, and smokes, one might have to wait quite a long time before obtaining another expectant mother with these characteristics. In fact, during the time available for conducting the study, one might never obtain a matching subject.

Obviously, this difficulty is avoided by pairing only on those few characteristics that are *most* relevant to the outcome. This implies, however, knowledge of a hierarchy of relevant characteristics. Sometimes this can be done, but all too often the establishment of this hierarchy can consume more of the available resources than the proposed study.

In summary, pairing is a technique frequently used in medical investigations. Its goal is to create homogeneity within pairs or heterogeneity between pairs. Intuitively, pairing seems to offer the advantage of controlling some of the extraneous sources of variability. A comparison of the treatment with the control in the same individual, or in two individuals who are as alike as possible in several crucial aspects, eliminates in part some of the biological and other sources of variation, and thereby permits a more precise comparison.

The comparison of means for paired observations is simple and reduces to the methods already discussed. The key to the analysis is that concern is only with the *difference* for each pair.

Letting d denote the differences for each of n paired observations, the test is based on $\bar{d}$, the *mean of the sample differences*. (Note that one can easily verify that the mean of the sample differences is the same as the difference of the sample means.) The null hypothesis states that the population mean difference is zero. Denoting the population difference as $\delta = \mu_T - \mu_C$ gives $H_o: \delta = 0$. This is now the one-sample-mean situation of the preceding section but the observations are now differences between pairs and the mean is the mean difference.

To perform the test, it must first be known whether σ_d, the standard deviation of the differences in the population, is or is not known. If it is known, then the test can be based on the normal distribution using the critical ratio:

$$z = \frac{\bar{d} - 0}{\sigma_d/\sqrt{n}}$$

(The subscript d with σ is used as a reminder that it is the SD of population *differences*.)

If the population standard deviation of the differences is *not* known (which is the more frequent situation), the test utilizes the sample standard deviation of the differences (denoted by s_d) and is based on the t distribution with $n - 1$ df. Here the critical ratio is

$$t_{n-1} = \frac{\bar{d} - 0}{s_d/\sqrt{n}}$$

where

$$s_d = \sqrt{\frac{\Sigma(d - \bar{d})^2}{n - 1}}$$

Note that the df are one less than the number of *pairs*.

Example 4.16. The use of the t test for paired samples is illustrated with data obtained from an investigation of the effects of two drugs on blood pressure in hypertensive patients [117] (Table 4.3).

Each of 11 hypertensive patients was administered several drugs on different occasions. The results of concern are for a placebo drug (see p. 263) compared with hydrochlorothiazide. Each patient first received the placebo. One month later they each received hydrochlorothiazide. Blood pressure was recorded similarly on these two occasions. The data presented are systolic blood pressures. The test of significance asks the following question: On the basis of these experimental results, is there any evidence of a difference in mean systolic blood pressure during the use of these two drugs? The concern is with a two-tailed test, i.e., if it is significant, the interest is in the two alternatives: either the placebo is higher than hydrochlorothiazide treatment or the placebo is lower than hydrochlorothiazide treatment.

This is clearly a self-pairing situation, so interest focuses on the difference for each subject. The first series of

Table 4.3. Comparison of paired means: effect of placebo and hydro-chlorothiazide on systolic blood pressure of 11 hypertensive patients (systolic blood pressure in mm Hg)

Patient	Placebo	Hydrochloro-thiazide	Difference, d	
FB	211	181	30	
IF	210	172	38	
PG	210	196	14	
HF	203	191	12	
RR	196	167	29	
LP	190	161	29	
BK	191	178	13	
IF	177	160	17	
MK	173	149	24	
MT	170	119	51	
JM	163	156	7	
	Sum		264	(1)
	Mean		24.0	$(2) = (1)/11$
	Sum of squares		8,050	(3)
	$(\text{Sum})^2/n$		6,336	$(4) = (1)^2/11$
	Sum of squares about mean		1,714	$(5) = (3) - (4)$
	s_d^2		171.4	$(6) = (5)/10$

Test of Significance:

$$t_{10} = \frac{\bar{d} - \delta_0}{\sqrt{s_d^2/n}} = \frac{24.0 - 0}{\sqrt{171.4/11}} = \frac{24.0}{3.95} = 6.08; \text{ statistically significant } (P < .01)$$

95 Percent Confidence Limits on Difference:

$$\bar{d} \pm t_{n-1,.05} \sqrt{s_d^2/n} = 24.0 \pm (2.228)(3.95) = 15.2 \text{ to } 32.8 \text{ mm Hg}$$

calculations at the foot of Table 4.3 yields the sample mean and the sample variance of the differences.

Before performing the test, note that inspection of the data reveals the hydrochlorothiazide value to be lower than the placebo value for each of the 11 patients, i.e., all 11 differences are positive, and a good portion are of substantial magnitude. On this basis, one would anticipate that the test of significance would yield a statistically significant result. The test confirms this expectation with a t ratio of 6.07, which, from Appendix Table A3, cuts off less than 1 percent in two tails, i.e., $P < .01$.

Generally, it is desirable to inspect one's data and to anticipate the result of a test of significance. If there is much discrepancy between the "eyeball" guess and the test result, the investigator or, alas, often too late, the reader should carefully review the procedure for either an arithmetical error or, worse yet, an error such as performance of an inappropriate test (e.g., analysis of paired data as if they were from independent samples). In one sense, a statistical test of significance is merely a formal verification of a conclusion the investigator has already reached by inspection of his data.

The statistically significant result obtained in the example above indicates that chance or sampling variation is a highly unlikely explanation of the observed difference between the placebo and hydrochlorothiazide. Hence, the conclusion is that there is sufficient evidence of a real difference. In attributing this difference to the effects of the drugs, some criticism can be raised concerning the design of the experiment. Note that the placebo was always the first treatment. Hence, a natural tendency for the blood pressure of hypertensives to decrease over time cannot be distinguished from an effect of hydrochlorothiazide. The test of significance merely indicates that chance variation is an unlikely explanation. More information is needed to distinguish between a drug effect and a naturally occurring secular trend.

Redesigning the experiment such that one-half the subjects received the placebo followed by hydrochlorothiazide, while the other half received hydrochlorothiazide followed by the placebo, would have eliminated such criticism. Any secular trend would be averaged out in obtaining the mean difference in drug response. In this experiment, the drugs were two of several given to each patient. It was not logistically feasible to administer the drugs in different order. Furthermore, the investigator's experience with these and many other hypertensive patients convinced him that blood pressure levels of hypertensives are stable over time, and a natural time trend is not a plausible explanation of the significant results.

The moral to be gained is that with self-pairing comparisons, when feasible, it is preferable to vary the order of administering the drugs or procedures so as to balance out any possible disturbing time trend. Such an experimental arrangement is called a *cross-over* design. When the order cannot be varied, there must be solid and convincing prior evidence that such time trends are not plausible. The latter is often extremely difficult to establish.

Finally, as before, the interest is not always in a test of significance, and sometimes confidence limits are more appropriate. The 95 percent confidence limits on the difference between the placebo and hydrochlorothiazide are calculated in Table 4.3. These indicate that, based on the sample observations, there is 95 percent certainty that the difference between the placebo and hydrochlorothiazide with regard to the mean systolic blood pressure in the underlying population of hypertensive patients is somewhere between 15.2 and 32.8 mm Hg. Note that zero is not within the 95 percent confidence limits. Likewise, one would find that zero is not within the 99 percent confidence limits. This indicates the compatibility of the test of significance and the confidence limit statement.

Independent Samples

In many situations one does not know the relevant factors for pairing, or there may just not be any such factors. Futhermore, pairing can be administratively difficult and time consuming. Often, there may be several or many individuals who are available for study but who cannot be used because of the inability to find suitable matches for the relevant characteristics. Many times, the conceivable benefits from pairing are just not worth the time and effort involved. The alternative is to have two independent samples of observations, i.e., a series of treatment observations obtained independently of a series of control observations. The following notation is employed for the populations and the available sample information:

Item	Treatment group	Control group
	Population:	
Mean	μ_T	μ_C
SD	σ_T	σ_C
	Sample:	
Number of observations	n_T	n_C
Mean	$\bar{x}_T$	$\bar{x}_C$
SD	s_T	s_C

Note that with independent samples, the numbers of treatment and control observations need not be the same (i.e., n_T is not necessarily equal to n_C).

The test of significance asks the same question as with paired data: If the null hypothesis of identical population means is true (i.e., if $\mu_T - \mu_C = 0$), what is the chance of a discrepancy in sample means $x_T - x_C$ as large as or larger than what was observed?

It is worthwhile to note here that the general format for conducting the test of significance is the same as before, namely, the calculation of a critical ratio whose numerator is the difference between a "something" calculated from a sample and the value for that "something" in the underlying population as specified by the null hypothesis and whose denominator is the standard error of the sample "something." Previously, when dealing with a single mean, the "something" was a single mean. With paired data, the "something" was the mean of the differences for each pair. In the present situation, the "something" is the difference in means. In the next chapter, the "something" is a single proportion (see Table 5.1) or the difference in two proportions (p. 164), and in Chapter 6, the "something" is the slope of a straight line (p. 199). This general format underlies a great deal of statistical methods for performing tests of significance.

In the present situation, the sample "something" is the difference in independent sample means, $\bar{x}_T - \bar{x}_C$, and the null hypothesis statement for the corresponding underlying population "something" is $\mu_T - \mu_C = 0$. It remains to determine the denominator, i.e., the standard error of the difference in sample means, which is denoted as $SE(\bar{x}_T - \bar{x}_C)$.

Further mathematical manipulation of the laws of probability as applied to random variables (p. 76) reveals a basic rule in dealing with sums or differences of independent random variables: the standard error of the sum or difference is the square root of the sum of the squares of the standard errors of each variable. Application to the present situation gives

$$SE(\bar{x}_T - \bar{x}_C) = \sqrt{[SE(\bar{x}_T)]^2 + [SE(\bar{x}_C)]^2}$$

Since $SE(\bar{x}) = \sigma/\sqrt{n}$, this yields

$$SE(\bar{x}_T - \bar{x}_C) = \sqrt{\frac{\sigma_T^2}{n_T} + \frac{\sigma_C^2}{n_C}}$$

If the population SDs, σ_T and σ_C, are known (which is rare), the test is based · on the normal distribution and is thereby achieved by calculating the critical ratio:

$$z = \frac{\bar{x}_T - \bar{x}_C - 0}{\sqrt{\frac{\sigma_T^2}{n_T} + \frac{\sigma_C^2}{n_C}}}$$

If the population SDs are not known (which is the more common situation), it will be necessary to obtain an estimate of the denominator by using the sample standard deviations. As before, when sample values s are substituted for σ, one must use the t distribution rather than the normal. Consequently, what follows is referred to as the t *test for the comparison of two independent means*.

Before proceeding, there is yet another difficulty that concerns the population SDs, σ_T and σ_C. The t test for independent means that proliferates in the medical literature rests on the additional assumption that the SDs in the underlying populations are equal, i.e., that $\sigma_T = \sigma_C$. When, the SDs are unequal, however, theoretical difficulties in developing a proper test are entailed. Several approximate methods are available to deal with this situation, but these are beyond the scope of the present text. The interested reader is referred to others [2, 29, 101].

Thus, this text assumes hereon that $\sigma_T = \sigma_C = \sigma$ (say). One may ask whether this is a reasonable assumption. The rationale is that, in many situations, the application of a new treatment to one group with the other group left as a control will tend, if at all, to affect the mean value and leave the variability unchanged. Experience has borne this out. It is also possible to test the assumption of equal variability in the two groups. One may encounter t tests for independent means that are preceded by a test of homogeneity of variability in the two groups. This test of homogeneity is also beyond the scope of this text and may be found in the texts mentioned above.

With a common SD of σ for each of the treatment and control populations, it may be seen that the standard error of the difference in means becomes

$$SE(\bar{x}_T - \bar{x}_C) = \sqrt{\sigma^2\left(\frac{1}{n_T} + \frac{1}{n_C}\right)}$$

It remains to obtain an estimate of σ^2, based on sample results. There are two sources for such an estimate: the sample variance in the treated group, s_T^2, and that in the control group, s_C^2. Naively, one might suggest a simple average of the two. This may be seen to be inappropriate; since the sample sizes may differ substantially in the two groups, one sample variance might be a much more reliable estimate of σ^2 than the other. Thus, a weighted average of s_T^2 and s_C^2 seems appropriate, with the weights depending somehow on the reliability of each sample variance.

Mathematically, it turns out that the optimal weights are the df in each sample variance, namely, $n_T - 1$ and $n_C - 1$. The resulting combined estimate of σ^2 is called the *pooled estimate of common variance*:

$$\text{Pooled } s^2 = \frac{(n_T - 1)s_T^2 + (n_C - 1)s_C^2}{(n_T - 1) + (n_C - 1)}$$

Recalling the basic formula for defining variance (p. 31), this pooled estimate of common variance may be written in the more convenient computational form:

$$\text{Pooled } s^2 = \frac{\Sigma(x_T - \bar{x}_T)^2 + \Sigma(x_C - \bar{x}_C)^2}{n_T + n_C - 2}$$

Thus, the pooled s^2 results from adding together in the numerator the sums of squares about the mean for each group, and in the denominator, adding the df for each group. The resulting "pooled s^2" itself carries $n_T + n_C - 2$ df. Thus, the independent samples t test consists of the t ratio:

$$t_{n_T + n_C - 2} = \frac{\bar{x}_T - \bar{x}_C}{\sqrt{s^2\left(\dfrac{1}{n_T} + \dfrac{1}{n_C}\right)}}$$

where s^2 is as defined above and t contains $n_T + n_C - 2$ df.

Example 4.17. Data of Martin et al. illustrate the independent samples t test [73]. This study concerned quantification of the changing "inputs" over the course of time in the hospitalization of patients with myocardial infarction. "Inputs" were defined as units of services, such as days of hospitalization, drugs, numbers of laboratory tests, procedures, and x-rays. The study was conducted in a large, voluntary community hospital wherein the investigators sampled records of patients admitted with myocardial infarction in four designated years that spanned a 30-year time period (the designated years were 1939, 1949, 1959, and 1969). The data chosen for illustration here concern the years 1959 and 1969, and they are restricted to patients classified as having had a mild attack (the definition of "mild" is elaborated in the paper). There were 19 patients in 1959 and 26 in 1969 who were classified as having had a mild attack. The data presented in Table 4.4 pertain to the number of electrocardiograms (ECGs) that

Table 4.4. Independent-samples t test: number of ECGs among patients hospitalized with mild myocardial infarctions in 1959 compared with 1969

Number of ECGs	Number of patients		
	1959	1969	
x	f_1	f_2	
0	—	—	
1	1	—	
2	2	—	
3	3	1	
4	8	2	
5	2	8	
6	3	6	
7	—	4	
8	—	3	
9	—	1	
10	—	—	
11	—	—	
12	—	1	
Total: Σf	19	26	(1)
Σfx	74	160	(2)
Mean: $\bar{x}$	3.89	6.15	$(3) = (2)/(1)$
Σfx^2	322	1070	(4)
$(\Sigma fx)^2/\Sigma f$	288.2	984.6	$(5) = (2)^2/(1)$
$\Sigma f(x - \bar{x})^2$	33.8	85.4	$(6) = (4) - (5)$
s^2	1.88	3.42	$(7) = (6)/[(1) - 1]$
SD, s	1.37	1.85	$(8) = \sqrt{(7)}$

patients in these two study years received during the course of their hospitalization. The body of Table 4.4 presents the frequency distributions of the number of ECGs for the two samples of patients from 1959 and 1969, respectively. The calculations at the foot of each distribution outline the determination of the means, sums of squares about the mean, variances, and SDs for the two samples (the formulas in Table 2.9 for grouped data are applicable).

Inspection indicates a sharp increase in the mean number of ECGs over the decade; the 1969 mean is approximately 50 percent higher than that for 1959. The question now is whether this difference is or is not above and beyond what one might expect by chance variation. Thus, the concern is with a test of significance to compare the mean number of ECGs in 1959 with that in 1969.

The null hypothesis specifies no difference in the underlying population means for 1959 and 1969. Since the investigators were as concerned with detecting a possible statistically significant increase as they were a decrease, they chose to employ a two-sided test. The unequal sample sizes in each group and the procedure by which the samples were obtained clearly indicate an independent-samples situation. The fact that the variances (or SDs) in the underlying populations are unknown indicates that one must employ an estimated variance from the sample data. Hence, the independent-samples t test is the appropriate analytical technique.

From the sums of squares about the means for each group (see the foot of Table 4.4) one first calculates the pooled variance as

$$\text{Pooled } s^2 = (33.8 + 85.4)/(19 + 26 - 2) = 119.2/43$$

$$= 2.77$$

Then one may calculate the t ratio as

$$t_{43} = \frac{6.15 - 3.89}{\sqrt{2.77\left(\frac{1}{19} + \frac{1}{26}\right)}} = \frac{2.26}{0.502} = 4.50$$

Since the 43 df for t are in excess of 30, one may, for all practical purposes, employ tables of the normal distribution and thus substitute z for t. Appendix Table A2 indicates that $z = 3.00$ cuts off .001 in two tails of the normal curve. Thus, 4.50 cuts off less than this, and clearly $P < .001$. The conclusion is that the difference in means is statistically significant ($P < .001$). Hence, chance or sampling variation does not offer a reasonable explanation of the observed difference in sample mean ECGs between 1959 and 1969.

Had the focus been on confidence limits rather than a test of significance, one would calculate 95 percent confidence limits on the true difference in population means as

$$(6.15 - 3.89) \pm 1.96\sqrt{2.77\left(\frac{1}{19} + \frac{1}{26}\right)}$$

$$= 2.26 \pm (1.96)(0.502)$$

$$= 1.28 \text{ to } 3.24 \text{ ECGs per patient}$$

Hence, the statement that the true mean increase in the underlying populations from 1959 to 1969 lies somewhere between 1.3 and 3.2 ECGs per person has a chance of 95 percent or 19 in 20 of being correct.

Again, one must warn the reader that the test of significance performed above merely rules out chance in explaining the sample difference in means. The reader is entitled to expect from the investigator reasonable evidence that other factors, such as patient selection, were unlikely to have contributed substantially to the observed sample discrepancy.

In addition to the increased mean number of ECGs, the study revealed similar sharp and statistically significant (at least at the 1 percent level) increases in the mean numbers of x-rays, bacteriological and chemical tests, sedation doses, and days of oxygen therapy. Yet, there was no statistically significant, or important, increase in the mean length of hospital stay. With quantification of this increased "input" during hospitalization, perhaps the most noteworthy study result was that the one "output" item investigated, namely, the death rate during hospitalization, revealed no statistically significant change between 1959 and 1969.

Summary

Table 4.5 summarizes the inference methods, namely, tests of significance and confidence limits, for the comparison of two means.

DETERMINATION OF SAMPLE SIZE

"How big a sample do I need?" This ranks among the most frequent questions the investigator poses to the statistician. There is no simple answer. The statistician, in turn, requires further specification concerning the risks that the investigator is willing to tolerate in the inferences he intends to draw. Depending on whether the interest is in a test of significance or in a confidence limit statement, the statistician requires whatever information, save for n, that lets him use the relevant formulas contained in this chapter.

For a test of significance on a single mean, mention has already been made of the three essential ingredients: an α or type I error associated with the null hypothesis mean μ_0, a β or type II error associated with the alternative hypothesis mean μ_1, and finally n. Thus, the specification of α for a μ_0 and β for a μ_1 leads to the determination of n. The α error specification gives the critical ratio

$$z_\alpha = \frac{\bar{x} - \mu_0}{\sigma/\sqrt{n}}$$

where z_α denotes the upper α percent point of the normal distribution, while the β specification gives

$$z_\beta = \frac{\bar{x} - \mu_1}{\sigma/\sqrt{n}}$$

where z_β denotes the lower β percent point of the normal distribution. Solving for n in these two equations yields

$$n = \left[\frac{(z_\alpha - z_\beta)\sigma}{\mu_1 - \mu_0} \right]^2$$

Table 4.5. Summary of inference for the comparison of two means

Situation	Tables	Test of significance	95% confidence limits
Paired Samples:			
Population SD of differences known	Normal	$z = \dfrac{\bar{d} - \delta_0}{\sigma_d/\sqrt{n}}$	$\bar{d} \pm 1.96\, \sigma_d/\sqrt{n}$
Population SD of differences unknown	t with $n-1$ df	$t_{n-1} = \dfrac{\bar{d} - \delta_0}{s_d/\sqrt{n}}$	$\bar{d} \pm t_{n-1,.05}\, s_d/\sqrt{n}$
Independent Samples:			
Population SDs known	Normal	$z = \dfrac{(\bar{x}_T - \bar{x}_C) - \delta_0}{\sqrt{\dfrac{\sigma_T^2}{n_T} + \dfrac{\sigma_C^2}{n_C}}}$	$(\bar{x}_T - \bar{x}_C) \pm 1.96\sqrt{\dfrac{\sigma_T^2}{n_T} + \dfrac{\sigma_C^2}{n_C}}$
Population SDs unknown but assumed to be approximately equal (use pooled s^2)	t with $n_T + n_C - 2$ df	$t_{n_T+n_C-2} = \dfrac{(\bar{x}_T - \bar{x}_C) - \delta_0}{\sqrt{s^2\left(\dfrac{1}{n_T} + \dfrac{1}{n_C}\right)}}$	$(\bar{x}_T - \bar{x}_C) \pm t_{n_T+n_C-2,.05}\sqrt{s^2\left(\dfrac{1}{n_T} + \dfrac{1}{n_C}\right)}$
		where $s^2 = [\Sigma(x_T - \bar{x}_T)^2 + \Sigma(x_C - \bar{x}_C)^2]/(n_T + n_C - 2)$	
Population SDs unknown and unequal	Not covered in this text; see more advanced texts for appropriate methods.		

Note the additional ingredient in the expression: the population SD, σ. Thus, in addition to specification of the two error levels, one must have some idea of the underlying variability in the measurements under consideration. Often, in planning studies, a pilot investigation is conducted, one of whose primary goals is the determination of a reasonable estimate of σ.

Example 4.18.   As an example of the determination of sample size, consider the preceding systolic blood pressure data on the evaluation of an antihypertensive drug (Example 4.16). These data illustrated the t test for paired samples, but restriction to the differences for each pair reduced the situation to one of testing a single mean, namely the mean difference of pairs. Suppose a new drug becomes available and will be tested against a placebo in a manner similar to that of hydrochlorothiazide. How large a sample of hypertensive patients is needed?

The investigator specifies that he will perform a two-tailed test at the 5 percent level of the null hypothesis, which is that there is no difference in population means. This indicates $\mu_0 = 0$ and $z_\alpha = 1.96$ (the point cutting off 5 percent in two tails of the standard normal distribution).

He further specifies that if the true difference is as much as 10 mm Hg, he wishes to risk only a 5 percent chance of failing to reject his null hypothesis of no difference. This indicates $\mu_1 = 10$ and $z_\beta = -1.65$ (the point cutting off 5 percent in the lower tail of the standard normal distribution). To complete the calculation, the investigator needs an estimate of σ_d. The hydrochlorothiazide-treatment data gave an $s_d^2 = 171.4$, and, presuming no other similar data were available, the investigator would use as a rough approximation $\sigma_d = \sqrt{171.4} = 13.1$.

He then determines his required sample size as

$$n = \left[\frac{(1.96 + 1.65)13.1}{10 - 0} \right]^2 = 22.4$$

or 23 hypertensive patients. This is, of course, a rough approximation, but it is sufficient for most practical purposes. It is rough in that the results depend on the adequacy of the approximation to σ_d, and, in practice, the testing will be accomplished with the t distribution rather than the normal distribution.

Note that in the calculations, the two-tailed specification for the test affects only the z_α value. The one-tailed normal curve value is used for z_β regardless of whether the test is specified as one- or two-tailed. Also remember that β always refers to the lower tail of the normal curves so that for $\beta < .50$, z_β is negative.

The logical structure of the formula for n may be seen to be reasonable by considering what happens as the error level specification changes. If the investigator wishes more protection against wrong decisions, lowering either his α error, β error, or both results in a higher z_α or z_β value and, consequently, a larger n. If he retains the same error levels but specifies an alternative mean with his β error closer to the null hypothesis population mean (in other words, if $\mu_1 - \mu_0$ decreases), then n increases. Finally, the sample size is directly related to σ. The greater the inherent variability in the measurement under consideration, the larger is the sample size required.

One determines the sample size for the comparison of two independent means in a similar manner. There usually are the further specifications of equal variability in the two groups, $\sigma_T = \sigma_C = \sigma$ (say), and of equal division of subjects between experimental and control groups, $n_T = n_C = n$ (say). The α error specification for the null hypothesis of no population difference, $\mu_T - \mu_C = 0$, and the β error specification for a particular population difference of interest, $\mu_T - \mu_C = \delta_1$ (say), yield two equations in two unknowns which, when solved, give

$$n = 2\left[\frac{(z_\alpha - z_\beta)\sigma}{\delta_1}\right]^2$$

Note that the result is the sample size in each group; the total sample size for the study is $2n$.

If the inference is to be a confidence limit statement, the sample size can be derived from the specification of the width of the interval. Consider the situation involving a single mean.

Example 4.19.   The data on the pulse rates of 10 medical students might be considered as a pilot study for a larger investigation. Suppose it is desired to determine pulse rates in the larger study such that a 95 percent confidence interval on the mean will be ± 2 beats per minute. How many students are needed?

The normal distribution may be used because here an approximation is adequate, despite the fact that the actual determination of the confidence interval might involve the t distribution. The 95 percent confidence limit on a mean then gives $\pm 1.96\sigma/\sqrt{n} = \pm 2$. Thus, $n = (1.96\sigma/2)^2$. The results of the pilot study of 10 gave 8.67 beats per minute as the sample SD. Using this, one would calculate $n = (1.96 \times 8.67/2)^2 = 72.2$, or 73 medical students are needed.

For the comparison of two means, the specification of the width of the interval at some particular level of confidence permits the use of the formulas in Table 4.5. Again, one assumes a normal distribution and uses z values in place of t. In addition, note that in each situation it is necessary to have some idea of the magnitude of σ, the inherent population variability.

This author's experience in dealing with medical investigators in the determination of sample size indicates that it is usually a matter of collective bargaining between the investigator and the statistician. When the investigator is asked to choose the specifications and error levels, the resulting *n* which the statistician calculates usually shocks the investigator. His retort is that he can't possibly collect that many cases. Often this leads to an indication of the size of sample that the investigator contemplated was manageable. One can then determine the degree of protection against wrong decisions afforded by that size sample. One hopes it is possible to reach a compromise between the desired degree of protection and what the investigator considers to be a feasible sample size for him to handle.

COMPARISON OF THREE OR MORE MEANS

It appears natural to extend the results of this chapter to the comparison of three or more means. Techniques are available for handling these comparisons, although these go far beyond the scope of this text and are generally termed *analysis of variance* (see other texts [2, 12, 29, 101]). The techniques discussed in this chapter will encompass most of the studies involving comparisons of means that the reader will encounter in the medical literature.

EXERCISES

1. Referring back to question 10 in Chapter 3,
    A. What is the chance that among 100 medical students selected at random, their mean National Board score will be 525 or higher? A class of 100 in a particular medical school, all of whom took the National Boards, achieved a mean score of 525. Is there cause for celebration at this medical school?
    B. At the time the National Boards changed their scoring system, the size of the class at a medical school increased from 64 to 100 students. What mean score in the old system for the school with 64 students is equivalent to 525 in the new system with 100 students?
    C. How large must a class be so a mean National Board score of 525 or higher for the class would be achieved by chance only 5 percent of the time?

2. Referring back to question 13 in Chapter 3,
    A. What is the chance that among 4 healthy males selected at random, their mean serum uric acid level is outside the range of 4.0 to 7.0 mg per 100 ml?
    B. How many healthy males must be selected so there is a 95 percent or better chance that their mean serum uric acid level is within the range of 4.9 to 5.9 mg per 100 ml?

3. Referring back to the cholesterol data of question 14 for Chapter 3,
    A. Consider a random sample of 36 healthy males without a coronary event from the general population. What is the chance that their

average initial cholesterol level would be 215 mg per 100 ml of serum or below?

B. An investigation of 36 healthy male prisoners without a coronary event revealed their initial cholesterol level to average 215 mg per 100 ml of serum. Do your results in part A supply evidence that male prisoners tend to have lower cholesterol levels than males of the general population? Can you suggest reasons for lower cholesterol levels among prisoners?

4. As part of an experiment, each mouse in a random sample of 25 is to be injected with a drug at a dose level of 0.004 mg per gram of body weight. For this mouse strain, it is known that the weight is approximately normally distributed with a mean of 19 g and an SD of 4 g.
   A. If the investigator secures a total of 2 mg of the drug, what is the chance he will run short?
   B. How much of the drug should he secure in order to run a risk of 1 percent or less of running short?

5. In a study of 49 healthy men, the 95 percent confidence limits on mean vital capacity were 4.62 to 4.94 liters. If the vital capacity in the underlying population is approximately normally distributed, what range encompasses 90 percent of healthy men?

6. The SD of serum uric acid levels in healthy males was 1.03 mg per 100 ml. An investigator is planning a study involving serum uric acid levels in males.
   A. How large a sample of men does he need in order that the 95 percent confidence limits on his mean serum uric acid level are ±0.20 mg per 100 ml?
   B. For each of the following specifications, indicate whether more, less, or about the same number of men as determined in part A are needed:
      (1) 99 percent confidence limits on the mean to be ± 0.20 mg per 100 ml
      (2) 95 percent confidence limits on the mean to be ± 0.30 mg per 100 ml
      (3) 99 percent confidence limits on the mean to be ± 0.26 mg per 100 ml

7. In a drug trial of a new antihypertensive agent, a sample of 25 known hypertensive patients will be given the drug and their blood pressure will be measured before and after drug administration. The investigator will claim the new agent is effective if a one-tailed test of significance at the 5 percent level rejects the null hypothesis that the mean decrease in systolic blood pressure is 5 mm Hg. Prior experience indicates that the SD of the systolic blood pressure decrease is 17 mm Hg among patients given an antihypertensive agent.

A. How large a mean decrease must he observe in his sample of 25 patients to lead to the conclusion that the new agent is effective (i.e., leading to rejection of the null hypothesis)?

B. If, in reality, the new agent reduces the systolic blood pressure by 15 mm Hg on the average when used in a large population of hypertensives, what is the chance that the test in part A with a sample of 25 hypertensive patients would fail to reject the null hypothesis, i.e., would lead to the conclusion that the new agent was not effective? (This chance is the type II error.)

C. The type I error is defined as the chance of rejecting the null hypothesis when the null hypothesis is true, and it is 5 percent in the above situation. If the experimenter wishes to reduce both the type I and II errors, how, if at all, may he achieve this?

D. If the experimenter wishes to have a type I error of 1 percent for the null hypothesis of a 5 mm Hg decrease and a type II error of 5 percent for the alternative hypothesis of a 15 mm Hg decrease, how many patients are needed? Also, what is the value for the observed mean that divides between rejecting and not rejecting the null hypothesis (i.e., the value such that for any observed mean above this value, he would reject the null hypothesis, whereas for any observed mean below this value, he would not reject the null hypothesis)? (*Hint*: Using the information given by the type I and type II error specifications, set up two equations in the two unknowns n and c, where n is the required sample size and c is the required point for the mean that distinguishes between rejecting and not rejecting the null hypothesis.)

E. Without performing any calculations, state for each of the following situations whether more, fewer, or the same number of patients are required as in the test in part D:

   (1) type I error of 1 percent for 5 mm Hg; type II error of 1 percent for 15 mm Hg

   (2) type I error of 1 percent for 5 mm Hg; type II error of 5 percent for 10 mm Hg

   (3) type I error of 1 percent for 5 mm Hg; type II error of 5 percent for 20 mm Hg

   (4) type I error of 1 percent for 10 mm Hg; type II error of 5 percent for 20 mm Hg

8. A class experiment in pharmacology consisted of distributing packets of "instant coffee" to medical students. The contents of the packet were to be mixed with hot water and drunk shortly before bedtime. The students received packets on two occasions: one time the packet contained a placebo and the other time it contained coffee with caffeine. Among other measurements, the students took their pulse rates (in beats per minute) before consuming the instant coffee and then again afterward. The students were classified as to whether they were coffee drinkers

(those who usually consumed two or more cups of coffee per day) or noncoffee drinkers (those who usually consumed one or fewer cups of coffee per day). For each student, the decrease in pulse rate was obtained (i.e., the pulse rate before minus the pulse rate after). The results for the 16 noncoffee drinkers and the 22 coffee drinkers are tabulated below:

	16 Noncoffee drinkers			22 Coffee drinkers		
	Caffeine	Placebo	Difference	Caffeine	Placebo	Difference
Total	70	15	55	64	56	8
Mean	4.4	0.9	3.5	2.9	2.5	0.4
Sum of squares about mean	708	107	538	436	371	783

A. Perform the appropriate tests of significance on the mean change in pulse rates corresponding to the following hypotheses:
   (1) Among the coffee drinkers, the response is the same for caffeine and the placebo.
   (2) Among noncoffee drinkers, the response is the same for caffeine and the placebo.
   (3) The caffeine response is the same for coffee and noncoffee drinkers.
   (4) The placebo response is the same for coffee and noncoffee drinkers.
   (5) The difference between the caffeine and placebo responses is the same for coffee and noncoffee drinkers.

B. Obtain 95 percent confidence limits on the mean difference between the caffeine and placebo responses:
   (1) for coffee drinkers
   (2) for noncoffee drinkers

C. Approximately how many coffee and noncoffee drinkers, respectively, are needed in order to have 95 percent confidence limits on the mean difference between the caffeine and placebo responses of ± 1.0 beats per minute?

9. In planning a study of lung function in teenagers, an investigator conducted a pilot study among students in a classroom at the local high school. For the 20 boys in the classroom, the mean vital capacity was 3.195 liters and the sum of squares about the mean was 5.27.

A. Assuming these results are typical, approximately how large a sample of boys is needed so that the 95 percent confidence limits on mean vital capacity will be ± 0.10 liters?

B. There were 5 girls in the class and their mean vital capacity was 2.575 liters. The SD of the vital capacity for these 5 girls was not reported, but the investigator stated that a comparison of mean vital capacity for the 20 boys and 5 girls was just barely significant with a two-tailed test at the 2 percent level. What is the SD of vital capacity for the 5 girls?

10. A study of hypertension and diet in a small fishing village involved the daily determination of sodium dietary intake over a one-week period. For each study subject, the daily values were averaged to yield a mean for the week. There were 7 hypertensive female participants, age 40 to 59 years, and the mean and SD of their sodium intake values (i.e., the mean and SD of their 7 means for the week) were 123.0 and 19.7 mEq per day, respectively.

    A.   In the village there were 7 female study participants in this same age group, all of whom had normal blood pressure. The mean and SD of the means for the week for these 7 normotensive women were 113.0 and 28.4 mEq per day, respectively. Are there sufficient data to perform the appropriate test of significance to compare the sodium intake of hypertensive women with normotensive women in this age group? If so, conduct the test; if not, indicate the additional information needed and outline how one would conduct the test.

    B.   The 7 hypertensive females participated in a second and similar dietary survey six months later. On this second occasion, the corresponding mean and SD of their sodium-intake means for the week were 142.6 and 27.5 mEq per day, respectively. Are there sufficient data to perform the appropriate test of significance to compare the sodium intake of these hypertensive women in the two times the study was conducted? If so, conduct the test; if not, indicate the additional information needed and outline how one would conduct the test.

    C.   Suppose that instead of the mean and SD of 7 means for the week in each group of 7 women, the investigator calculated the mean and SD of all 49 observations (i.e., the values for each of 7 women on each of seven days of the week). How, if at all, would the means and SDs of the 49 observations differ from the means and SDs presented in the preceding parts of this question? Why is it inappropriate to use the mean and SD on a sample size of 49 in conducting tests of significance such as those asked for in parts A and B?

Chapter 5
Inference on Proportions

The methodology of statistical inference can be extended to enumeration-type data, namely, the *analysis of proportions*. The principles of inference are identical with those developed for means in the preceding chapter. This chapter is concerned chiefly with tests of significance and with confidence limit statements on proportions. In analogy with Chapter 4, inference on a single proportion will be considered first, then the comparison of two proportions, and finally the comparison of more than two proportions. As before, the normal distribution plays a large role in the methodology.

A SINGLE PROPORTION

Binomial Distribution

The binomial distribution provides the foundation for the analysis of enumeration data and proportions Recall from Chapter 3 (p. 76) that the binomial distribution concerns n independent trials with a constant probability π of success on each trial. The chance of x successes in n trials was obtained as

$$\frac{n!}{x!\,(n-x)!}\,\pi^x(1-\pi)^{n-x},$$

Example 5.1.   Consider 10 tosses of a fair coin. What is the chance of:
  A.   two or fewer heads?
  B.   eight or more heads?
  C.   two or fewer or 8 or more heads?
  Answers:
  A.   The specification of a fair coin indicates $\pi = \frac{1}{2}$. Thus, what is the chance of 0, 1, or 2 successes when $n = 10$ and $\pi = \frac{1}{2}$?

$$\Pr(0,\,1,\,\text{or }2) = (\tfrac{1}{2})^{10} + 10(\tfrac{1}{2})(\tfrac{1}{2})^9 + \frac{10 \times 9}{2 \times 1}(\tfrac{1}{2})^2(\tfrac{1}{2})^8$$
$$= (1 + 10 + 45)/2^{10} = 56/1024$$

  B.   In a similar manner, what is the chance of 8, 9, or 10 successes?

$$\Pr(8,\,9,\,\text{or }10) = \frac{10 \times 9}{2 \times 1}(\tfrac{1}{2})^8(\tfrac{1}{2})^2 + 10(\tfrac{1}{2})^9(\tfrac{1}{2}) + (\tfrac{1}{2})^{10}$$
$$= (45 + 10 + 1)/2^{10} = 56/1024$$

(Note that the answers to A and B are identical, which follows from the symmetry of the binomial distribution when $\pi = \frac{1}{2}$.)

C.   The chance of 2 or fewer or 8 or more successes is obtained from the application of the additive law of probability to the answers for A and B:

$$Pr(0, 1, 2, 8, 9, \text{ or } 10) = \frac{56}{1024} + \frac{56}{1024} = \frac{112}{1024} = .109$$

Example 5.2.   Now consider the following situation. In a clinical trial to compare two analgesics denoted as A and B, each of 10 patients who suffered from chronic headache received the analgesics A and B on two separate occasions. At random, half the patients received A on the first occasion, then B. The other half received B on the first occasion, then A. Each patient was asked to indicate which drug he preferred, i.e., which he found more effective in relieving his headache symptoms. Patients were coerced into making a preference; they were not allowed to indicate that they preferred both or that they preferred neither. (The situation in which results can be "ties," namely, success on both drugs or failure on both drugs, is dealt with later in this chapter; see p. 172.) A simple compilation of results revealed that eight preferred A and two preferred B.

The essential question is whether these data provide sufficient evidence that patients prefer A more often to B in the relief of chronic headache. Could such a result obtain purely by chance? Interest thus focuses on a test of significance.

First, what is the null hypothesis? In this situation the obvious null hypothesis claims that in the underlying population from which the sample of 10 patients was chosen, drugs A and B are equally preferable. In other words, with the definition of π as the probability in the population of a preference for drug A ($1 - \pi$ is then the probability of preference for drug B), the null hypothesis states $\pi = \frac{1}{2}$, namely, that A and B are equally preferable.

According to Chapter 4, the other ingredients needed to conduct the test of significance are (1) the specification of the significance level and (2) an indication of whether it is to be one- or two-sided. Suppose that 5 percent is considered a small enough chance. Also, the investigator is as interested in the conclusion that patients prefer A significantly more often than B as he is in the conclusion that patients prefer B significantly more often than A; therefore a two-sided test is used.

The rationale for the test is identical to the test on a mean. If the null hypothesis is true, what is the chance of sample observations being as discrepant as or more discrepant than what was observed? The question must be asked in either direction from the null hypothesis value because of the two-tailed nature of the test. This is equivalent to asking what is the chance—when $\pi = \frac{1}{2}$ and $n = 10$—of 8, 9, or 10 (one-tail) or 0, 1, or 2 (other tail) A preferences or successes. Thus, when the null hypothesis is true, the question is identical with question C regarding the 10 tosses of a fair coin in Example 5.1; therefore, Pr(0, 1, 2, 8, 9, or 10 A preferences) $= .109$. The result is not statistically significant ($P > .05$). This means that if the null hypothesis were true, the observed result could well arise purely by chance. Hence, there is no reason to doubt the validity of the null hypothesis. This does *not* mean the null hypothesis has been proved true; as discussed in Chapter 4, it means only that these experimental results do not provide sufficient evidence to doubt the validity of the null hypothesis, i.e., that A and B are equally preferable.

The above test is called an *exact test* since the probability was determined exactly by use of the binomial distribution. An alternative approximate test, however, can be developed which is based on the fact that under certain circumstances the normal distribution can closely approximate the binomial.

Normal Approximation to the Binomial Distribution

Figure 5.1 illustrates the binomial distribution with $\pi = .4$ for $n = 5, 10, 20$, and 40. Inspection of Figure 5.1 reveals that, as n increases, the binomial distribution increasingly resembles a normal distribution. The rule generally employed states that when each of $n\pi$ and $n(1 - \pi)$ is of the magnitude of 5 or more, the normal distribution can safely be used as an alternative to the binomial.

In essence, the similarity of the normal and binomial distributions is not a new result, but it is a special case of the third property of the sampling distribution of means (see p. 101), namely, that the sampling distribution of means resembles the normal distribution. If one defines a large population in which each observation consists of either "success" scored as 1 or "failure" scored as 0, then it may easily be shown that the mean of the population corresponds merely with the population proportion of successes, that is, $\mu = \pi$. Further, the standard deviation in the population can be calculated as $\sigma = \sqrt{\pi(1 - \pi)}$. Now consider repeat samples of size n from this population.

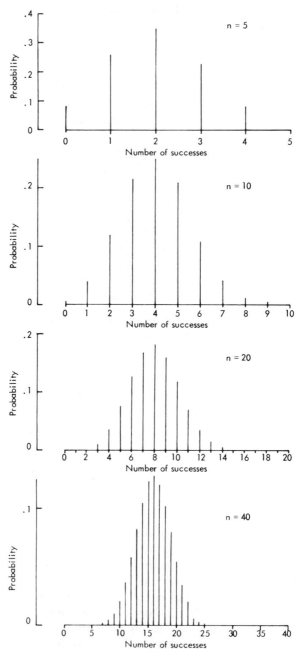

Figure 5.1
Binomial distribution with $\pi = .4$ and $n = 5, 10, 20,$ and 40.

Each sample consists, of course, of a series of observations of 1s and 0s; the mean for the sample is merely the *proportion* of 1s in the sample, which is denoted as *p*. Application of the three properties of the sampling distribution of means gives:

1. The mean of sample means (or proportions in this case) from repeat samples of size n is that of the population mean, namely, π.
2. The standard error of the mean is $\sigma/\sqrt{n}$, namely, $\sqrt{\pi(1 - \pi)/n}$.
3. The shape is approximately normal provided n is sufficiently large—in this case, $n\pi \geq 5$ and $n(1 - \pi) \geq 5$ are the requirements for sufficiently large n.

With the binomial distribution as a special case of the sampling distribution of means, its standard deviation is best referred to as a *standard error*. Hence, the *standard error of a sample proportion* is defined as $\sqrt{\pi(1 - \pi)/n}$.

The above argument pertains to the *proportion* success, *p*, in a sample of *n*. The initial question concerning the tosses of a coin dealt with the *number* of successes, *x*, in a sample of *n*. Since $np = x$, one can easily go from *proportion* success to the *number* of successes by multiplying by *n*. It is important to remember, however, that the standard errors of the proportion success and the number of successes also differ by a factor of *n*. In other words, having shown that the standard error of the *proportion* of successes is $\sqrt{\pi(1 - \pi)/n}$, the standard error of the *number* of successes becomes $n\sqrt{\pi(1 - \pi)/n} = \sqrt{n\pi(1 - \pi)}$. It is well to remember this distinction between the two standard errors.

To use the tables of the normal distribution, one needs to calculate critical ratios. With such ratios, if one employs the *number* of successes in the numerator, one must employ in the denominator the corresponding standard error of the *number* of successes. Among the inexperienced, the use of an improper standard error is a common mistake.

To avoid dealing with decimals, some prefer to express results as *percentage* success, which is denoted here as 100*p*. Correspondingly, the standard error of the *percentage* success becomes $100\sqrt{\pi(1 - \pi)/n}$. These three forms for expressing the outcomes of the binomial distribution—number, proportion, and percentage success—are summarized in Table 5.1. The critical ratios for number, proportion, and percentage success are, of course, identical.

Note in the numerators of the critical ratios the quantities $\frac{1}{2}$, $1/(2n)$, and $100/(2n)$ respectively for number, proportion, and percentage success. These quantities represent the *correction for continuity*. The correction for continuity emanates from the fact that a smooth, continuous normal curve approximates the discrete binomial distribution. On the smooth normal curve, the number of successes, *x*, actually corresponds with the interval on the abscissa, $x - \frac{1}{2}$ to $x + \frac{1}{2}$ successes. Thus, if asking about *x* or more successes, one does better to ask for the area in the smooth normal curve above $x - \frac{1}{2}$. Figure 5.2 illustrates the continuity correction for $n = 10$, $\pi = \frac{1}{2}$, and $x = 2$ or fewer or 8 or more successes.

Table 5.1. Summary of the expression of the results in binomial distribution

Outcome	Result in sample of n	Population mean	Standard error	Critical Ratio[a]	
				Upper tail	Lower tail
Number of successes	x	$n\pi$	$\sqrt{n\pi(1-\pi)}$	$z_c = \dfrac{x - n\pi - \frac{1}{2}}{\sqrt{n\pi(1-\pi)}}$	$z_c = \dfrac{x - n\pi + \frac{1}{2}}{\sqrt{n\pi(1-\pi)}}$
Proportion success	$p = x/n$	π	$\sqrt{\pi(1-\pi)/n}$	$z_c = \dfrac{p - \pi - 1/(2n)}{\sqrt{\pi(1-\pi)/n}}$	$z_c = \dfrac{p - \pi + 1/(2n)}{\sqrt{\pi(1-\pi)/n}}$
Percentage success	$100p$	100π	$100\sqrt{\pi(1-\pi)/n}$	$z_c = \dfrac{100p - 100\pi - 100/(2n)}{100\sqrt{\pi(1-\pi)/n}}$	$z_c = \dfrac{100p - 100\pi + 100/(2n)}{100\sqrt{\pi(1-\pi)/n}}$

[a] Normal curve is applicable only when $n\pi \geq 5$ and $n(1-\pi) \geq 5$.

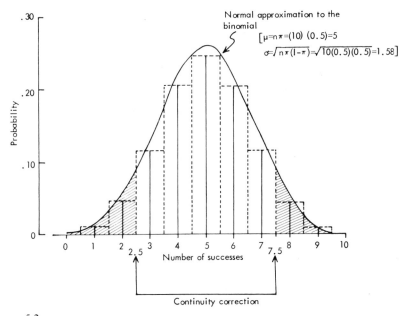

Figure 5.2
Continuity correction with the binomial distribution: determination of the chance of two or fewer or eight or more successes when $n = 10$ and $\pi = .5$.

The continuity correction for number of successes consists merely of arbitrarily reducing the magnitude of the numerator of the critical ratio by one-half. Thus, for the upper tail, $\frac{1}{2}$ is subtracted, and for the lower tail, $\frac{1}{2}$ is added. The subscript c accompanying the z of a critical ratio indicates that the continuity adjustment has been made.

When dealing with values of $n\pi$ and $n(1 - \pi)$ that are well above 5, the continuity correction has a negligible effect. Except for questions involving the determination of the approximate sample size, however, it is wise to employ the continuity correction routinely. Its use will not hinder the calculations, and when $n\pi$ and $n(1 - \pi)$ hover close to the critical value of 5, its use will ensure a normal curve that provides a better fit to the binomial distribution.

If one considers now the example that deals with the comparison of two analgesics, it may be seen that $n\pi = n(1 - \pi) = (10)(\frac{1}{2}) = 5$. Thus, one could alternatively employ the normal approximation to the binomial to conduct the test of significance. The chance of 8 or more successes is approximately the same as the area above $x = 8$ (or 7.5, with the continuity correction) in the normal curve, whose mean is $n\pi = (10)(\frac{1}{2}) = 5$ and whose SD is $\sqrt{n\pi(1 - \pi)} = \sqrt{10(\frac{1}{2})(\frac{1}{2})} = 1.58$. One therefore calculates the critical ratio as:

$$z_c = \frac{x - n\pi - \frac{1}{2}}{\sqrt{n\pi(1 - \pi)}} = \frac{8 - 5 - \frac{1}{2}}{\sqrt{10(\frac{1}{2})(\frac{1}{2})}} = \frac{2.5}{1.58} = 1.58$$

Since it is a two-sided test (the reader may verify for himself that 2 or fewer successes gives, with the continuity correction, $z_c = -1.58$), the two-tailed normal table (Appendix Table A2) yields .114 as the approximate required chance. This agrees quite well with the exact result of .109 determined previously, the discrepancy occurring at the third decimal. In this situation the normal approximation method provides an entirely satisfactory alternative.

As n gets larger, it becomes increasingly more cumbersome to calculate and sum the terms of the binomial, so the normal approximation presents a particularly attractive alternative for conducting tests of significance involving proportions. Extensive tables of the binomial exist, such as those calculated by the National Bureau of Standards [81]. These, however, are not readily available and tend to be used more by statisticians than by experimenters. In practice, most of the inferences concerning proportions that appear in the medical literature are based on the normal approximation to the binomial distribution.

Other Aspects of Significance Testing

Using the normal approximation to the binomial, one can answer other questions regarding tests of significance that involve the inverse use of the formulas given in Table 5.1. For example, by specifying the significance level and the null hypothesis, one can determine the number of successes that are needed to achieve statistical significance.

Example 5.3.   Consider a trial of two analgesics, A and B, conducted similarly to that described before, but with the participation of an anticipated 100 patients with chronic headache. If the investigator tests the null hypothesis that the analgesics are equally preferable and he employs a two-sided test at the 5 percent level, how many preferences of each kind must he observe in order to reject the null hypothesis?

As before, $\pi = \Pr(A$ preference$)$ and the null hypothesis claims $\pi = \frac{1}{2}$. Since $n\pi = n(1 - \pi) = (100)(\frac{1}{2}) = 50$, which is well above 5, the normal distribution can safely be used. The two-sided test at the 5 percent level means 5 percent in two tails of the normal distribution, namely, z values of ± 1.96. The critical ratio for "number of successes" in Table 5.1 gives, for the upper tail,

$$1.96 = \frac{x - (100)(\frac{1}{2}) - \frac{1}{2}}{\sqrt{(100)(\frac{1}{2})(\frac{1}{2})}}$$

Solving for x yields $x = (1.96)(5) + 50 + 0.5 = 60.3$. For the lower tail, $z = -1.96$ results in $x = (-1.96)(5) + 50 - 0.5 = 39.7$. Thus, 61 or more A preferences would lead to the conclusion that A is preferred significantly more often than B ($P < .05$). Also, 39 or fewer A preferences would lead to the conclusion B is preferred significantly more often than A ($P < .05$).

So far, the numerical examples have involved $\pi = \frac{1}{2}$. Of course, this need not be so, and interest may center on testing hypotheses involving values of π other than $\frac{1}{2}$. Consider the following example concerning an epidemic of atypical pneumonia among troops returning from Italy during World War II.

Example 5.4.   Among U.S. troops stationed at an Air Force base in southern Italy toward the close of World War II, there occurred an epidemic of atypical pneumonia in which 40 percent of the several hundred men in one squadron contracted the disease. During the investigation of the epidemic, illness attack rates were calculated according to the assigned duties on the base. In one instance, among 25 men who belonged to the ground crew working in communications, 14 (or 56 percent) contracted the disease. Is there evidence that the communications ground crew had a higher attack rate than the entire squadron? Considering that the overall attack rate was 40 percent, was this observed attack rate of 56 percent among these 25 men something out of the ordinary? Or, could such a sample attack rate arise purely by chance? Consider a test of significance with these data.

The null hypothesis states that the communications ground crew had the same attack rate as the underlying population, namely, $\pi = .4$. If the null hypothesis of a population attack rate of 40 percent is true, what is the chance of finding in a sample of 25 an attack rate of 56 percent or higher?

Suppose that 5 percent is deemed a small enough chance and that interest centers on a two-tailed test. (The latter specification indicates that the investigator, before examining his sample data, had as much interest in the possibility the communications ground crew had a higher attack rate than the entire squadron as in their having a lower rate.)

It may easily be seen that the conditions for application of the normal distribution as an approximation to the binomial are met, namely, $n\pi = (25)(.4) = 10$ and $n(1 - \pi) = (25)(.6) = 15$. Application of the critical ratio for percentages (Table 5.1) gives

$$z_c = \frac{56 - 40 - 100/(2 \times 25)}{100\sqrt{(.4)(.6)/25}} = \frac{14}{9.8} = 1.43$$

From the two-tailed normal tables, the required probability is .153. Thus, the observed rate in the sample can well be explained by chance or sampling variation. Hence, the communications ground crew attack rate is compatible with that of the entire squadron ($P > .05$).

Confidence Limits

To obtain 95 percent confidence limits on a proportion, one proceeds analogously to the development of confidence limits on a mean. One would solve for π in the relation

$$\pm 1.96 = \frac{p - \pi - 1/(2n)}{\sqrt{\pi(1 - \pi)/n}}$$

The equation is not as easy to solve as that for a mean (p. 126), since π occurs both in the numerator and denominator of the right-hand expression. Algebraic manipulation would reveal that a quadratic equation in π can be derived. From college algebra, one would employ the solution for a quadratic equation to yield the required limits. For most practical purposes, however, the above equation, upon neglecting the continuity factor, may be rewritten as

$$\pi = p \pm 1.96\sqrt{\pi(1 - \pi)/n}$$

Then, with substitution of the sample p for the population π and $q = 1 - p$ for $1 - \pi$, the right-hand side, or 95 percent confidence limits, becomes

$$p \pm 1.96\sqrt{pq/n}$$

Of course, in order to apply these confidence limits, the normal approximation to the binomial must be appropriate.

Example 5.5. Consider the observed 56 percent attack rate of atypical pneumonia among a sample of 25 men. What are the 95 percent confidence limits on the underlying population attack rate?

Answer:

$$.56 \pm 1.96\sqrt{(.56)(.44)/25}$$
$$= .56 \pm .195$$
$$= .365 \text{ to } .755$$

Thus, one has 95 percent certainty that, in the underlying population, the attack rate is somewhere in the range of 36.5 to 75.5 percent.

For comparison, the application of the more complex confidence limit determination that involves the solution of a quadratic equation yields 35.4 to 75.1 percent. Both methods depend on the normal approximation to the binomial. One may also obtain the exact determination of 95 percent confidence limits by the use of published tables of the binomial distribution. Such limits for the data at hand are 34.9 to 75.6 percent. Clearly, the approximate limits obtained initially appear to be quite sufficient and agree well with the other more accurate determinations.

Determination of Sample Size

There are several ways in which one may answer the question, "How large a sample do I need?" when inference concerns a single proportion. One way is analogous to that for means whereby one specifies α and β error levels for the particular null and alternative hypotheses denoted as π_0 and π_1, respectively. As before, z_α and z_β denote the upper α percent and lower β percent of the normal distribution. The critical ratio for proportions in Table 5.1 gives, upon neglecting the continuity correction, the two equations:

$$z_\alpha = \frac{p - \pi_0}{\sqrt{\pi_0(1 - \pi_0)/n}}$$

$$z_\beta = \frac{p - \pi_1}{\sqrt{\pi_1(1 - \pi_1)/n}}$$

Solving for n yields

$$n = \left[\frac{z_\alpha \sqrt{\pi_0(1 - \pi_0)} - z_\beta \sqrt{\pi_1(1 - \pi_1)}}{\pi_1 - \pi_0} \right]^2$$

Example 5.6.   Consider the planning of a clinical trial to compare analgesics A and B in a manner similar to that described in previous examples. Each patient receives both analgesics on two separate occasions and ultimately indicates which he prefers. The investigator claims as his null hypothesis that A and B are equally preferable. He proposes to conduct a two-sided test at the 5 percent level. He states that if, in actuality, the proportion preferring A in the underlying population is as high as .8, then he wishes to risk only a 5 percent chance of failing to conclude that A is significantly preferable to B. (An alternative statement of this latter specification is that if the true preference rate for A is .8, then the investigator wishes to be 95 percent certain that his test will result in the conclusion. "A preferred significantly more often than B.") How many patients with chronic headache are needed?

Answer: With π defined as the probability of an A preference, the α error specification indicates $\pi_0 = .5$, and the two-sided test at 5 percent gives $z_\alpha = 1.96$. The β error specification indicates $\pi_1 = .8$, and the 5 percent error level gives $z_\beta = -1.65$. (Note that, as before, the two-tailed z value is used for z_α, whereas the one-tailed z value is used for z_β.) Hence,

$$n = \left[\frac{1.96\sqrt{(.5)(.5)} - (-1.65)\sqrt{(.8)(.2)}}{.8 - .5} \right]^2 = 29.9$$

or 30 patients with chronic headache are needed.

The following is another common procedure for the determination of sample size and is more applicable to surveys. The investigator specifies the magnitude of the difference he wishes to tolerate between the sample and population proportions, and he states the degree of certainty he wishes for the result to be within this discrepancy.

Example 5.7.   Consider a survey of school children in a community to determine the proportion immunized against measles. One can secure a list of all school children, but the list is too long and funds are insufficient to query every name on the list. It is decided to choose a random sample of names from the list, and, for each sample name, the child's family will be interviewed in order to determine his immunization status. How large a sample is needed? By chance, the percentage immunized among the sample will differ somewhat from the percentage immunized in the population. The investigator specifies his interest in a maximum discrepancy between sample and population percent immunized of ±4 percent (absolute percent). Further, he states that he wishes to be 99 percent certain that the discrepancy is within these limits.

Answer: The 99 percent certainty and the "±" for his discrepancy indicates 1 percent in two tails of the normal distribution, namely, $z = \pm 2.58$. The discrepancy of ±4 percent between the sample and population percentage gives $100p - 100\pi = 4$. The critical ratio for percentage success in Table 5.1 then yields

$$2.58 = \frac{4}{100\sqrt{\pi(1 - \pi)/n}}$$

Solving for n yields

$$n = (258/4)^2\pi(1 - \pi) = 4{,}160.25\,\pi(1 - \pi)$$

This result presents somewhat of a dilemma because, in order to determine n, one must know π, the unknown population proportion that one is trying to estimate!

One approach, which is exceedingly conservative, is based on the fact that the maximum value of the quantity $\pi(1 - \pi)$ is .25. (Application of differential calculus to the expression will easily verify this result.) Hence, no more than $n = (4{,}160.25)(.25) = 1{,}040$, or approximately 1,000 school children, are needed. The investigator would use this as his determination of sample size if he had no clue whatsoever as to what to expect for π.

More often, however, the results of previous experience or similar studies in other areas will enable the investigator to make a "ballpark" guess for the value of π. For instance, immunization studies among children in other communities might lead him to expect that roughly 80 to 90 percent of the children in this community were immunized. He would then calculate

$$n = (4,160.25)(.8)(.2) = 666$$

$$n = (4,160.25)(.9)(.1) = 374$$

Thus, a sample of somewhere between 400 and 700 children would suffice if the percent immunized is in this range.

COMPARISON OF TWO PROPORTIONS

As with the comparison of means, two situations pertain to the comparison of proportions: paired and independent samples. The criterion for recognizing paired samples is, of course, the same as before. Paired samples exist when each observation in one sample has a pair or mate in the other sample. Again, the types of pairing range from the individual as his own control to pairs created by the investigator (p. 132). It is convenient to deal first with the comparison of proportions in independent samples.

Independent Samples

Test of Significance

The notation, similar to that for comparison of independent means, is as follows:

Item	Treatment group	Control group	Total
	Population:		
Proportion success	π_T	π_C	—
	Sample:		
Sample size	n_T	n_C	$n_T + n_C$
Number of successes	x_T	x_C	$x_T + x_C$
Proportion success	$p_T = x_T/n_T$	$p_C = x_C/n_C$	$p = (x_T + x_C)/(n_T + n_C)$

For the sample data, the combined results in the two groups appear in the last column. These quantities are employed in the methods described below.

Almost always, the null hypothesis regarding the underlying population values claims identical proportion success, namely, $\pi_T = \pi_C$ or, equivalently, $\pi_T - \pi_C = 0$. The test of significance asks: If the null hypothesis is true and there is no difference in the population proportion success, what is the chance of finding a difference in the sample proportion success as large as or larger than that observed? As before, one must also specify a significance level and whether interest is in a one- or two-sided test.

Analogous to the test on a single proportion, there are two ways to proceed: (1) to develop an exact test based on the fact that each of the two samples follows the binomial distribution or (2) to develop an approximate test based on the normal approximation to the binomial distribution. This text considers only the second procedure, the approximate test. The exact test is described in other texts [2, 12, 82].

In practice, the exact test applies when the conditions for the appropriateness of the approximate test fail. The reader of the medical literature will occasionally encounter the exact test (it is usually termed "Fisher's exact test for the comparison of two proportions"). The inference, of course, is identical with that for the approximate test described here.

The approximate test is based on the principle described previously for the calculation of a critical ratio, z, namely, a numerator that consists of the difference between a sample "something" and the null hypothesis value for the "something" in the underlying populations and a denominator that consists of the standard error of the sample "something." In this case the "something" is the difference in two independent proportions. The sample difference is thus $p_T - p_C$, and the population difference, when the null hypothesis is true, is $\pi_T - \pi_C = 0$. It remains to determine the standard error of the difference in proportions, denoted as $\text{SE}(p_T - p_C)$. Using the rule employed in the argument for the comparison of two means (p. 138), it may be seen that

$$\text{SE}(p_T - p_C) = \sqrt{[\text{SE}(p_T)]^2 + [\text{SE}(p_C)]^2} = \sqrt{\frac{\pi_T(1 - \pi_T)}{n_T} + \frac{\pi_C(1 - \pi_C)}{n_C}}$$

Since the null hypothesis states that $\pi_T = \pi_C$, let π denote the common population proportion success, that is, $\pi_T = \pi_C = \pi$. Then

$$\text{SE}(p_T - p_C) = \sqrt{\pi(1 - \pi)\left(\frac{1}{n_T} + \frac{1}{n_C}\right)}$$

Unfortunately, π is unknown. What one needs is an estimate of π from sample results. There are two sample estimates of π (presuming the null hypothesis is true): p_T and p_C, the respective sample proportion successes. For purposes of performing the required inference, their best combination is a weighted average with weights proportional to the number of observations in each sample. Denoting the weighted average as p, then

$$p = \frac{n_T p_T + n_C p_C}{n_T + n_C}$$

or, more simply,

$$p = \frac{x_T + x_C}{n_T + n_C}$$

In other words, p is the ratio of the total successes in the combined treated and control samples to the total observations in the combined treated and control samples.

Substituting p for π (and, of course, $q = 1 - p$ for $1 - \pi$), it can be shown that the resulting critical ratio follows a normal distribution so that

$$z = \frac{p_T - p_C}{\sqrt{pq\left(\dfrac{1}{n_T} + \dfrac{1}{n_C}\right)}}$$

There is, however, an additional consideration derived from the fact that the critical ratio is based on smooth normal curves used as substitutes for discrete binomial distributions. A correction for continuity is therefore appropriate. The continuity correction affects only the numerator of the critical ratio. The continuity correction rule is that in the calculation of $p_T - p_C$, *reduce* the numerator of the larger sample proportion by $\frac{1}{2}$ and *increase* the numerator of the smaller sample proportion by $\frac{1}{2}$. Thus, if p_T is greater than p_C, the continuity correction substitutes

$$\frac{x_T - \frac{1}{2}}{n_T} - \frac{x_C + \frac{1}{2}}{n_C}$$

for $p_T - p_C$ in the critical ratio. The test then becomes

$$z_c = \frac{\dfrac{x_T - \frac{1}{2}}{n_T} - \dfrac{x_C - \frac{1}{2}}{n_C}}{\sqrt{pq\left(\dfrac{1}{n_T} + \dfrac{1}{n_C}\right)}}$$

where

$$p = \frac{x_T + x_C}{n_T + n_C} \quad \text{and} \quad q = 1 - p$$

(The subscript c on z denotes the inclusion of the continuity correction.) Note that the effect of the continuity correction is always to reduce the magnitude of the numerator of the critical ratio. In this sense, the continuity correction is conservative in that its use, compared with its not being used, will label somewhat fewer observed sample differences as being statistically significant.

Finally, one must remember that the use of the normal distribution is approximate and rests on the adequacy with which the normal represents the binomial distribution. A conservative rule of thumb for the appropriateness of the test is that *each* of the quantities $n_T p$, $n_T q$, $n_C p$, and $n_C q$ be 5 or more. One should verify that these conditions prevail before embarking on the calculation of a critical ratio. If they do not prevail, then the computation of Fisher's exact test is appropriate.

Example 5.8.   The first set of data in Chapter 2 (Table 2.1) provides an ideal illustration of the comparison of independent proportions. These data pertain to a clinical trial of the drug propranolol among patients with myocardial infarction. The two groups of patients are those treated with propranolol and a control group not receiving the drug. The dichotomous outcome consisted of each patient being alive on the 28th day following admission to the study or his having succumbed some time within this 28-day time period. The data are reproduced below along with the survival rates in each of the two groups and in the combined group.

Outcome	Propranolol group	Control group	Total
Survived 28 days	38	29	67
Did not survive	7	17	24
Total	45	46	91
Percent surviving	84.4%	63.0%	73.6%

Do these sample results provide sufficient evidence that propranolol increases the 28-day survival rate compared with a control? If, in fact, there were no difference in survival rates between the underlying propranolol-treated and control populations, is it likely that with the samples involved in this trial one could observe a discrepancy this large or larger purely by chance?

Suppose that the 5 percent significance level is adopted and that a two-sided test is desired.

Answer: First, is it appropriate to employ the test based on the normal distribution? Clearly, $p = 67/91 = .7363$, and $q = 1 - p = .2637$. Since $n_T = 45$ and $n_C = 46$, it may be seen that each of $n_T p$, $n_T q$, $n_C p$, and $n_C q$ will certainly be well above 5. Thus it is safe to use the test based on the normal distribution.

Since the survival rate of the propranolol-treated group is greater than that of the control group, the critical ratio with the continuity correction becomes

$$z_c = \frac{\dfrac{38 - 0.5}{45} - \dfrac{29 + 0.5}{46}}{\sqrt{(.7363)(.2637)\left(\dfrac{1}{45} + \dfrac{1}{46}\right)}} = \frac{.8333 - .6413}{\sqrt{.008536}}$$

$$= \frac{.1920}{.0924} = 2.08$$

The two-tailed normal tables give a probability of .038.

The conclusion is that the propranolol-treated patients have a statistically significantly higher 28-day survival rate compared with the control group without propranolol treatment ($P < .05$). In other words, the observed difference in survival rates cannot be explained by chance or sampling variation.

As has been noted previously, the reader is warned that the statistically significant result merely rules out chance alone as explaining the difference. It does not necessarily imply that the increased survival can be attributed to propranolol treatment. The reader must assure himself that the design and the conduct of the investigation were sufficiently stringent so that no doubts concerning bias and selective factors could have arisen. In this particular study, such questions did arise and resulted in considerable controversy. These issues are discussed more fully in Chapter 10. There is, however, no disputing the fact that the results were statistically significant and this is the focus of the present argument.

Confidence Limits

Rather than a test of significance, the comparison of two proportions may entail the determination of confidence limits on the difference in population proportion success. Using the normal approximation, approximate 95 percent confidence limits on $\pi_T - \pi_C$ result from calculating

$$p_T - p_C \pm 1.96\sqrt{\frac{p_T q_T}{n_T} + \frac{p_C q_C}{n_C}}$$

The slight difference in the confidence limit statement and the test of significance calculations pertains to the standard error of the difference in proportions, i.e., the terms under the square root sign. The test of significance employs the common p, which derives from the assumption that the null hypothesis is true. The confidence limit statement employs the individual p_T and p_C values. For the propranolol trial, 95 percent confidence limits on the difference in survival rates are

$$.844 - .630 \pm 1.96\sqrt{\frac{(.844)(.156)}{45} + \frac{(.630)(.370)}{46}}$$

$$= .214 \pm .175$$

$$= .039 \text{ to } .389$$

Thus, in the underlying populations from which these samples came, the difference in 28-day survival rates between the propranolol-treated and control patients is within the range of 3.9 to 38.9 percent, with 95 percent confidence.

Determination of Sample Size

Determination of sample size for the comparison of two independent proportions follows from the specification of α and β errors, respectively, for the particular null and alternative hypotheses on the true difference in population proportion success. Usually, one assumes further that the sample sizes in each group are to be the same, namely, $n_T = n_C = n$ (say). The null hypothesis, which claims no difference in population success rates ($\pi_T - \pi_C = 0$), together with the accompanying α error, yield the equation

$$z_\alpha = \frac{p_T - p_C - 0}{\sqrt{\pi(1 - \pi)\left(\dfrac{1}{n} + \dfrac{1}{n}\right)}}$$

The alternative hypothesis that specifies a particular difference in population success rates, say $\pi_T - \pi_C = \delta$, together with the accompanying β error, yield the equation

$$z_\beta = \frac{p_T - p_C - \delta}{\sqrt{\dfrac{\pi_T(1 - \pi_T)}{n} + \dfrac{\pi_C(1 - \pi_C)}{n}}}$$

Solving for n in the two equations gives

$$n = \left[\frac{z_\alpha \sqrt{2\pi(1 - \pi)} - z_\beta \sqrt{\pi_T(1 - \pi_T) + \pi_C(1 - \pi_C)}}{\delta}\right]^2$$

As with inference on a single proportion, the determination of sample size for the comparison of two independent proportions involves the unknown population success rates! Usually, however, one compares a treatment group with a control group. Most often the investigator, relying on his past experience, can produce a reasonably good estimate of the success rate anticipated in the control group. If he uses this estimate to represent both π_C and π in the above expression and if he then uses $\pi_T = \pi_C + \delta$, he will be able to calculate the required sample size.

Example 5.9. Consider a clinical trial for the comparison of a new drug with a control in the treatment of the acute phase of myocardial infarction. As with the propranolol example, suppose the chief response is 28-day survival. The null hypothesis—that there is no population difference in 28-day survival rates—will be tested with a two-sided test at the 5 percent level. If, in fact, the new drug increases the survival rate by 20 percent (in absolute percentage), the investigator wishes to risk a 10 percent chance of failing to conclude that the new drug is significantly better than the control. Alternatively, the latter specification could be stated as follows: if the new drug increases survival by as much as 20 percent, the investigator wishes 90 percent certainty that his test will conclude that the survival rate with the drug is significantly higher than that of the control. How large a sample is needed?

Answer: Past experience and the 63 percent control survival rate in the preceding data might lead the investigator to anticipate a control survival rate of 60 percent, that is, $\pi = \pi_C = .6$. His specification that the interest is in a 20 percent increase in survival yields $\pi_T = .6 + .2 = .8$. The two-tailed test at the 5 percent level gives $z_\alpha = 1.96$ from the two-tailed normal tables. The 10 percent chance prescribed for the β error gives $z_\beta = -1.28$ from the one-tailed normal tables. Thus,

$$n = \left[\frac{1.96\sqrt{2(.6)(.4)} - (-1.28)\sqrt{(.8)(.2) + (.6)(.4)}}{.2} \right]^2$$

$$= 117.4$$

or 118 in each of the treatment and control groups, for a total of 236 study participants.

If this is thought to be too large, n would decrease if there were less stringent error levels; i.e., higher α and β values, or if the alternative hypothesis were focused on a larger difference between the treatment and control population proportions.

For a more precise determination of required sample size in the comparison of independent proportions, tables are available elsewhere [18, 72].

Paired Samples

Example 5.10.   Colton, Gosselin, and Smith describe a study of the effects of caffeine on medical students that well illustrates the comparison of proportions in paired samples [21]. Second-year students were given packets of instant coffee on two separate occasions. On one occasion, the packet contained a placebo (lactose) mixed with Sanka; on the other occasion, caffeine (50 mg) mixed with Sanka. The two preparations were identical in appearance and taste. The students were assigned at random to the order in which the two preparations were administered and were unaware of the contents of the packets. Thus, approximately half the students had the placebo on the first occasion, followed by the caffeine mixture on the second, while the other half were given the mixtures in the reverse order. On each occasion, the students were instructed to dissolve the contents of the packet in hot water and to drink the beverage shortly before retiring. On the morning following ingestion of the drink, the students completed a questionnaire, one item of which asked, "Did it take you more time than usual to fall asleep?" The yes-no dichotomous response to this question on each of the occasions (placebo or caffeine) represents a self-pairing situation, with each student serving as his own control.

Students were classified as being coffee or noncoffee drinkers. A "noncoffee drinker" was arbitrarily defined as an individual whose usual habit is to consume one or fewer cups of coffee or tea or bottles of Coke per day. The data under consideration pertain to the 31 students classified as noncoffee drinkers. The following data summarize the responses to the question on whether it took the student longer than usual to fall asleep:

	Results in 31 noncoffee drinkers	
Response to question	After placebo	After caffeine
Yes	1	8
No	30	23
Total	31	31
Percent Yes	3.2%	25.8%

Thus, only 3 percent of the 31 noncoffee drinkers claimed it took them longer to fall asleep after the placebo, whereas 26 percent indicated it took longer to fall asleep after the caffeine mixture.

Do these data provide evidence that it takes longer for a noncoffee drinker to fall asleep after ingesting caffeine as compared with his taking a placebo?

Note that the above format for data presentation is analogous to the tabular format used in the comparison of two independent proportions. In fact, this format tempts the investigator to apply erroneously the methods of analysis for independent proportions. There may be a total of 62 observations, but there are only 31 subjects, each subject giving a response to both the placebo and the caffeine. The deficiency in the above format is that it entirely disregards the inherent paired nature of the observations. The data cannot be analyzed properly in this form; one needs to refer to the original paired observations and must somehow account for the pairing in the summary of results.

The reader is warned that disregard of the pairing in the analysis of the results of a paired experiment represents a major pitfall to medical investigators. Often, however, the inappropriate analysis of paired data as if they were from independent samples will not lead to any materially different conclusion from the proper paired analysis. Still, the method of data analysis should coincide with the manner in which the data were collected. Paired data deserve analysis by pairs; independent samples entail their appropriate analysis.

For proportions in paired samples, the basic data consist of each pair's responses in each of the two groups. With the data at hand, each pair is a subject and the responses are the dichotomous yes-no answers following the placebo and the caffeine ingestion. Each pair can result in only one of the four following possibilities:

Placebo yes, caffeine yes

Placebo yes, caffeine no

Placebo no, caffeine yes

Placebo no, caffeine no

The proper form of data summarization consists merely of a count of the number of each of the above responses. For the 31 students the results were:

Response to question following:		
Placebo	Caffeine	No. of students
Yes	Yes	0
Yes	No	1
No	Yes	8
No	No	22
	Total	31

These data can be rearranged in the following tabular format:

		Placebo response		
		Yes	No	Total
Caffeine	Yes	0	8	8
Response	No	1	22	23
	Total	1	30	31

In this format, each of the four entries in the body of the table corresponds with one of the possible paired responses. The table totals 31 paired responses or subjects. In addition, note that the Total *row* above (1, 30, 31) corresponds with the placebo response, and the Total *column* above (8, 23, 31) corresponds with the caffeine response, in the initial misleading table that disregarded the pairs.

It is now possible to conduct the appropriate test of significance for comparing the proportions. The key to the analysis involves discarding the tied pairs, namely, the yes-yes and no-no responses. The rationale for doing so is that a pair in which the responses are both yes or both no provides no information concerning the *comparison* of the two treatments under investigation. All information concerning the comparison is derived from the untied pairs: the yes-no and no-yes responses.

Thus, the analysis focuses solely on the nine untied pairs: one yes-no and eight no-yes observations. If the null hypothesis—that there is no difference between the placebo and caffeine—is true, then one would expect an even distribution of untied pairs, i.e., just as many yes-no as no-yes responses. Letting $\pi = $ Pr (untied pair is yes-no) amounts to testing the null hypothesis that among the total of n untied pairs, $\pi = \frac{1}{2}$. Thus, when the null hypothesis is true, the total of n yes-no and no-yes untied pairs is equivalent to the heads and tails in n tosses of a fair coin. The test consists of determining the chance, under the null hypothesis, of results as deviant as or more deviant than that observed. Equivalently, the test asks, "With nine tosses of a fair coin, what is the chance of eight or more heads?"

To complete the required specifications, suppose one indicates a two-sided test at the 5 percent level. One must then add the chance of deviation from expectation in the other tail, namely, the chance of one or fewer heads. The two-tailed test then becomes, with the use of the binomial distribution (p. 151),

$$\text{Pr}(0, 1, 8, \text{ or } 9) = (\tfrac{1}{2})^9 + 9(\tfrac{1}{2})(\tfrac{1}{2})^8 + 9(\tfrac{1}{2})^8(\tfrac{1}{2}) + (\tfrac{1}{2})^9$$

$$= 2(1 + 9)/2^9 = 20/512 = .039$$

The chance is less than the predetermined 5 percent so the result is statistically significant. In conclusion, noncoffee drinkers take a longer time than usual to fall asleep after drinking a mixture containing caffeine as compared with a placebo ($P < .05$).

Note that the above test was exact in that it employed the binomial distribution. An approximate test, based on the normal approximation to the binomial distribution, may also be used, provided the appropriate requirements are satisfied. With the example above, $n\pi = n(1 - \pi) = (9)(\tfrac{1}{2}) = 4.5$, so the normal approximation to the binomial cannot be used safely. The following example serves to illustrate the use of the normal approximation to the binomial distribution in the comparison of proportions in paired samples.

Example 5.11.　Sartwell et al. reported the results of the first American study that sought to corroborate the British studies linking thromboembolic disease with the use of oral contraceptives [97]. The study was conducted in a number of medical school–affiliated hospitals in several large northeastern American cities. Among participating hospitals, during a 3-

year period all married women from age 15 to 44 who were discharged with a diagnosis of idiopathic thromboembolism were identified. For each identified case, a control was selected.

Sartwell states:

> Controls were female patients discharged alive from the same hospitals in the same six-month time interval. In addition to these matching factors, they were individually matched to the thromboembolism cases on age (within the same five-year span), marital status, residence, race, parity (three classes: zero, one to two, three or more prior pregnancies) and hospital pay status (ward, semi-private or private). . . . The same exclusions . . . applied to the controls as to the cases. Controls for the most part were admitted for acute medical or surgical conditions, trauma including fractures and dislocations, and elective surgery such as nose and throat operations. . . .
>
> Both groups were interviewed to ascertain whether they had used oral contraceptives before the hospitalization.

The investigation is clearly paired, since the investigator determined the pairs and matched the women according to the characteristics described above. A total of 175 pairs of thromboembolic and control women was obtained. Their history of oral contraceptive usage is summarized as follows:

Oral contraceptive usage of thromboembolic and control pairs of women	Number of pairs
Used by both	10
Used by thromboembolic women only	57
Used by control women only	13
Used by neither	95
Total	175

The question is whether there is any difference between thromboembolic and control women in their oral contraceptive usage. The null hypothesis claims that in the underlying population thromboembolic and control women have an equal history of oral contraceptive usage.

Analysis requires the discarding of the tied pairs: the 10 pairs where both members indicated oral contraceptive usage and the 95 pairs where neither member indicated usage. There remains a total of $n = 70$ untied pairs. Letting $\pi = $ Pr (untied pair is usage by thromboembolic woman only), the null hypothesis claims $\pi = \frac{1}{2}$. Among the 70 untied pairs, there are 57 "successes," or, correspondingly, "heads." What is the chance of a result being this deviant or more so? Since $n\pi = n(1 - \pi) = (70)(\frac{1}{2}) = 35 > 5$, the normal distribution can be used safely as a substitute for the binomial.

The critical ratio for the number of successes (Table 5.1) gives

$$z_c = \frac{57 - (70)(\frac{1}{2}) - \frac{1}{2}}{\sqrt{70(\frac{1}{2})(\frac{1}{2})}} = \frac{21.5}{4.183} = 5.14$$

Using the two-tailed normal tables, the result is far beyond the range of the tables; clearly, $P < .001$. Thus, women discharged from the hospital with thromboembolic disease are significantly more likely than their matched controls to have used oral contraceptives prior to hospitalization ($P < .001$).

The adequacy of this evidence in establishing an association between oral contraceptives and thromboembolic disease is discussed in Chapter 11.

CHI-SQUARE TEST

For the comparison of two proportions in paired or independent samples, the chi-square test presents an alternative to the use of critical ratios of the preceding sections. As will be shown, the results of the chi-square calculations are identical with those of the z-value calculations in the preceding sections.

Why, then, use chi-square? First, many investigators find the chi-square method simpler and easier to understand and apply. Second, the chi-square method can be extended to the comparison of several proportions, whereas the critical ratio method cannot.

The general formulation of chi-square is

$$\chi^2(\mathrm{df}) = \sum_{\substack{\text{all} \\ \text{categories}}} (O - E)^2/E$$

where

O = observed count in a category

E = expected count in that category if the null hypothesis is true

Note that this formulation of chi-square applies only to *counts* of the number of observations in a category and not to measured quantities, ranks, percentages, or proportions. The misapplication of chi-square to data other than counts represents one of the common errors committed by investigators inexperienced in statistical methods. The "df" in parentheses indicates that chi-square, like the previously discussed t distribution, involves the concept of degrees of freedom (p. 32).

Comparison of Proportions in Independent Sample

The propranolol treatment trial in myocardial infarction can be summarized with the following fourfold table (so-called because there are four quantities within the body of the table):

		Treatment group		
		Propranolol	Control	Total
28-Day	Survived	38	29	67
Outcome	Died	7	17	24
	Total	45	46	91

The four cells or categories forming the body of the table correspond with the numbers 38, 29, 7, and 17. These are the observed counts (O).

How does one now determine the *expected* counts? Recall that the null hypothesis claims identical survival rates for propranolol-treated and control patients. This rate is, of course, unknown but it can be estimated from the sample results. Recall that the best estimate of the common survival rate is the rate in the combined total of the two samples, which, from the last column in the table, is 67/91.

When the null hypothesis is true, this estimate of the proportion surviving then gives, among the 45 propranolol-treated patients, an *expected* number surviving of $45(67/91) = 33.13$. Correspondingly, among the 46 control patients, the number *expected* to survive is $46(67/91) = 33.87$.

The same reasoning applies to the deaths, with 24/91 being the corresponding estimate from the combined samples of the mortality rate when the null hypothesis is true. Hence, the *expected* deaths among 45 propranolol-treated and 46 control patients are respectively $45(24/91) = 11.87$ and $46(24/91) = 12.13$.

Thus, for the four categories in the table, the *expected* counts are

		Treatment group		
		Propranolol	Control	Total
28-Day	Survived	33.13	33.87	67
Outcome	Died	11.87	12.13	24
	Total	45	46	91

Note in the above table of expected counts that the row and column totals are identical with those of the observed counts in the previous table. As a matter of fact, once one of the expected counts in the body of the table is determined, the others can be determined by appropriate subtractions, since the expected totals must be the same as the observed totals. For example, once one determines 33.13 expected propranolol-treated survivors, all other expected quantities follow by subtraction from the column totals of 45 and 46 and the row totals of 67 and 24. Not only does this simplify the determination of the expected quantities, but it indicates as well the number of df to accompany the chi-square calculation. Since the body of the table contains only one independent expected quantity, this chi-square calculation entails 1 df.

The chi-square, like the critical ratio, is an approximate method. A conservative rule of thumb for the validity of the chi-square calculation is that the expected count in each category be at least 5. The data at hand clearly fulfill this criterion. (The reader may verify that this criterion for the applicability of chi-square is identical with the previous criterion for the applicability of the normal critical ratio.)

One further aspect of chi-square depends on its being based on the normal approximation to the binomial, so there is the need for a continuity correction. The appropriate continuity modification consists of reducing the absolute magnitude of $O - E$ by one half. Thus, the chi-square, when applied to the comparison of two independent proportions, becomes

$$\chi_c^2(1\,\mathrm{df}) = \sum_{\substack{\text{four}\\\text{categories}}} (|O - E| - \tfrac{1}{2})^2/E$$

where the subscript c denotes that the continuity modification has been made and the notation $||$ indicates the absolute difference of O and E (the difference regardless of sign). The continuity correction of this chi-square formulation is called *Yates' correction*.

Note that, for the data at hand, $|O - E|$ is the same in each of the four categories, namely, 4.87. This is not an arithmetical accident. Substitution of letters for numbers will indicate that the constant $|O - E|$ values pertain to any fourfold table.

Thus, with factoring, the chi-square calculation becomes

$$\chi_c^2(1\,\mathrm{df}) = (|O - E| - \tfrac{1}{2})^2 \sum_{\substack{\text{four}\\\text{categories}}} (1/E)$$

$$= (4.87 - \tfrac{1}{2})^2 \left(\frac{1}{33.13} + \frac{1}{33.87} + \frac{1}{11.87} + \frac{1}{12.13} \right)$$

$$= (4.37)^2 (.2264) = 4.32$$

Appendix Table A4 presents the percentage points of the chi-square distribution for df 1 through 25. The first line of the table indicates that for the chi-square distribution with 1 df, the 5 percent point corresponds with 3.84, while the 1 percent point corresponds with 6.63. The chi-square figure calculated in the example falls between these two values. Hence, the calculated chi-square cuts off less than 5 percent and more than 1 percent of the chi-square distribution with 1 df. Stated algebraically, the result is $.01 < P < .05$. Thus, propranolol-treated patients have a significantly higher 28-day survival rate compared with control patients ($P < .05$).

The previous analysis of these data using the normal critical ratio gave $z_c = 2.08$. Note that $(2.08)^2 = 4.32$; that is, the square of the previous critical ratio calculation is identical with the chi-square calculation. Note further that if one takes the 10, 5, 1, and 0.1 percent points in two tails of the normal distribution (1.65, 1.96, 2.58, and 3.09, respectively) and squares them, one obtains the corresponding percentage points of the chi-square distribution with 1 df (approximately $1.65^2 = 2.71$, $1.96^2 = 3.84$, $2.58^2 = 6.63$, and $3.29^2 = 10.83$). Thus, the chi-square distribution with 1 df is none other than the square of the standard normal distribution, using the two-tailed normal percentage points. Hence, the two tests are arithmetically identical. In fact, with substitution of letters for numbers to give the following fourfold table,

	T Group	C Group	Total
With characteristic	a	b	a + b
Without characteristic	c	d	c + d
Total	a + c	b + d	N = a + b + c + d

the algebraically adept reader may verify the equivalence of the present chi-square calculation and the previous normal critical ratio calculation.

Finally, with the use of the above algebraic notation for a fourfold table, the chi-square calculation may also be shown to be equivalent to

$$\chi_c^2(1\,\mathrm{df}) = \frac{(|ad - bc| - N/2)^2 N}{(a + c)(b + d)(a + b)(c + d)}$$

This formula for chi-square appears in many statistical texts. This author, however, prefers the initial chi-square formula since it is easier to recall and its calculation more directly reflects the rationale underlying the chi-square test.

One of the disadvantages of the chi-square approach is that it does not permit the calculation of confidence limits; another is that its formulation does not readily permit the determination of required sample size. However, the chi-square test outlined in this section pervades the medical literature, and it is probably the statistical test of significance that the physician will most frequently encounter in his general medical reading.

Comparison of Proportions in Paired Samples

Chi-square may also be applied to the comparison of proportions in paired samples. The initial analysis proceeds as before. The numbers of each type of pair are counted, and the tied pairs are discarded. The numbers of each of the two categories of untied pairs constitute the observed counts.

As before, the null hypothesis claims an equal chance for each of the two categories of untied pairs. Consequently, when the null hypothesis is true, the *expected* counts are merely one-half the total number of untied pairs.

The chi-square calculation, being an approximate method, is not always valid. As before, a conservative rule for its applicability is that the expected counts each be 5 or more. There is also a continuity modification which, like the preceding chi-square calculation, consists of reducing the absolute magnitude of $O - E$ by one half.

Finally, with only two categories and with the requirement of the equivalence of the total observed and expected counts, the determination of an expected count in one category automatically determines the expected count in the other category. Hence, the chi-square calculation in this situation also entails 1 df.

Example 5.12.   The calculation is illustrated with the data on oral contraceptives and thromboembolic disease previously analyzed by the critical ratio method:

Oral contraceptive usage of thromboembolic and control pairs of women	Observed counts (O)	Expected counts (E)
Used by both	10: Tied pairs; discard	
Used by thromboembolic woman only	57 ⎫ Total of	$70/2 = 35$
	⎬ 70 untied	
	⎪ pairs	
Used by control woman only	13 ⎭	$70\;2 = 35$
Used by neither	95: Tied pairs; discard	
Total	175	

$$\chi_c^2(1\mathrm{df}) = \sum_{\substack{\text{two}\\ \text{categories}}} (|O - E| - \tfrac{1}{2})^2/E$$

$$= \frac{(|57 - 35| - \tfrac{1}{2})^2}{35} + \frac{(|13 - 35| - \tfrac{1}{2})^2}{35} = \frac{2(21.5)^2}{35} = 26.41$$

Appendix Table A4 indicates that with 1 df, 10.83 cuts off 0.1 percent of the distribution. The calculated chi-square exceeds this value, so $P < .001$. Hence, as before, thromboembolic women are significantly more likely than their matched controls to have used oral contraceptives ($P < .001$).

Note that here, as with independent samples, the chi-square is the square of the previous normal critical ratio, that is, $26.41 = (5.14)^2$. Hence, this chi-square test for comparison of proportions in paired samples is identical to the previous critical ratio test. With substitution of letters for numbers as follows,

| Untied pairs | Number of pairs | |
	Observed (O)	Expected (E)
$+$ $-$	r	$(r + s)/2$
$-$ $+$	s	$(r + s)/2$
Total	$r + s$	$r + s$

the algebraic identity of the two approaches can be established. Furthermore, it may be seen that an equivalent algebraic formula for chi-square in comparing matched proportions is

$$\chi_c^2(1\,\mathrm{df}) = \frac{(|r - s| - 1)^2}{r + s}$$

which is a formula that appears in many statistics texts.

Comparison of Several Proportions

As has been mentioned, the chi-square approach to the comparison of proportions is easily extended to the simultaneous comparison of several proportions. This section concerns the comparison of more than two proportions in *independent* samples. The situation concerning the comparison of more than two proportions in *paired* samples is not dealt with in this text. The data in Chapter 2 (p. 12) on thromboembolic disease and blood group serve to illustrate this extension of chi-square. The data appear in what is called a $2 \times k$ contingency table, namely, a table of counts of observations arrayed in two columns and k rows. (Note that the fourfold table previously discussed consisted of two rows and two columns and is therefore also designated as a 2×2 contingency table.) The observed counts for the thromboembolic disease and blood groups are reproduced as follows:

| | Observed (O) counts | | |
Blood group	Thromboembolic women	Healthy women	Total
A	32	51	83
B	8	19	27
AB	6	5	11
O	9	70	79
Total	55	145	200

The null hypothesis claims an identical distribution by blood group for thromboembolic and healthy women. Alternatively, the null hypothesis may be specified as the claim that within each of the four blood group types, there is a constant proportion of thromboembolic women. In the total study the proportion of thromboembolic women is $55/200 = 0.275$, and the proportion of healthy women, $1 - 0.275 = 0.725$. Hence, if the null hypothesis of equal proportions by blood group is true, the expected number of thromboembolic women in each blood group results from multiplication of the total women in each blood group by 0.275. The expected number of healthy women in each blood group results correspondingly from multiplication of the total in each blood group by 0.725. The expected quantities calculate as:

| Blood group | Expected (E) counts | | Total |
	Thromboembolic women	Healthy women	
A	$83 \times 0.275 = 22.825$	$83 \times 0.725 = 60.175$	83
B	$27 \times 0.275 = 7.425$	$27 \times 0.725 = 19.575$	27
AB	$11 \times 0.275 = 3.025$	$11 \times 0.725 = 7.975$	11
O	$79 \times 0.275 = 21.725$	$79 \times 0.725 = 57.274$	79
Total	55	145	200

Note that, as before, the row and column totals of the observed and expected counts are identical. Hence, some of the expected counts may, alternatively, be derived by subtraction from the fixed row and column totals. It may be seen that once one determines the expected counts of thromboembolic women in blood groups A, B, and AB (i.e., the first three entries in the first column), all remaining expected counts result by subtraction. Therefore, this chi-square calculation will entail 3 df. In general, a $2 \times k$ contingency table carries $k - 1$ df for the chi-square calculation. (Of course, the previous 2×2 table with 1 df is a special case of this rule.)

An alternative procedure for the calculation of the expected quantities is worth noting and is perhaps more easily remembered. The expected count for any cell or category is derived by multiplying the row and column totals for the cell and then dividing by the total number of observations, which is 200 for the data under consideration here. For example, with thromboembolic women in blood group A, the corresponding row and column totals are 83 and 55, respectively, so the expected count for this cell is $83 \times 55/200 = 22.8$. With healthy women in blood group O, the expected count is $79 \times 145/200 = 57.3$.

For chi-square with more than 1 df, there is no need for a continuity correction. The value of $(O - E)^2/E$ for each of the eight cells in the table is as follows:

Blood group	Contribution to chi-square	
	Thromboembolic women	Healthy women
A	3.69	1.40
B	0.04	0.02
AB	2.93	1.11
O	7.45	2.83

Summation of these eight quantities gives a total chi-square of 19.47. The chi-square table with 3 df indicates that the calculated chi-square cuts off less than 0.1 percent of the distribution, hence $P < .001$. Thus, there is a statistically significant difference in the blood group distributions of thromboembolic and healthy women.

Inspection of the contribution of each blood group to the chi-square calculations reveals that blood group O contributes $7.45 + 2.83 = 10.28$ to the total chi-square figure of 19.47. Thus, the significance of the resulting chi-square test derives mainly from the discrepancy in blood group O. Inspection of the observed data reveals a distinct deficit of the thromboembolic women of blood group O compared with healthy, control women. Analysis of these data was but one piece of the accumulated evidence that led the investigators to conclude that female contraceptive users in blood group O are less prone than their contraceptive-user counterparts of other blood types to develop thromboembolic disease.

The chi-square test can also be extended without difficulty to an $r \times c$ contingency table, i.e., a set of category or cell counts arranged in r rows and c columns. Expected counts are formed as before by multiplication of corresponding row and column totals followed by division by the total for the entire table. The df for chi-square become $(r - 1)(c - 1)$. For details, the reader is referred to other texts [2, 101].

Chi-square also has other uses, such as testing for goodness of fit (the data in Table 2.5 are well set up for a chi-square goodness-of-fit test), performing inferences concerning the variance of a normal distribution, and testing for compliance of data with theoretical binomial and Poisson distributions. The previously mentioned texts provide details on these and other uses of chi-square.

SUMMARY

Table 5.2 summarizes the various methods of inference concerning proportions.

Table 5.2. Summary of inference on proportions

Situation	Methodology	Relevant statistical tables	Text references
A single proportion	1. Exact: Use of binomial distribution	Not in this text; calculate by hand	151–153
	2. Approximate: Normal approximation to the binomial distribution with continuity correction	Areas in the normal curve (Appendix Tables A1 and A2)	153–158
	3. Approximate: Chi-square with 1 df and continuity correction (*Note*: Methods 2 and 3 are algebraically identical)	Chi-square with 1 df (Appendix Table A4)	169–172
Comparison of two proportions in independent samples	1. Exact: Fisher's exact test (Not covered in this text)		
	2. Approximate: Critical ratio of difference in proportions (with continuity correction) relative to standard error of difference	Areas in normal curve (Appendix Tables A1 and A2)	163–167
	3. Approximate: Chi-square with 1 df and Yates' continuity correction (*Note*: Methods 2 and 3 are algebraically identical)	Chi-square with 1 df (Appendix Table A4)	175–177
Comparison of two proportions in paired samples	(*Note*: Each method below hinges on discarding the tied pairs and analyzing only the untied pairs) 1. Exact binomial distribution with $\pi = \frac{1}{2}$	Not in this text; calculate by hand	169–172

	2. Approximate: Normal approximation to the binomial with $\pi = \frac{1}{2}$ and continuity correction	Areas in normal curve (Appendix Tables A1 and A2)	172–174
	3. Approximate: Chi-square with 1 df and continuity correction (*Note*: Methods 2 and 3 are algebraically identical)	Chi-square with 1 df (Appendix Table A4)	177–179
Comparison of more than two proportions in independent samples	Approximate: Chi-square with $k - 1$ df where k denotes the number of sample proportions	Chi-square with $k - 1$ df (Appendix Table A4)	179–181
Comparison of more than two proportions in matched samples	Not covered in this text		

183

EXERCISES

1. Among susceptible individuals exposed to a particular infectious agent, 36 percent generally develop clinical disease.
   A. Among a school group of 144 persons suspected of exposure to the agent, only 35 developed clinical disease. Is this result within chance variation? If not, what possibilities may offer an explanation?
   B. An investigator reports that among a school group suspected of exposure to the agent, 28 percent developed clinical disease. This result, when compared with a null hypothesis rate of 36 percent, was just significant at the 1 percent level with a two-tailed test. How large was the group?

2. An investigator wishes to estimate the percentage of inhabitants of a city who are inoculated against polio. He plans to take a sample survey of the population and would like his sample estimate to be correct within ±3 percent with a 99 percent chance. (This means that if his estimate is 75 percent, he wants to be 99 percent certain that the correct figure in the population is between 72 and 78 percent.) From his previous experience, the investigator feels that the percentage of the population inoculated against polio is likely to be between 70 and 80 percent.
   A. If he can draw a random sample of individuals, how large a sample should he take?
   B. If instead, he takes a sample of *families* and surveys everybody in the family, then state, giving your reason, whether he would need more, less, or about the same number of persons as in part A.
   C. If the survey were to be done in your home area, state specifically how you might go about drawing a random sample of *families*.

3. Experience reveals that the complications rate for a particular operative procedure is 20 percent. A surgeon who has developed a new operative technique that he believes may reduce the complications rate plans to utilize this new technique on a sample of his patients. He will test the null hypothesis that the complications rate with the new technique is 20 percent and he will perform a two-tailed test of significance at the 5 percent level.
   A. If, using his new technique, he operates on a sample of 100 patients, how many must have complications if he is to reject his null hypothesis and conclude that the new technique has a significantly lower complications rate?
   B. If the actual complications rate with the new technique is 10 percent, what is the chance that in a sample of 100 he will fail to reject his null hypothesis of a 20 percent rate? (Note that this question asks for the type II error.)

C.   Suppose that the investigator retains a type I error of 5 percent for a two-tailed test of his null hypothesis and that he also specifies that, if the complications rate with the new technique is actually 10 percent, he wants his type II error to be 5 percent. How many patients must he treat with the new technique?

D.   What are the defects in this procedure for evaluating the new technique? What factors other than the effectiveness of the new technique might contribute to explain a statistically significant result?

4.   A clinical trial among 25 patients consisted of administering to each patient a new drug and a standard drug on two different occasions. At the end of the trial, each patient indicated which drug he preferred. (Ties were not allowed; each patient was coerced into indicating a preference.) The investigator tested the null hypothesis of equal preference of the two drugs with a two-tailed test. He stated that he determined his sample size so that if the actual probability of preference for the new drug was .8, he would risk a type II error of 5 percent. He did not indicate his type I error (i.e., the significance level for testing the null hypothesis of equal preference). What was the type I error?

5.   A clinical trial comparing a new treatment with a standard treatment for a disease consisted of 25 matched pairs of patients: one member of each pair received the new treatment and the other member received the standard treatment. The patient's and the physician's assessments at the conclusion of the trial were utilized to arrive at a verdict as to whether there was or was not improvement in the patient's condition. Among the 25 patients who had received the new treatment, 20 were judged to have demonstrated improvement; among the 25 patients who had received the standard treatment, 15 were judged to have demonstrated improvement. In addition, among the 25 pairs of patients, there were 13 in which both pair members demonstrated improvement.

A.   Complete the table below relating to the number of pairs of patients:

		New treatment		
		Improvement	No improvement	Total
Standard	Improvement	————	————	————
Treatment	No improvement	————	————	————
	Total	————	————	25

B.   Test the null hypothesis that the proportion exhibiting improvement is the same for the new treatment as for the standard treatment.

6.   A retrospective study of death certificates was directed to the detection of a possible association between a particular occupation and a certain neoplastic disease. Among the death certificates filed in a geographic area over several years' time, all those which listed the neoplastic disease in question as the primary cause of death were selected. There were some 1,500 such death certificates. For each of these 1,500 death certificates, a matched control death certificate was selected. The matching consisted of these factors: age within five years, race, sex, county of residence, and date of death within four weeks. Among the control death certificates, any cause of death except the neoplastic disease in question was acceptable. The occupation of the decedents was examined for each of the case and control death certificates. For only one matched pair had both the case and control members been listed in the occupation in question. There were 69 pairs in which the case pair member had been in the occupation while the control member had not. There were 30 pairs in which the control member had been in the occupation while the case pair member had not. In all the remaining 1,400 pairs, neither the case nor the control member had been in the occupation.

A.   Perform a test of significance of the null hypothesis that an equal proportion of case and control members had been in the occupation.

B.   Discuss the limitations or possible biases of this study format in providing evidence that this particular occupation is associated with increased risk of the neoplastic disease in question.

7.   A clinical trial to determine the effects of gamma-globulin in preventing posttransfusion hepatitis was undertaken among patients undergoing chest surgery for tuberculosis. This patient group was selected because they would be likely to receive a number of transfusions at operation and they would be available for follow-up study in the hospital for several months. The study was conducted in three cities. In each city, half the patients were given gamma-globulin while the other half served as untreated controls. In one city, the allocation of patients to treatment groups was by alternate weeks, i.e., in the first week, all tuberculosis patients undergoing chest surgery that week received gamma-globulin, the next week all patients undergoing surgery were untreated controls, and so on. In the other two cities, patients were assigned to the treatment and control groups on a strictly alternate basis. Patients were followed for at least two months, the follow-up including monthly tests of liver function. Almost all patients were followed for three or more months, two-thirds for four or more months, and almost one-half for 6 or more months. A patient was considered to have hepatitis if there was normal liver function before transfusion but subsequent abnormal values of liver function

tests could be found on at least two occasions after transfusion. Of the total of 774 patients who received gamma-globulin, 12 developed hepatitis, whereas among 816 untreated control patients, 33 developed hepatitis.

A. Perform an appropriate test of significance to compare the rates of hepatitis in the gamma-globulin treated group and the untreated control group.

B. As the design and follow-up have been described, do you have any criticism of the procedures and suggestions for improvement?

C. The following table gives for the untreated controls the number of patients and cases of hepatitis in each of the three cities:

| City | Control group | |
	Number of patients	Cases of hepatitis
A	587	22
B	146	9
C	83	2
Total	816	33

Perform an appropriate test of significance to compare the hepatitis case rates among the controls in the three cities.

D. If there were statistically significant differences in the hepatitis case rates for controls in the three cities, what possibilities might you explore to explain such a result?

8. A study whose purpose was to determine the incidence of cardiovascular diseases in castrated women began with the location of the records at a particular hospital of all women under 45 years old who underwent bilateral oophorectomy (usually with hysterectomy). The hospital's records over a 20-year period were reviewed and 424 cases were located. As a control group, a similar review process, with the same age restriction and over the same time interval, located 462 records of women who had only hysterectomy, with or without removal of one ovary. An attempt was made to trace the women in the castrate group (bilateral oophorectomy) and in the control group (hysterectomy with or without removal of one ovary) and to encourage as many as possible in each group to undergo a complete cardiovascular evaluation. Examinations were completed on 100 of the castrated women and 110 of the controls. These examinations revealed definite arteriosclerotic cardiovascular disease in 17 among the 100 castrated women examined and in 4 among the 110 control women examined.

A. Consider the following procedure for a chi-square test to compare the rates of arteriosclerotic cardiovascular disease in the castrated and control women examined:

Overall proportion with disease in two groups combined:

$$(17 + 4)/(100 + 110) = 21/210 = .100$$

	Castrate group	Control group
Observed with disease (O):	17	4
Expected with disease (E):	$(100)(.10) = 10$	$(110)(.10) = 11$

$$\chi_c^2(1 \text{ df}) = \sum \frac{(|O - E| - \frac{1}{2})^2}{E}$$

$$= \frac{(|17 - 10| - \frac{1}{2})^2}{10} + \frac{(|4 - 11| - \frac{1}{2})^2}{11}$$

$$= \frac{6.5^2}{10} + \frac{6.5^2}{11} = 8.07, \ P < .01$$

State whether you agree or disagree with the above calculation for the chi-square test. If you disagree, recalculate chi-square correctly and perform the test of significance.

B. With a statistically significant result, would this study provide suitable evidence that female castration results in increased risk of arteriosclerotic cardiovascular disease? Indicate what factors, if any, may offer possible sources of selection or bias in these results.

9. A clinical trial consists of the random assignment of 40 patients to treatment and control groups so that there are 20 in each group. The investigator will test the null hypothesis of equal success rates in the two groups with a two-tailed test at the 5 percent level. If among his 20 control patients he observes 12 successes, how many successes must he observe among his 20 treatment patients in order to conclude that the success rate is significantly higher in the treatment group compared with the control group?

Chapter 6
Regression and Correlation

Many medical investigations center on the establishment of a relationship between two variables. For example, in the laboratory, how does an animal's response to a drug change as the dosage of the drug changes? In the clinic, is there a relation between two physiological or biochemical determinations measured in the same patients? In the community, what is the relation between various indices of health and the extent to which health care is available? In the field of medical education, what relation exists among achievement test scores and measures of academic performance? All these questions concern the relationship between two variables, each measured on the same units of observation, be they animals, patients, communities, or medical students. Regression and correlation constitute the statistical techniques for investigating such relationships.

Table 6.1. Age and systolic blood pressure among 33 adult females

Age (yr)	Systolic BP (mm Hg)	Age (yr)	Systolic BP (mm Hg)	Age (yr)	Systolic BP (mm Hg)
22	131	41	139	52	128
23	128	41	171	54	105
24	116	46	137	56	145
27	106	47	111	57	141
28	114	48	115	58	153
29	123	49	133	59	157
30	117	49	128	63	155
32	122	50	183	67	176
33	99	51	130	71	172
35	121	51	133	77	178
40	147	51	144	81	217

To illustrate the techniques, Table 6.1 presents data on age and systolic blood pressure among 33 women. These data were acquired in an epidemiological survey of hypertension among several fishing villages in Newfoundland. The 33 observations in Table 6.1 represent a random sample of one-fifth of the female participants in one of the villages. The objective with these data is to examine the relation between two variables, in particular, to determine what happens to systolic blood pressure as age increases.

DISTINCTION BETWEEN REGRESSION AND CORRELATION

Regression and correlation have much in common, yet each represents somewhat different approaches to the analysis of a set of data. Their chief distinction is that with *regression* the relationship between the two variables is not symmetrical. One studies the change in the mean value of one variable (termed the *dependent variable*) as the other variable (termed the *independent variable*) changes. In *correlation*, no such distinction is possible. With correlation, both variables are viewed as dependent. (Note that the present usage of "dependent" and "independent" differs from that in the context of the probabilities of dependent and independent events, as in Chapter 3.)

Regression, in its purest form, pertains to the situation in which the investigator chooses the values of the independent variable. A classic example is in the laboratory when the experimenter predetermines the doses of an agent to be administered to laboratory animals. He administers these doses and observes some measure of response. His chief interest is with regression analysis for determination of a dose-response relationship, where the dose is the independent variable and the response is the dependent variable. The assay of many pharmacological and biological substances depends on just such a procedure and the use of regression analysis for the quantification of the dose-response relationship.

At the other extreme, many studies in the health care field tend to involve correlation. The investigator is unable to pick an independent variable: each of the two variables is beyond his manipulation; each may be affected by a wide variety of other variables. His interest with correlation analysis is in the quantification of the degree to which the two variables tend to be related.

This does not mean that all observational studies are concerned with correlation as opposed to regression. Even though the investigator has not himself chosen the values of one of the variables, his interest in their relationship may indicate regression analysis. If his two variables are denoted as x and y and if he asks, "What happens to y as x changes?," then he has implied x for his independent and y for his dependent variable. His analysis thus points to regression techniques. The data in Table 6.1 on age and systolic blood pressure are a case in point. Clearly, the investigator did not choose the ages of the women in the study. He obtained a random sample of the women in the village and observed their ages and blood pressures. The ages in Table 6.1 were beyond his control; they represent what existed in the village at that time. However, when he asks, "What happens to blood pressure as age increases?," he indicates his interest in the regression of blood pressure on age.

If he were to phrase his question, "Do blood pressure and age tend to be related?," then his analysis would point in the direction of correlation. The distinction is subtle. Obviously, there are many instances in which it is not clear whether regression or correlation is intended. Under certain circumstances, they lead—as will be shown later—to closely related analyses. However, it is well to remember that, should there be any suggestion that one of the variables is independent while the other is dependent, then regression techniques would more often be most profitably employed. In the discussion that follows, regression methods are considered first.

LINEAR REGRESSION

Scatter Diagrams

Before conducting any analysis, it is wise for an investigator to plot his data and inspect the nature of the relationship. The *scatter diagram* represents a convenient plot; it consists of a graph whose abscissa represents one variable and whose ordinate represents the other. Each observation, consisting of an x and y value, is represented by a dot on the graph at the point (x, y). If regression is intended, it is customary to denote the abscissa as the independent and the ordinate as the dependent variable. Figure 6.1 presents the scatter diagram for the 33 observations of age and blood pressure in Table 6.1. The points exhibit a wide scatter, but they distinctly reveal an increase in systolic blood pressure as age increases.

Linear regression, as the adjective indicates, concerns the fitting of a straight line to a scatter of points such as that in Figure 6.1. Many readers, no doubt, have had some experience in the laboratory when a line or curve needed to be fitted to a plot of experimentally observed points. The simplest and most obvious procedure is to fit by eye. Although an "eyeball" fit has much merit

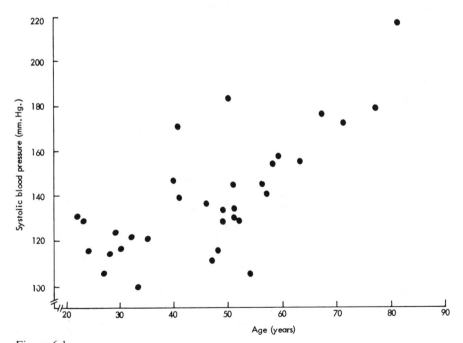

Figure 6.1
Scatter diagram of age and systolic blood pressure for adult females in a small fishing village in Newfoundland.

in its simplicity and it often does suffice for the experimenter's purpose, it suffers the distinct disadvantage of a lack of objectivity. Different observers, when confronted with the same scatter diagram, would fit different lines. No doubt, an investigator, were he to fit a line by eye to the same scatter of points on two different occasions, would likewise fit different lines. A further disadvantage of an "eyeball" fit is that sampling variation cannot be determined, and the line is thereby not amenable to the methods of statistical inference.

Method of Least Squares

Intuitively, there appears to be some merit in obtaining a mathematically derived best-fitting line. At the very least, such a line would be unique, and it would be possible to develop methods of statistical inference. One such method that has great intuitive appeal as well as a firm statistical basis is the *method of least squares*. The line determined by the method of least squares is such that the sum of the squares of deviations of the observed points about the line is a minimum. It is important to note that the deviations of the points about the line are measured *parallel* to the ordinate. That is, for each point on the scatter diagram, the deviation is obtained by dropping a line from the point and parallel to the y-axis until the fitted line is reached. For the data in Figure 6.1, Figure 6.2 illustrates the line fitted by least squares and the deviations of the 33 observed points about the line.

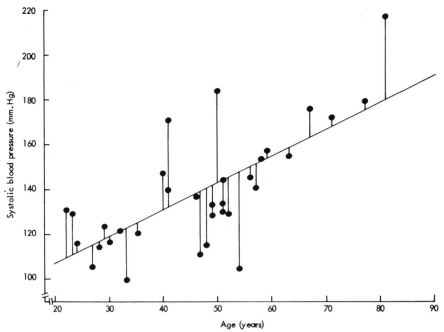

Figure 6.2
Linear regression line and deviations from the fitted line for the data in Figure 6.1.

The reason for defining the deviations in this manner concerns the notion that "regression of y on x" indicates that x, the independent variable, is considered fixed and y, the dependent variable, is considered subject to experimental variation. Thus, with x fixed, deviations and least squares apply only to the variation for the y values.

For a particular x, if y denotes the observed ordinate and Y the point on the fitted line, the deviation is $y - Y$. The principle of least squares then requires minimization of the quantity

$$\Sigma (y - Y)^2$$

The equation of a straight line is

$$Y = a + bx$$

where a is the intercept and b the slope of the line. Hence, the principle of least squares when applied to linear regression requires the determination of the values of the intercept, a, and the slope, b, that minimize the expression

$$\Sigma (y - a - bx)^2$$

One might employ differential calculus to locate a minimum. One would obtain the partial derivatives of the above expression with respect to a and b and then set the derivatives equal to zero. This would result in two equations in the two unknowns a and b. The reader adept with calculus may verify that this procedure leads to the solutions

$$b = \frac{\Sigma (x - \bar{x})(y - \bar{y})}{\Sigma (x - \bar{x})^2}$$

$$a = \bar{y} - b\bar{x}$$

Thus, the above equations yield the slope and intercept for the regression line fitted by least squares. In the equation for b, the denominator is a familiar sum of squares of deviations about the mean. As before (for example, p. 33), it may alternatively be written in the more computationally convenient form

$$\Sigma (x - \bar{x})^2 = \Sigma x^2 - (\Sigma x)^2/n$$

The numerator of b, however, is new and represents the sum of cross-products of deviations about the mean for the xs and ys. Analogously to a sum of squares of deviations, the sum of cross-products of the deviations has an alternative form that is also preferable for computation, namely,

$$\Sigma (x - \bar{x})(y - \bar{y}) = \Sigma xy - (\Sigma x)(\Sigma y)/n$$

It may be seen that a cross-product term is derived from a sum-of-squares term upon the replacement of each squared value with an appropriate cross-product value. Thus, in the above computational form for the sum of cross-products, x^2 is replaced with xy and $(\Sigma x)^2$ with $(\Sigma x)(\Sigma y)$.

The equation for the intercept is best expressed in terms of the slope, as above. With this expression for a, the least-squares regression line can be alternatively written as

$$Y = a + bx = \bar{y} + b(x - \bar{x})$$

Many researchers prefer the latter expression. It may be seen that with this format the least-squares regression line goes through the point $(\bar{x}, \bar{y})$, the point corresponding with the means of the x and y values.

The top portion of Table 6.2 indicates the calculation of the least-squares

Table 6.2. Calculation of the least-squares regression line for the data in Table 6.1

Raw Sums, Sums of Squares, and Sum of Cross-Products:

$$n = 33$$

$$\Sigma x = 1{,}542 \qquad \Sigma y = 4{,}575$$
$$\Sigma x^2 = 79{,}716 \qquad \Sigma y^2 = 656{,}481$$
$$\Sigma xy = 223{,}144$$

Means:

$$\bar{x} = \Sigma x/n = 1{,}542/33 = 46.73$$
$$\bar{y} = \Sigma y/n = 4{,}575/33 = 138.64$$

Sums of Squares and Cross-Products about the Mean:

$$\Sigma(x - \bar{x})^2 = \Sigma x^2 - (\Sigma x)^2/n = 79{,}716 - (1{,}542)^2/33 = 7{,}662.6$$
$$\Sigma(y - \bar{y})^2 = \Sigma y^2 - (\Sigma y)^2/n = 656{,}481 - (4{,}575)^2/33 = 22{,}219.6$$
$$\Sigma(x - \bar{x})(y - \bar{y}) = \Sigma xy - (\Sigma x)(\Sigma y)/n = 223{,}144 - (1{,}542)(4{,}575)/33 = 9{,}366.7$$

Least-Squares Regression Line:

$$\text{Slope} \quad b = \frac{\Sigma(x - \bar{x})(y - \bar{y})}{\Sigma(x - \bar{x})^2} = \frac{9{,}366.7}{7{,}662.6} = 1.222 \text{ mm Hg per year of age}$$

$$\text{Intercept} \quad a = \bar{y} - b\bar{x} = 138.64 - (1.222)(46.73) = 81.54 \text{ mm Hg}$$

$$\text{Equation of line} \quad Y = a + bx = 81.54 + 1.222x \text{ or}$$
$$Y = \bar{y} + b(x - \bar{x}) = 138.64 + 1.222(x - 46.73)$$

SD of Points about the Fitted Line and Standard Errors of Slope and Intercept:

$$s^2_{y \cdot x} = \frac{1}{n-2}\left\{ \Sigma(y - \bar{y})^2 - \frac{[\Sigma(x - \bar{x})(y - \bar{y})]^2}{\Sigma(x - \bar{x})^2} \right\}$$

$$= \frac{1}{31}\left\{ 22{,}219.6 - \frac{[9{,}366.7]^2}{7{,}662.6} \right\} = \frac{10{,}769.8}{31} = 347.4129$$

$$s_{y \cdot x} = \sqrt{s^2_{y \cdot x}} = \sqrt{347.4129} = 18.64$$

$$SE(b) = \sqrt{s^2_{y \cdot x}/\Sigma(x - \bar{x})^2} = \sqrt{347.4129/7{,}662.6} = 0.2129$$

$$SE(a) = \sqrt{s^2_{y \cdot x}\left[\frac{1}{n} + \frac{\bar{x}^2}{\Sigma(x - \bar{x})^2}\right]} = \sqrt{347.4129\left[\frac{1}{33} + \frac{(46.73)^2}{7{,}662.6}\right]} = 10.47$$

Table 6.2. (*Continued*)

Tests of Significance and Confidence Limits on Slope:

$$\text{Null hypothesis} \quad \beta = 0$$

$$t_{31} = \frac{b - 0}{\text{SE}(b)} = \frac{1.222}{0.2129} = 5.74 \quad P < .001$$

95 percent confidence limits on β

$$b \pm t_{31,.05}\,[\text{SE}(b)] = 1.222 \pm (1.96)(0.2129)$$
$$= 1.222 \pm 0.417$$
$$= 0.81 \text{ to } 1.64 \text{ mm Hg per}$$
$$\text{year of age}$$

Confidence Limits on Predicted Mean Blood Pressure for Given Age:

Width of 95 percent confidence limits

$$t_{31,.05}\,\sqrt{s_{y\cdot x}^2\left[\frac{1}{n} + \frac{(x - \bar{x})^2}{\Sigma(x - \bar{x})^2}\right]} = 1.96\,\sqrt{347.4129\left[\frac{1}{33} + \frac{(x - \bar{x})^2}{7{,}662.6}\right]}$$

Predicted Mean

$x - \bar{x}$	$Y = \bar{y} + b(x - \bar{x})$	$(x - \bar{x})^2/7{,}662.6$	Width of 95% conf. lim.	95% conf. lim. on predicted mean of ys
0	138.64	0	6.36	132.28 , 145.00
$+10$	150.86	.013050	7.61	143.25 , 158.47
-10	126.42	.013050	7.61	118.81 , 134.03
$+20$	163.08	.052201	10.49	152.59 , 173.57
-20	114.20	.052201	10.49	103.71 , 124.69
$+30$	175.30	.1175	14.04	161.26 , 189.34
-30	101.98	.1175	14.04	87.94 , 116.02

regression line for the data on systolic blood pressure and age in Table 6.1. The slope is 1.222 mm Hg per year of age and the intercept is 81.54 mm Hg. The line is plotted in Figure 6.2. There is no other line that can be drawn through the points that will have a smaller sum of squares of deviations. The reader may note that the line goes through the point "46.73 years, 138.64 mm Hg," which corresponds with $(\bar{x},\bar{y})$. The results could be summarized by the line $Y = 81.54 + 1.222x$ or $Y = 138.64 + 1.222(x - 46.73)$.

In a least-squares regression line, the intercept represents the predicted mean of the dependent variable, y, when the independent variable, x, is zero. In this particular example, there is no interest in the predicted mean blood pressure of 81.54 mm Hg for women of zero age.

The more important quantity is usually the slope, which is interpreted as the estimated mean change in the dependent variable for a unit change in the independent variable. Thus, in the example at hand, blood pressure increases an average of 1.2 mm Hg for each year of age over the range of age studied.

Inference with Regression Lines

Underlying Concepts

The discussion has been purely descriptive up to this point. The formulas for calculating the slope and intercept of the least-squares regression line are analogous, in this sense, to the calculation of a mean or a proportion in a single sample. The next step consists of discussing inference with regard to the least-squares regression line. This requires the concept that the sample of the n observation pairs of (x, y) values comes from some larger population. For inference, one needs to envision repeat samples of n observation pairs from this larger population. With each sample, one would compute a least-squares regression line. In the underlying population, there is a particular linear regression relationship of the y on the x values that is, of course, unknown. What conclusions may be drawn concerning the unknown population relationship based upon the relationship determined by the least-squares fitted line for the sample? The slope and intercept of a least-squares regression line are quantities calculated in a sample just as the mean and proportion were in Chapters 4 aud 5. In order to perform tests of significance or to obtain confidence limits with regard to regression, it will be necessary to consider the sampling variation of the quantities involved. Thus, inference with a regression line requires the determination of the standard errors of the slope and intercept.

Following the previous notation that employed Greek letters to denote population values, the regression relation in the underlying population is expressed as

$$Y_{pop} = \alpha + \beta x$$

Further, the appropriate assumptions for regression analysis specify that in the underlying population, for a given x, the values of the dependent variable y are normally distributed with a mean of $\alpha + \beta x$ and a standard deviation of σ. In other words, for each x, one conceives of an underlying population of an infinite number of possible y values. The frequency distribution of these y values tends to resemble the normal distribution. As one proceeds from one x to another, the underlying normally distributed populations of y values have means that fall on the straight line $Y_{pop} = \alpha + \beta x$. Figure 6.3 represents this model, with the normal distributions coming up from the x, y plane of the graph.

With this model, a sample observation pair (x, y) consists of fixing an x value and then selecting a sample of one from the normally distributed population of y values for that x. The y selected is unlikely to be at the mean of the distribution and hence will not fall on the population regression line. For n points at different x values, each sample point will deviate somewhat from the mean, and thus a scatter of points about the straight line $Y_{pop} = \alpha + \beta x$ will be obtained. The least-squares line that is fitted to the observed sample of n points, $Y = a + bx$, is an estimate of the population regression

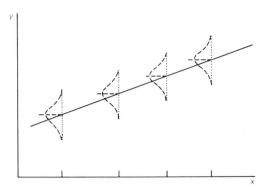

Figure 6.3
The statistical assumptions underlying linear regression analysis.

line, $Y_{\text{pop}} = \alpha + \beta x$. One might conceive of many repeat samples of n observation pairs with each sample of n obtained for the same fixed values of x. In each of these samples, a different y would be selected from the normal distribution of the ys for the same fixed xs, and the least-squares regression line would be calculated. The resulting slopes and intercepts then describe, over the many samples selected, the sampling distributions of the slope and intercept of the regression line. The SD of the slope and intercept from one sample of n to another yields, as discussed on page 108, the standard errors of the slope and intercept. Although it is beyond the scope of this text, it may be shown that these standard errors are

$$SE(b) = \frac{\sigma}{\sqrt{\Sigma\,(x - \bar{x})^2}}$$

$$SE(a) = \sigma\sqrt{\frac{1}{n} + \frac{\bar{x}^2}{\Sigma\,(x - \bar{x})^2}}$$

These are the essential quantities needed to conduct statistical inferences.

In the above discussion, one assumption deserves attention. This is the assumption that the normal distributions of the ys for each x have the same SD, σ, no matter what the value of x may be. This assumption of equal variability of the ys throughout the range of xs is known as *homoscedasticity*. There are occasions when this assumption does not hold, and the reader is referred to more advanced texts for methods of regression analysis of such data; these methods entail what is called a *weighted regression* analysis. However, there are many instances in which the homoscedasticity assumption is reasonable, and the "unweighted" regression methods described here give entirely satisfactory results.

Estimates of Standard Errors of the Slope and Intercept

The difficulty in applying the standard errors of the slope and intercept as described above is that almost invariably σ will be unknown. One employs, analogously to the methods underlying the t test, an estimate of σ obtained from the sample. This estimate consists of the SD of the observed points about the fitted line. In other words, the estimate of σ is based on the sum of squares $\Sigma (y - Y)^2$, the quantity that was minimized with the least-squares procedure. Using the principle of degrees of freedom as it was employed in calculating the sample SD (p. 32), it may be shown that the n deviations about the line contain $n - 2$ df. In other words, once $n - 2$ deviations about the line are specified, the last two result automatically from the requirement that the line have the calculated intercept a and slope b. Thus, the required estimate of σ is obtained as

$$s_{y \cdot x} = \sqrt{\Sigma (y - Y)^2/(n - 2)}$$

This sample estimate of σ is called the *standard deviation from regression*, or, in some textbooks, the *standard error of estimate*. The subscript $y \cdot x$ is used to denote the fact that the estimate pertains to deviations of the points about the fitted regression line of y on x.

It is rather tedious to calculate each predicted Y on the fitted least-squares line and the deviation $y - Y$. It may be shown that, by substitution of $Y = a + bx$ and the values for a and b of the least-squares line given previously (p. 193), the sum of squares of the deviations can alternatively be written as

$$\Sigma (y - Y)^2 = \Sigma (y - \bar{y})^2 - [\Sigma (y - \bar{y})(x - \bar{x})]^2/\Sigma (x - \bar{x})^2$$

Thus, the estimated standard deviation from regression is most conveniently calculated as

$$s_{y \cdot x} = \sqrt{\frac{\Sigma (y - \bar{y})^2 - [\Sigma (x - \bar{x})(y - \bar{y})]^2/\Sigma (x - \bar{x})^2}{n - 2}}$$

This involves the already familiar sums of squares and cross-products of deviations about the mean. The calculation of $s_{y \cdot x}$ for the data on blood pressure and age is shown in Table 6.2.

With this result, the estimated standard errors of the sample slope and intercept become

$$\text{Est SE}(b) = \frac{s_{y \cdot x}}{\sqrt{\Sigma (x - \bar{x})^2}} = \sqrt{s_{y \cdot x}^2/\Sigma (x - \bar{x})^2}$$

$$\text{Est SE}(a) = s_{y \cdot x} \sqrt{\frac{1}{n} + \frac{\bar{x}}{\Sigma (x - \bar{x})^2}} = \sqrt{s_{y \cdot x}^2 \left[\frac{1}{n} + \frac{\bar{x}^2}{\Sigma (x - \bar{x})^2} \right]}$$

The calculations of the estimated standard errors of the slope and intercept of the blood pressure–age data are also shown in Table 6.2.

In order to perform inferences, the one additional piece of information that is needed is the mathematically derived result that the t distribution applies to the slope and intercept of regression analysis.

Test of Significance and Confidence Limits on a Slope

The slope is generally the more important of the two regression values. It carries the basic information on the relationship between x and y, namely, the average change in y for unit change in x. For a test of significance, the null hypothesis consists of the specification of a particular value, say β_0, for the slope of the underlying population regression line of y on x. The test of significance then becomes

$$t_{n-2} = \frac{b - \beta_0}{\text{Est SE}(b)}$$

The form is, as before (p. 137), the deviation between the sample and null hypothesis population values relative to the standard error of the quantity involved. The $n - 2$ df for t are derived from the $n - 2$ df in the $s_{y \cdot x}^2$ figure that is employed in the estimated SE(b). Frequently, the null hypothesis specifies $\beta_0 = 0$, namely, that there is no slope or no relation between y and x in the underlying population. In this case, the test of significance on the slope asks: If there is no slope or no relation between y and x in the underlying population, what is the chance that a sample of observations at the particular x values chosen would yield a sample slope as large as or larger than that observed? For the data on systolic blood pressure and age, a two-tailed test of zero population slope, as shown in Table 6.2, yields a t value of 5.74 with 31 df. The tables of t (in this case the normal tables can be used since the df exceed 30) indicate $P < .001$. Thus, if there were no relation between blood pressure and age in the underlying population, there would be less than one chance in a thousand of finding a sample slope as large as or larger than that observed. The slope is statistically significant, and therefore one rejects the null hypothesis of no relation between blood pressure and age in the underlying population.

The 95 percent confidence limits on the slope are obtained as

$$b \pm t_{n-2, .05}[\text{Est SE}(b)]$$

and are shown in Table 6.2 for the data on blood pressure and age. The limits are interpreted as follows: based on the sample, the chances are 19 in 20 that, in the underlying population, the slope of the regression line of blood pressure on age is somewhere within the range of 0.8 to 1.6 mm Hg per year of age.

Test of Significance and Confidence Limits on the Intercept

When interest centers on the intercept, similar calculations are made using the t distribution. A test of significance of the null hypothesis that the population regression line has intercept α_0 is

$$t_{n-2} = \frac{a - \alpha_0}{\text{Est SE}(a)}$$

while the 95 percent confidence limits on α are

$$a \pm t_{n-2, .05}[\text{Est SE}(a)]$$

In drawing inferences regarding the intercept, one should note first whether the intercept falls within the range of the observed data points. When the data points cluster far beyond $x = 0$, the determination of the intercept involves considerable extrapolation of the straight line. As indicated later (p. 202), such extrapolation is at the least risky, and, more often, totally unwarranted. Fortunately, however, in situations where the data points cluster at a considerable distance from the intercept, there is usually little or no interest in inferences regarding the intercept. Such is the case with the age and blood pressure data. In this study, there was no interest in the predicted mean blood pressure of females at age zero. Hence, inference regarding the intercept is not illustrated with the data at hand.

Confidence Limits on Predicted Mean y Values

If, however, one considers the alternative expression for the least-squares line, $Y = \bar{y} + b(x - \bar{x})$, there is often interest in obtaining the 95 percent confidence limits on one or more predicted Y values. These predicted Y values represent the mean of the distribution of the ys for a given x. The 95 percent confidence limits on the underlying population mean for a given x are obtained by adding to and subtracting from $Y = \bar{y} + b(x - \bar{x})$ the quantity

$$t_{n-2, .05} \sqrt{s_{y \cdot x}^2 \left[\frac{1}{n} + \frac{(x - \bar{x})^2}{\Sigma (x - \bar{x})^2} \right]}$$

The calculation of several of these 95 percent confidence limits is shown in Table 6.2, and the results are graphed in Figure 6.4. The curved lines in Figure 6.4 represent 95 percent confidence limits on the regression line. In one sense, any straight line that can be drawn within the curved limits of Figure 6.4 represents a population regression relationship that would be compatible with the sample of 33 observed pairs of (x,y) values at the 5 percent significance level.

The fact that the limits about the line in Figure 6.4 are curved may be understood by considering the term under the square root sign in the above expression. Clearly, the last term in the expression is zero when $x - \bar{x} = 0$ or when $x = \bar{x}$. This means the limits are narrowest at the point $(\bar{x}, \bar{y})$. In other words, at the center of the observed points, there is greatest confidence on the predicted mean of the ys. As x departs from $\bar{x}$ in either direction, the last term increases in magnitude and the confidence limits widen. This means there is less certainty regarding the mean of the ys as one departs from the center of the observed points.

Limits on Predicted Individual y Values

Sometimes, instead of predicting the *mean y* for a given x as above, interest centers on the prediction of an *individual y* for a given x. The predicted values

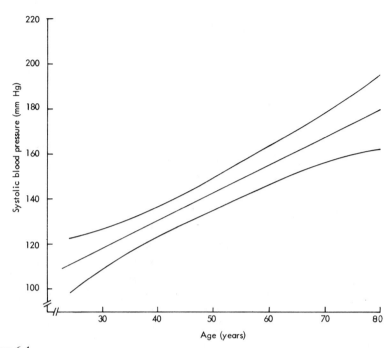

Figure 6.4
The 95 percent confidence limits on the predicted mean systolic blood pressure for the fitted regression line in Figure 6.2.

are the same as above, namely, $Y = \bar{y} + b(x -- \bar{x})$. The determination of confidence limits, however, is different. One must now account for the variation of the ys about their mean, i.e., the normal distribution about the regression line having SD $= \sigma$ as illustrated in Figure 6.3. The 95 percent limits on a predicted individual y value for given x are obtained by adding to and subtracting from $\bar{y} + b(x - \bar{x})$ the quantity

$$t_{n-2,\, .05} \sqrt{s_{y \cdot x}^{2} \left[1 + \frac{1}{n} + \frac{(x - \bar{x})^{2}}{\Sigma\, (x - \bar{x})} \right]}$$

Note the similarity of the above expression to that for confidence limits on a mean y. There is the additional term, "1," within the bracketed expression under the square root sign. Thus, the limits on a predicted *individual y* value are wider than those on the predicted *mean y* value. The limits on a predicted *individual y* value will also be curved. The reader will most often encounter confidence limits on *mean y* in the medical literature. It is well to remember, however, that there are these two forms of limit statements that apply to a least-squares regression line. Occasionally, the purposes of the regression analysis will entail prediction of an individual y for given x, and then these latter limits are appropriate. With the data on blood pressure and age, the only interest was with the prediction of *mean* blood pressure for a given age.

As such, the 95 percent limits on an *individual* woman's blood pressure for a given age were not calculated with these data.

Interpretation

In the interpretation of inferences resulting from linear regression analysis, there are two important limitations that deserve emphasis. The first is that the inference is applicable only within the experimental range covered by the values of the independent variable, *x*. It would be most dangerous to extrapolate the fitted regression line beyond this range. For example, with the data on blood pressure and age, it would be unwise to extend the regression line below age 20 and suggest that a linear blood pressure–age relationship pertains to adolescents and children. In fact, if one extends the line to $x = 0$, that is, to the ordinate or intercept of the regression line, one can see that it is quite anomalous to predict a mean blood pressure for females of 81.52 mm Hg at age zero. The observed points correspond with ages from roughly 20 to 80 years; one cannot extrapolate safely beyond this range.

The second limitation pertains to the adequacy of a linear fit. There may actually be a very distinct relationship between the *x* and *y* variables, but one that is not linear. An inference from regression analysis that suggests the lack of a slope does not mean the lack of a relationship. The relationship may be other than that described by a straight line. For example, Figure 6.5 indicates an exact mathematical relationship between *x* and *y* that is determined by the quadratic equation

$$y = (x - 4)^2 + 1$$

All seven points shown in the figure lie on the quadratic curve. Since there is no linear trend to the points, it may be seen at the foot of Figure 6.5 that the least-squares slope of a fitted regression line is zero. Hence, lack of slope does not indicate lack of a relationship; it indicates only the lack of a *linear* relationship.

On the other hand, even when there is strong evidence for a slope in regression analysis, one cannot conclude that the linear relationship entirely explains the relationship between *y* and *x*. The relationship may be much more complicated, but one that includes a distinct linear trend as one component. For example, Figure 6.6 indicates an exact mathematical relationship between *x* and *y* that is determined by the quadratic equation

$$y = (x - 4)^2 + 2x$$

All seven points in the figure lie on the quadratic curve. The last term in the equation, however, indicates that the relationship between *x* and *y* has a linear component. The calculations at the foot of the figure show the least-squares slope to be $b = 2$. Thus, one cannot construe the presence of a slope as the establishment of a direct linear relationship between *x* and *y*. The relationship may be more than linear; the presence of a slope indicates that, at the very

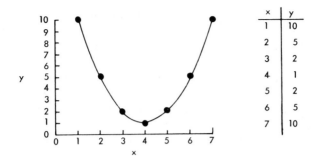

x	y
1	10
2	5
3	2
4	1
5	2
6	5
7	10

Calculation of b

$$\Sigma x = 28 \qquad \Sigma x^2 = 140 \qquad \Sigma(x - \bar{x})^2 = 140 - 28^2/7 = 28$$

$$\Sigma y = 35 \qquad \Sigma y^2 = 259$$

$$\Sigma xy = 140 \qquad \Sigma(x - \bar{x})(y - \bar{y}) = 140 - (28)(35)/7 = 0$$

$$b = \Sigma(x - \bar{x})(y - \bar{y})/\Sigma(x - \bar{x})^2 = 0/28 = 0$$

Figure 6.5
Scatter diagram and the calculation of the slope for hypothetical data where x and y have a direct quadratic relationship.

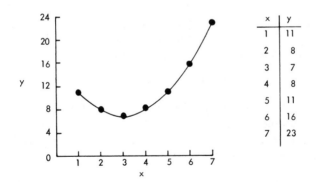

x	y
1	11
2	8
3	7
4	8
5	11
6	16
7	23

Calculation of b

$$\Sigma x = 28 \qquad \Sigma x^2 = 140 \qquad \Sigma(x - \bar{x})^2 = 140 - (28)^2/7 = 28$$

$$\Sigma y = 84 \qquad \Sigma y^2 = 1204$$

$$\Sigma xy = 392 \qquad \Sigma(x - \bar{x})(y - \bar{y}) = 392 - (84)(28)/7 = 56$$

$$b = \Sigma(x - \bar{x})(y - \bar{y})/\Sigma(x - \bar{x})^2 = 56/28 = 2$$

Figure 6.6
Scatter diagram and the calculation of the slope for hypothetical data where x and y have a quadratic relationship that includes a linear component.

203

least, there is a linear component. For the data on blood pressure and age, no doubt the relationship is quite complex and entails more than a linear regression. (The interested reader is referred to Oldham for an account of the blood pressure–age relationship [82].) The analysis conducted indicates that, whatever the relationship, it includes a distinct linear component. One can safely conclude that, at the least, systolic blood pressure among adult females rises an average of about 1 mm Hg per year of age. In many instances, the establishment of this minimal linear relationship between the dependent and independent variables suffices for the aims of the investigation.

BEYOND LINEAR REGRESSION

Polynomial and Multiple Regression

The above discussion raises the issue of the fitting of relationships other than those described by straight lines. There are techniques available for doing so. Briefly, to fit any type of polynomial of the form

$$Y = a + bx + cx^2 + dx^3 + \cdots$$

one only has to extend the principle of least squares and consider the minimization of

$$\Sigma \, (y - Y)^2 = \Sigma \, (y - a - bx - cx^2 - dx^3 - \cdots)^2$$

Application of differential calculus will yield the appropriate equations that, when solved, will give the least-squares values of $a, b, c, d, \ldots$.

One might also consider the fitting of a linear relationship in which more than one independent variable is involved, namely,

$$Y = a + b_1 x_1 + b_2 x_2 + b_3 x_3 + \cdots$$

This situation concerns *multiple linear regression*. For example, one might consider the multiple linear regression of female systolic blood pressure (y) on age (x_1), height (x_2), and weight (x_3). Again, the principle of least squares would involve the determination of values of $a, b_1, b_2, b_3, \ldots$ that minimize

$$\Sigma \, (y - Y)^2 = \Sigma \, (y - b_1 x_1 - b_2 x_2 - b_3 x_3 - \cdots)^2$$

The details of polynomial and multiple regression may be found in more advanced texts (for example, [2] and [101]).

Nonlinear Regression

Although techniques are also available for fitting more complex mathematical forms, these are more difficult to apply and usually entail considerable computation. Much is known, however, about the fitting of straight lines. Often some manipulation of the data will make them more amenable to linear regression analysis. For example, the relationship

$$y = ac^{bx}$$

will, upon taking logarithms, give

$$\log y = \log a + bx \log c$$

Defining new values as follows

$$y' = \log y, a' = \log a, b' = b \log c$$

gives the linear relationship

$$y' = a' + b'x$$

to which the linear regression techniques can be applied. In other words, one fits a linear regression of $\log y$ on x.

As another example, the upper portion of Figure 6.7 indicates a sigmoid curve relationship. Such curves are common in pharmacology, where the abscissa x represents a series of doses (or, more usually, the logarithm of the doses) administered to groups of laboratory animals. The ordinate y represents the percentage of animals responding in each group to the dose (the response in many such investigations is death). At very low doses, no animal responds. A dose level is reached at which the animals begin to respond, and the percentage responding rises until at all high doses all animals respond. The bottom portion of Figure 6.7 displays the relationship obtained by using in place of y the value

$$y' = \log \frac{y}{100 - y}$$

The result is a straight-line relationship between y' and x. This particular change of the ordinate is called the *logit transformation*. Thus, the relationship between dose and response can be determined statistically by the fitting of a linear regression line of logit response on log dose. Armitage [2] provides the details of fitting such a regression line.

Tests of Assumptions Underlying Linear Regression

One final point with regard to regression is that techniques exist that permit one to test the adequacy of the linear fit and to examine the validity of the assumption of equal variability about the line. These techniques apply when there is more than one observed y value for each x. With regard to equal variability along the line, replicate y observations at each x enable one to calculate and compare the SDs of the ys at each x. The proper test of equal variability is called *Bartlett's test of homogeneity of variance*. The reader will find it described in the more advanced texts cited above.

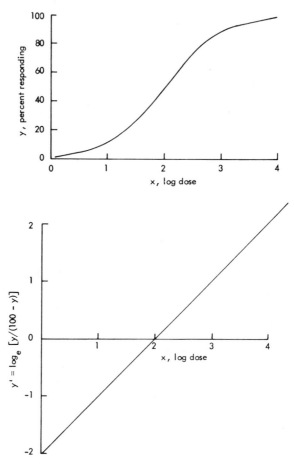

Figure 6.7
A sigmoid-shaped dose-response curve (top) and its transformation to a straight line upon taking logit response (bottom).

With regard to the adequacy of the linear fit, one technique involves analysis of variance. Briefly, the variation of the mean values of the y observations at each x is split into two components: the variation explainable by the fitted regression line and a residual variation of the means about the regression line. One can then determine whether the variation of the means about the regression line is beyond what can be explained by chance. If it is, then this result points to a relationship between y and x that involves more than merely a linear component. If it is not, the regression line represents an adequate fit.

By grouping the data on blood pressure and age within 10-year age groups, this more detailed analysis can be obtained. With such a grouping, the six blood pressure values for women in their twenties are considered as six replicate observations at the midpoint of the interval, i.e., 25 years; the four observations for women in their thirties are considered as four replicate observations at age 35 years, and so on. With such grouping, the fitted regression line changes little; it is

$$Y = 138.64 + 1.28(x - 47.42)$$

The analysis of variance of the regression line indicated that the linear regression fits the data well. In other words, there was no suggestion from such analysis of a relationship much beyond that of a straight line.

Another technique that is rapidly gaining popularity is the *analysis of residuals*. This consists of calculating the $y - Y$ values for each data point. Often, a simple plotting will reveal clumps of residuals of like sign, which indicates systematic deviation from a linear fit. Other perturbations among the residuals can be detected and will pinpoint a poorly fitting linear regression line.

CORRELATION

Definition

As stated before, when one cannot designate at least one variable as being independent, then correlation is the appropriate method for describing the relationship between two mutually dependent variables. The *coefficient of correlation* describes the degree of relationship between x and y and is calculated as

$$r = \frac{\Sigma (x - \bar{x})(y - \bar{y})}{\sqrt{\Sigma (x - \bar{x})^2 \Sigma (y - \bar{y})^2}}$$

It is sometimes known as the *product moment correlation*, or *Pearson's coefficient of correlation*, after Karl Pearson.

All terms in r are familiar. The numerator is the sum of cross-products about the mean (see p. 193), whereas the denominator is the square root of the product of the sum of squares of deviations about the mean for each of the two variables. As before, the computationally more convenient forms are

$$\Sigma (x - \bar{x})(y - \bar{y}) = \Sigma xy - (\Sigma x)(\Sigma y)/n$$
$$\Sigma (x - \bar{x})^2 = \Sigma x^2 - (\Sigma x)^2/n$$
$$\Sigma (y - \bar{y})^2 = \Sigma y^2 - (\Sigma y)^2/n$$

Properties

Inspection of the formula for r indicates that the correlation coefficient has no units. Whatever units are used for the x and y variable cancel out when dividing the numerator by the denominator of r. It may also be shown, although it is not obvious on inspection, that the minimum value for r is -1 and the maximum value is $+1$. Thus, with any set of data, the calculated correlation coefficient must lie somewhere between $+1$ and -1.

It is a simple algebraic exercise to show that, when there is an exact linear relationship between x and y, the correlation coefficient is either $+1$ or -1, the sign depending on whether the slope of the line is positive or negative. (This applies to all lines except those perpendicular to the abscissa or perpendicular to the ordinate, i.e., those with either zero or infinite slope.) This situation is described as *perfect correlation*: perfect positive correlation occurs when the slope is positive; perfect negative correlation, when the slope is negative.

As the points on a scatter diagram begin to deviate from a perfect straight line, the correlation coefficient departs from $+1$ or -1. Thus, the closeness with which points on a scatter diagram resemble a straight line determines the magnitude of the correlation coefficient. A correlation coefficient of zero means there is no relationship between the two variables.

Table 6.3 presents two sets of data: (1) course grades (with scoring A = 4 to D = 1) in pathophysiology and the National Board (Part I) subscores in

Table 6.3. Relationship between medical school course grades and National Board subscores (*Top:* Pathophysiology grade and National Board (Part I) subscore in pathology for 38 students; *Bottom:* Surgery grade and National Board (Part II) subscore in surgery for 31 students)

Pathophysiology Course Grade vs. National Board Subscore in Pathology:

	x	y		x	y		x	y
Course grade	Score	Board score	Course grade	Score	Board score	Course grade	Score	Board score
C−	1.7	86	E	0.0	82	A	4.0	95
C−	1.7	83	D	1.0	85	C	2.0	81
C+	2.3	88	D+	1.3	83	B	3.0	88
B+	3.3	87	E	0.0	70	D	1.0	83
C	2.0	78	C	2.0	84	A	4.0	87
A	4.0	94	C	2.0	77	A	4.0	93
B	3.0	87	B−	2.7	83	B−	2.7	87
B	3.0	85	B	3.0	85	C+	2.3	84
B−	2.7	86	C+	2.3	85	B−	2.7	88
C+	2.3	86	C+	2.3	81	C	2.0	88
C	2.0	88	A	4.0	94	B−	2.7	89
C	2.0	82	C−	1.7	75	C	2.0	75
D	1.0	80	A	4.0	92			

Calculation of correlation coefficient, r:

$n = 38$ $\Sigma x = 89.7$ $\Sigma x^2 = 251.15$

$\Sigma y = 3,224$ $\Sigma y^2 = 274,616$

$\Sigma xy = 7,763.1$

$\Sigma(x - \bar{x})^2 = 251.15 - 89.7^2/38 = 39.41$

$\Sigma(y - \bar{y})^2 = 274,616 - 3,224^2/38 = 1,085$

$\Sigma(x - \bar{x})(y - \bar{y}) = 7,763.1 - (89.7)(3,224)/38 = 152.8$

$$r = \Sigma(x - \bar{x})(y - \bar{y})/\sqrt{\Sigma(x - \bar{x})^2\Sigma(y - \bar{y})^2}$$
$$= 152.8/\sqrt{(39.41)(1,085)} = 152.8/206.8 = 0.74$$

Table 6.3 (*Continued*)

Surgery Course Grade vs. National Board Subscore in Surgery:

Course grade	x Score	y Board score	Course grade	x Score	y Board score	Course grade	x Score	y Board score
B	3.0	86	A−	3.7	83	B	3.0	87
C	2.0	87	B	3.0	84	B	3.0	79
A	4.0	81	B	3.0	88	A−	3.7	88
C+	2.3	88	B	3.0	84	B+	3.3	88
B+	3.3	96	B−	2.7	81	B+	3.3	81
B	3.0	84	B+	3.3	85	B	3.0	79
B+	3.3	92	C	2.0	83	C	2.0	80
B	3.0	88	B+	3.3	84	B	3.0	83
B+	3.3	84	B−	2.7	80	A	4.0	86
C+	2.3	82	B	3.0	85	B+	3.3	79
						C	2.0	90

Calculation of correlation coefficient, r:

$n = 31$ $\quad$ $\Sigma x = 92.8$ $\qquad$ $\Sigma x^2 = 286.66$

$\qquad\qquad$ $\Sigma y = 2,625$ $\qquad$ $\Sigma y^2 = 222,757$

$\qquad\qquad\qquad\qquad\qquad$ $\Sigma xy = 7,861.1$

$\Sigma(x - \bar{x})^2 = 286.66 - 92.8^2/31 = 8.86$

$\Sigma(y - \bar{y})^2 = 222,757 - 2,625^2/31 = 479$

$\Sigma(x - \bar{x})(y - \bar{y}) = 7,861.1 - (92.8)(2,625)/31 = 3.04$

$$r = \Sigma(x - \bar{x})(y - \bar{y})/\sqrt{\Sigma(x - \bar{x})^2 \, \Sigma(y - \bar{y})^2}$$
$$= 3.04/\sqrt{(8.86)(479)} = 3.04/65.15 = 0.05$$

pathology for a group of 38 medical students, and (2) course grades in surgery and National Board (Part II) subscores in surgery for another group of 31 medical students. Figure 6.8 exhibits the corresponding scatter diagrams. For each set of data, the calculations at the foot of the table illustrate the determination of the correlation coefficient. Pathophysiology grades and National Board (Part I) pathology subscores have a correlation of .74; surgery grades and National Board (Part II) subscores in surgery have a correlation of .05.

The reconciliation of an "eyeball" inspection of a scatter diagram with a calculated correlation coefficient might begin with inspection of the extreme values for each variable. The association of the extreme values of one variable with extremes of the other indicates correlation. One would also consider the tightness of the ellipse formed by the points in the center of the diagram. The tighter and thinner the ellipse, the higher is the value of *r*. Generally, correlations between −.30 and +.30 remain nearly impossible to detect by eye upon inspection of the scatter diagram.

For the data on the pathophysiology grades and the National Board pathology subscores, the points can be enclosed by a fairly tight ellipse and

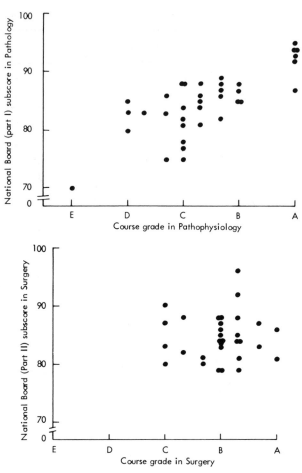

Figure 6.8
Scatter diagrams for course grades in pathophysiology versus National Board (Part I) subscores in pathology (top) and course grades in surgery versus National Board (Part II) subscores in surgery (bottom).

the extremes tend to be associated. Hence, inspection would lead one to expect a reasonably high correlation coefficient, as was confirmed by the calculations. For the data on the surgery grades and the National Board surgery subscores, there are no such tendencies among the points in the scatter diagram. Thus, inspection leads one to anticipate little or no correlation, as was also confirmed by the calculations.

Interpretation

The interpretation of a correlation coefficient depends mainly on the particulars of the investigation and the extent of one's background in the subject-matter under study. Previous experience in the field usually serves as a basis of comparison in determining whether a particular correlation coefficient is noteworthy. As a very crude rule of thumb, however, the following general guidelines may be helpful. Correlations from 0 to .25 indicate little or no relationship, those from .25 to .50 indicate a fair degree of relationship, those from .50 to .75 a moderate to good relationship, and those above .75 a very good to excellent relationship. Thus, by these criteria, the first set of data displays good correlation and the second displays virtually no correlation.

Sometimes one encounters correlations of .95 or higher. When such correlations arise, particularly in the biological field and where human data are involved, one should immediately be suspect. Correlations this high are almost too good to be true. In practice, when correlation this high occurs, it is usually evident long before the plotting of the scatter diagram or the calculation of r. When unanticipated extremely high correlations are found, it is wise to query whether the strong relationship might be an artifact. For example, one should not be surprised to find a high correlation between medical students' grades in medicine and their grade point averages during their clinical years. The medicine grade enters into the determination of the grade point average, and this grade usually receives the greatest weight in the calculations. Thus, the artifact is the correlation of the medicine grade with itself. In a similar manner, one would expect a high correlation between any test subscore and the average score for the entire exam. In general, it is unwise to correlate one quantity with another quantity that has the first as a component. This can lead to spuriously high correlations.

Inference

As with regression, inference on a correlation coefficient involves the concept of the observed sample of (x, y) points originating from some larger population. In the population, the correlation between x and y is denoted as ρ. With the correlation coefficient in the sample data calculated as r, what conclusions can be drawn regarding the unknown population correlation ρ?

This section considers the test of significance of the null hypothesis $\rho = 0$, namely, that there is no correlation between x and y in the underlying population. The test consists of determining the compatibility of a sample r with the null hypothesis population $\rho = 0$. Thus, with no correlation in the population, what is the chance of finding a sample correlation as extreme as or more so than that observed?

The performance of the test of significance entails an additional assumption concerning the data. This is that the population approximately follows the *bivariate normal distribution*. The bivariate normal distribution is an extension of the already familiar bell-shaped normal curve to three dimensions. Figure 6.9 illustrates two bivariate normal distributions. The two-dimensional bell-shaped normal distribution becomes, in three dimensions, a bell-shaped mound for the bivariate normal distribution. The two axes or coordinates forming a plane on the landscape represent the possible (x, y) population values. As with the two-dimensional normal curve, the three-dimensional normal surface can be represented by a specific mathematical equation.

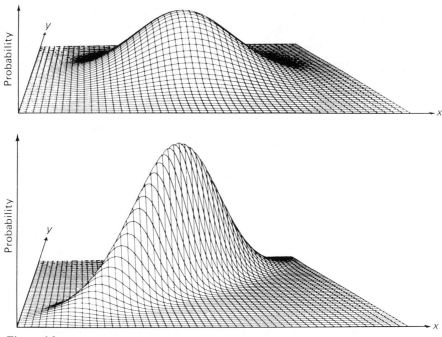

Figure 6.9
Bivariate normal surfaces with $\rho = 0$ (top) and $\rho = .9$ (bottom). (From *Biometry: The Principles and Practice of Statistics in Biological Research* by Robert R. Sokal and F. James Rohlf. W.H. Freeman and Company. Copyright © 1969.)

Although it is not necessary to present the equation here, it is useful to indicate what quantities are necessary to depict a particular surface. Recall that the two-dimensional normal curve was mathematically determined by two quantities: its mean, μ, and SD, σ. The bivariate normal surface is mathematically determined by *five* quantities: a mean and SD for the x variable (μ_x and σ_x), a mean and SD for the y variable (μ_y and σ_y), and, lastly, the correlation coefficient ρ for x and y.

The two surfaces in Figure 6.9 have the same means and SDs on their x and y axes; they differ only in their correlation ρ. The top surface has $\rho = 0$; the bottom has $\rho = .9$. One may infer that as ρ increases from zero, with other quantities remaining unaltered, the bivariate normal surface changes from a symmetrical mound to an increasingly narrow ridge. If one considers slices of the bivariate normal surface taken parallel to the horizon, at $\rho = 0$ the slices correspond to circular sections. As ρ increases, the sections become increasingly thinner and more elongated ellipses. At the extreme of $\rho = 1$, the surface degenerates into a plane standing perpendicular to the horizon. A slice of this plane parallel to the horizon yields a straight line.

For the particular situation in which $\rho = 0$ in the underlying bivariate normal population, it has been mathematically derived that the quantity

$$t_{n-2} = \frac{r}{\sqrt{1 - r^2}} \sqrt{n - 2}$$

follows the t distribution with $n - 2$ df. Thus, a test of the null hypothesis $\rho = 0$ follows from the calculation of t in the above formula and the use of the t tables.

Had correlation rather than regression been intended for the data in Table 6.1, it may be seen that

$$r = \frac{\Sigma\ (x - \bar{x})(y - \bar{y})}{\sqrt{\Sigma\ (x - \bar{x})^2\ \Sigma\ (y - \bar{y})^2}} = \frac{9,366.7}{\sqrt{(7,662.6)(22,219.6)}} = .718$$

A test of the null hypothesis $\rho = 0$ then becomes

$$t_{31} = \frac{.718}{\sqrt{1 - (.718)^2}} \sqrt{31} = 5.74$$

which gives $P < .001$. Thus, if there were no correlation in the underlying population, these sample results would occur by chance alone less than one time in a thousand. One concludes that there is a statistically significant correlation between systolic blood pressure and age.

The reader may note that the above t ratio value is identical with the t ratio of Table 6.2 for the significance test of zero slope in the regression analysis of blood pressure versus age. This is no numerical accident. The t ratio for the test $\rho = 0$ in correlation analysis is algebraically identical to the t ratio for the test $\beta = 0$ in the regression analysis of y on x. Thus, a test of significance of zero correlation is identical to the test of significance of zero slope in regression analysis. With regard to the present data, it matters not whether one chooses to pursue regression or correlation analysis for the test of significance.

To simplify the above t test for a correlation coefficient, tables have been calculated that give the sample correlation required to achieve statistical significance at some particular level. Appendix Table A5 presents these values. Once one calculates r in the sample, one may alternatively use Appendix Table A5 directly to test the significance of the correlation. The values tabulated are for two-tailed tests at the 5 and 1 percent significance levels. For example, with a sample of 12 observation pairs giving 10 df for the calculated r, Appendix Table A5 indicates that a sample r in excess of .576 (or below $-.576$) would result in statistical significance at the 5 percent level. At the 1 percent level, the sample correlation must exceed .708 (or be below $-.708$) in order to achieve statistical significance.

Cautions in Interpretation

As with regression analysis, similar warnings pertain to the limitations in the interpretation of a correlation coefficient.

First, the correlation coefficient applies only to a *linear* relationship between x and y. In Figure 6.5 the correlation coefficient is zero. Hence, the lack of correlation does not necessarily mean the lack of a relationship; it means merely the lack of a linear relationship.

Second, one must not extrapolate an observed correlation beyond the observed ranges of the x and y variables.

The third point is the cliché, "Correlation does not mean causation." Correlation indicates that two variables tend to be related. One may directly influence or "cause" the other to vary, but it is also possible that some other variable, or a whole host of other variables, may influence the two that are correlated. Thus, x and y may be correlated, but mainly because they are each strongly influenced by z. For example, among the states in the U.S., the infant mortality rate and the number of physicians per capita exhibit a strong negative correlation. One cannot conclude, however, that raising of a state's physician-to-population ratio will decrease infant mortality. Among others, the following variables likely relate both to physicians per capita and infant mortality rate: per capita income, level of education, the availability of hospital and medical facilities and auxiliary medical personnel, population density, degree of urbanization, general nutritional status, adequacy of housing, and sanitation level.

Often one encounters what seem to be nonsense or spurious correlations between two variables that logically appear to be totally unrelated to one another. These often arise with correlations taken over time, usually over a period of several years, for various indices. For example, Snedecor and Cochran cite a nonsense correlation of $-.98$ between the annual birth rate in Great Britain and the annual production of pig iron in the United States from 1875 to 1920 [101]. Clearly, general social, economic, and technological trends strongly influence both variables and aid in producing the high correlation. Another example, cited by Wallis and Roberts [111], concerns a positive correlation over time between the number of stork's nests and the number of births in northwestern Europe. Apart from a romantic interpretation, they suggest the more prosaic explanation that population increases result in an increase in the number of buildings which thereby provides more places for storks to nest. Another possibility is that among the many nonsense-type correlations that are run, it is only those that turn out high that receive attention. This is not to deny that high correlations—even those that initially appear to be of the nonsense type—deserve further study and explanation.

In medicine, much more than correlation is necessary to establish causation. Correlation, however, is a useful and widely employed technique. It can provide an important and strong link in a chain of evidence leading to establishment of causation (see also the discussion on p. 271).

Further aspects

With correlation coefficients, one may also calculate confidence limits. One may also compare correlation coefficients in two or more different populations. Sometimes, when there are more than two variables under study, interest focuses on what are called *multiple* and *partial correlation* techniques. These methods are beyond the scope of this text and the reader is referred to other texts such as [2] and [101].

EXERCISES

1. One concern in a study of different regimens in the management of diabetes was weight loss during the course of therapy. The following data pertain to the question of whether the amount of weight loss is related to initial weight. For 16 newly diagnosed adult diabetic patients who received phenformin (DBI) to manage their diabetic state, the following table gives their initial weight at the start of therapy and their weight loss one year after therapy began. (The value of -3 pounds indicates, of course, a gain rather than a loss in weight.)

x Initial weight (lb)	y Weight loss at 1 yr (lb)
225	15
235	44
173	31
223	39
200	6
199	16
129	21
242	44
140	5
156	12
146	-3
195	19
155	10
185	24
150	-3
149	10

$\Sigma x = 2{,}902$ $\Sigma y = 290$
$\Sigma x^2 = 546{,}542$ $\Sigma y^2 = 8{,}636$

A. Test the null hypothesis that there has been no change in weight at one year.

B. Plot a scatter diagram relating the initial weight to the weight loss at one year.

C. Calculate the slope and intercept for the least-squares regression line of weight loss at one year on initial weight. (Note that to simplify your calculations, the raw sums and sums of squares are presented. You will need to calculate for yourself the sum of cross-products.) Draw the least-squares regression line on your scatter diagram.

D. Test the null hypothesis that there is no relation between the initial weight and the amount of weight loss at one year.

E.   For diabetics with an initial weight the same as yours, calculate the 95 percent confidence limits on their predicted *mean* weight loss at one year after DBI therapy.

F.   For an *individual* diabetic with an initial weight the same as yours, calculate the 95 percent limits on his predicted weight loss at one year after DBI therapy.

G.   Clarify the distinction in the interpretation of the limits calculated in Part E and F.

2.   The following table gives four measures of academic performance for a sample of 12 medical students: grade-point averages in the preclinical and clinical years, and the National Board scores for Parts I and II.

w	*x*	*y*	*z*
Grade-point average[a]		National board scores	
Preclinical	Clinical	Part I	Part II
2.1	2.3	80	84
3.0	2.6	89	89
2.2	2.8	83	78
3.4	3.6	95	92
3.6	3.0	96	94
2.5	2.2	86	85
2.9	2.4	92	88
2.9	2.7	89	86
2.0	2.7	86	82
3.4	2.9	94	90
2.5	2.1	87	84
2.5	2.4	92	83
$\Sigma w = 33.0$	$\Sigma x = 31.7$	$\Sigma y = 1,069$	$\Sigma z = 1,035$
$\Sigma w^2 = 93.90$	$\Sigma x^2 = 85.61$	$\Sigma y^2 = 95,497$	$\Sigma z^2 = 89,495$
$\Sigma wx = 88.63$	$\Sigma yz = 92,395$	$\Sigma wy = 2,965.2$	$\Sigma xz = 2,744.6$

[a] Scoring is A = 4 to D = 1.

A.   Plot a scatter diagram and determine by eye the degree of relationship for the following:

(1)   Preclinical grade-point average and National Board Part I score (*w* and *y*).

(2)   Clinical grade-point average and National Board Part II score (*x* and *z*).

(3)   Preclinical grade-point average and clinical grade-point average (*w* and *x*).

(4)   National Board Part I score and National Board Part II score (*y* and *z*).

B. For each relationship in part A, compute the correlation coefficient. Do the numerical values of the correlation coefficients reconcile with the assessment by eye in part A?

C. Test each of the correlations in part B for statistical significance. State, in your own words, the interpretation of a statistically significant correlation.

Chapter 7
Nonparametric Methods

In recent years, what have come to be known as *nonparametric methods* (or, equivalently and more precisely, *distribution-free methods*) have gained popularity and are now frequently employed by medical investigators. In one sense these methods represent alternatives to the traditional methods of statistical analysis that have constituted most of this book. There are occasions when a body of data does not conform with the assumptions underlying traditional statistical methods but does conform with the assumptions underlying nonparametric methods. This is because nonparametric methods generally entail fewer assumptions concerning the nature of the data. When there are such gross violations of the assumptions that traditional methods do not apply, nonparametric methods can often be employed with impunity. Even when data do conform with all the assumptions underlying traditional methods, the nonparametric methods hold up rather well and result in essentially the same conclusions.

Three of the most frequently employed nonparametric methods are (1) the *signed rank test* for the comparison of two groups in paired samples, (2) the *rank sum test* for the comparison of two groups in independent samples, and (3) *rank correlation*. The discussion centers on the advantages and disadvantages of nonparametric techniques and the rationale for their use.

SIGNED RANK TEST

The Wilcoxon signed rank test, named after Wilcoxon who initially proposed it [115], concerns the difference between two groups in paired samples and is the nonparametric analog of the paired-sample t test (p. 134). As with the t test, the signed rank test examines only the difference for each pair. The null hypothesis for the signed rank test claims that, in the underlying population, there is a median difference among pairs of zero. Recall that the t test has the null hypothesis that the population *mean* difference is zero. When the data come from an underlying, approximately normal distribution, the mean and median are identical, so the t test and signed rank tests have identical null hypotheses in this case.

Table 7.1 illustrates the signed rank test with data concerning the comparison of tensile strengths of tape-closed versus sutured wounds on rats. The data are taken from a report by Forrester and Ury that was intended to popularize the signed rank test among medical investigators [42]. The data in Table 7.1 pertain to a group of 10 rats who were sacrificed on the 150th day of their healing period. Each rat had had wounds on his back; one of these wounds was tape closed and the other was sutured. The experiment was of a paired nature, with each rat serving as his own control. Responses consisted of tensile strengths of each type of wound on each rat after the animal was sacrificed. The differences in tensile strength (in pounds per square inch) for each rat appear in the second column of Table 7.1. (The data in Table 7.1 represent only a portion of the experiment; the authors also presented similar results for groups of 10 rats sacrificed at 10, 20, 40, 60, 80, and 100 days.)

The signed rank test proceeds as follows: for each difference, the sign is ignored (column 3 of Table 7.1), and the observations are ranked from low to high (column 4). A difference of zero is ignored in the rankings; that is, zero differences are discarded from the analysis and the sample size is reduced by the number of zero differences. Table 7.1 shows that a zero difference was found with rat 3. Consequently, the analysis discarded the datum from rat 3, and the sample size for the test became nine instead of ten. One then assigns a plus or minus sign to each rank according to the sign of the original difference (column 5). Thus, the data from rats 2 and 5, having negative differences, receive negative signs for their ranks. All the data from other rats receive positive signs for their ranks. The test consists of examination of the sum of the positive or of the negative signed ranks. At the foot of the table, it may be seen that the sum of the negative signed ranks is 3; that of the positive signed ranks is 42. The test proceeds by referring either of these sums to an

Table 7.1. Wilcoxon signed rank test: Tensile strength of tape-closed versus sutured wounds on rats

Rat	Difference in tensile strength (tape-suture)(lb/sq.in.)	Difference with sign disregarded	Rank	Signed Rank
1	372	372	5	5
2	−107	107	2	−2
3	0	0	—	—
4	564	564	7	7
5	−70	70	1	−1
6	649	649	8	8
7	199	199	4	4
8	198	198	3	3
9	738	738	9	9
10	452	452	6	6

Sum of negative signed ranks: 3
Sum of positive signed ranks: 42
Sample size (n): 9
Result from Appendix Table A6: $P < .02$

Data from Forrester and Ury [42].

appropriate table of critical levels. Appendix Table A6 contains critical levels for a two-sided signed rank test with sample sizes up to 25 differences. It may be seen that with $n = 9$ a sum of signed ranks of 3 or 42 corresponds with

$P = .02$. Thus, the difference between the two groups is statistically significant ($P = .02$). In other words, tape-closed wounds have a significantly greater tensile strength then sutured wounds at the 150th day of healing.

In the conduct of the test—though this did not occur with the data presented—one should note that if observations have identical absolute differences, then one averages the ranks for these ties. For example, if the data for rats 7 and 8 had displayed a difference of 199 lbs per sq. in. for each, they would have tied for ranks 3 and 4. Thus, each would have received the average of the two ranks, i.e., a rank of 3.5.

As another illustration, one may apply the signed rank test to the data in Chapter 4 (Table 4.3) on hydrochlorothiazide treatment versus a placebo in patients with hypertension. In this example, all 11 differences are positive. Hence, the negative ranks have a sum of zero, while the sum of positive ranks becomes the sum of the integers 1 through 11, namely 66. Appendix Table A6 reveals that with $n = 11$ the results achieve significance, at least at the 1 percent level. The 0.1 percent values for the signed rank test have not been tabulated in Appendix Table A6, so one cannot state whether the results achieve significance at that level as well. In any event, the signed rank test and the previous paired-sample t test represent two entirely appropriate and alternative methods for conducting the test of significance.

RANK SUM TEST

For the comparison of two groups in independent samples, the Wilcoxon rank sum test represents the nonparametric analog of the independent-samples t test (p. 139). The rank sum test has the null hypothesis that the underlying population distributions are identical.

Data provided by West may be used to illustrate the test [113]. Among the letters to the editor of *The Lancet* following Forrester and Ury's paper on the signed rank test, West called attention to the rank sum test for two samples and presented data on the length of remission between attacks of endogenous and of neurotic depression, with the two samples being independent. All subjects were out-patients attending a psychiatric clinic. The data are presented in Table 7.2.

The test proceeds by combining both samples, ordering the observations from low to high, and then assigning a rank to each observation. This procedure is illustrated at the foot of Table 7.2, where the observations and ranks for the endogenous depression patients are italicized. For tied observations, one assigns the corresponding average rank to each tie. Table 7.2 contains three observations of 105 days (two in the endogenous group and one in the neurotic depression group) that correspond with ranks 4, 5, and 6; each of the three received rank 5. There were two observations of 140 days corresponding with ranks 8 and 9; each received rank 8.5. The test consists of summing the ranks in the group having the smaller sample size. Since, for the data under consideration, the two samples are of equal size (12 observations in each group), one may use either the rank sum of 140 among the patients with endogenous depression or 160 among the patients with neurotic depression. The rank sum is referred directly to the table of critical values for the rank sum test that is given in Appendix Table A7. This table gives the 5, 1, and 0.1 percent critical values of the rank sum test for almost all sample sizes that total 30 or fewer observations in the two groups combined. For $n_1 = n_2 = 12$, Appendix Table A7 indicates that a sum of ranks of 115 or less or 185 or more produces significance at the 5 percent level. The sum of ranks in each of the two samples in Table 7.2 falls between 115 and 185, so the conclusion becomes "not statistically significant," since $P > .05$. In other words, the samples fail to provide evidence of a difference in distribution of length of remission for endogenous depression compared with neurotic depression.

Table 7.2. Wilcoxon rank sum test: Length of remission of endogenous versus neurotic depression

Length of Remission (days)	
12 patients with endogenous depression	12 patients with neurotic depression
109	546
214	844
1818	602
140	87
179	794
744	643
105	199
101	91
105	105
1547	479
529	1296
140	279

Ordering and ranks for total of 24 patients (the observations for patients with endogenous depressions are italicized):

Order: 87, 91, *101*, *105*, *105*, 105, *109*, *140*, *140*, *179*, 199, *214*
Rank: 1, 2, *3*, *5*, *5*, 5,   *7*, *8.5*, *8.5*, *10*, 11, *12*

Order: 279, 479, *529*, 546, 602, 643, *744*, 794, 844, 1296, *1547*, *1818*
Rank: 13, 14, *15*, 16, 17, 18, *19*, 20, 21, 22,   *23*,   *24*

Sum of ranks:
   Among 12 patients with endogenous depression: 140
   Among 12 patients with neurotic depression: 160
Result from Appendix Table A7:
   Not statistically significant ($P > .05$)

Data from West [113].

An alternative version of the Wilcoxon rank sum test is the Mann-Whitney test. The results, however, are identical with those of the Wilcoxon rank sum test. The Mann-Whitney test is not described in this text. Should the reader encounter the Mann-Whitney test and its "U-statistic" in the literature, he need only remember that the test is precisely the same as the Wilcoxon rank sum test described in this section. In fact, there is a direct algebraic relationship between the Mann-Whitney U-value and the sums of the ranks in each sample for the Wilcoxon test.

RANK CORRELATION

The third nonparametric technique that the reader might be likely to encounter is rank correlation. Rank correlation is an alternative to the correlation coefficient r used to determine the degree of relationship between two dependent variables (see p. 207). To distinguish between rank correlation and other types of correlation, the previously described correlation coefficient r (Chapter 6) is usually labeled *product moment correlation* and sometimes bears the additional label *Pearson's product moment correlation*. The nonparametric correlation described in this section is termed *Spearman's rank correlation.*

The calculation of Spearman's rank correlation is illustrated with the data of Table 2.4 concerning the relationship between grades and the evaluation of oral examination performance of 12 senior medical students. For each of the two variables, the n observations are ranked from high to low. The rankings for both the grade-point average and oral examination performance appeared in Table 2.4 (in fact, for the oral examination performance, the only available data were the ranks). For each student, one then calculates the difference in their ranks on the two variables to give 0, −3, 0, −4, −6, 4, 3, 1, 0, 0, 5, and 0. These differences, when squared, yield 0, 9, 0, 16, 36, 16, 9, 1, 0, 0, 25, and 0, which total 112. Denoting the sum of these squared differences in ranks as Σd^2, the rank correlation coefficient is defined as

$$r_S = 1 - \frac{6\Sigma d^2}{n(n^2 - 1)}$$

(The subscript S denotes "Spearman's rank correlation.")

For the 12 medical students, the rank correlation between the grade average and oral examination performance is

$$r_S = 1 - \frac{(6)(112)}{12(12^2 - 1)} = .608$$

which is a moderate degree of correlation.

Like the product moment correlation coefficient, the rank correlation coefficient may vary from −1 to +1; +1 indicates perfect agreement on ranks, 0 indicates no relationship, and −1 indicates a perfect inverse relationship among the ranks.

One may also conduct a test of significance of rank correlation; in particular, a test of the null hypothesis of zero rank correlation in the underlying population may be performed. Appendix Table A8 presents critical values for up to 30 observation pairs at the 5 and 1 percent levels for this test of significance. With 12 observations, Appendix Table A8 indicates .591 and .780 as the 5 and 1 percent values, respectively. The calculated r_S in the example above exceeds .591, but it fails to exceed .780. Thus, the result is statistically significant at the 5 percent level but not at the 1 percent level. This means that if there were no relationship in the underlying population, such a sample rank correlation result would occur by chance less than one time in twenty but more than once in a hundred. Thus, there is a statistically significant relationship between the grade-point average and oral examination performance ($.01 < P < .05$).

For the data on systolic blood pressure and age in Table 6.1, the reader may verify a rank correlation of $r_s = .659$. (In the calculation, tied values receive, as before, the average of their corresponding ranks. For example, the two 41-year-old women correspond with ranks 12 and 13 and thereby each receives rank 12.5; the three women with systolic blood pressure of 128 mm Hg correspond with ranks 12, 13, and 14 and thereby each receives rank 13.) The rank correlation agrees fairly well with the product moment correlation of $r = .718$ that was previously calculated (p. 213).

Kendall has proposed another measure of rank correlation, and his book may be consulted for details [63].

ADVANTAGES AND DISADVANTAGES OF NONPARAMETRIC METHODS

Simplicity of calculation and rapidity in the attainment of test results represent one advantage of nonparametric methods. In fact, many nonparametric methods, including those described here, were initially created to provide a rapid and approximate analysis as an alternative to the classic methods. As such, one eminent statistician labeled them "quick and dirty" methods. Careful and extensive investigations of their properties have revealed, however, that nonparametric methods measure up quite well with classic methods. They may be "quick," but no longer can they be called "dirty."

The examples in this section clearly demonstrate the ease of their calculation. Little time and effort is needed to rank a small series of observations. It should be pointed out, however, that with a large number of observations, ranking becomes an increasingly complex task; the ranking of a large number of observations may entail more computational effort than the calculation of the requisite sums and sums of squares for traditional analysis. Thus, ease of calculation pertains only to samples of relatively small size.

With the advent of electronic computers, the argument based on simplicity of calculation carries less weight than it did in the past. Also, ease of calculation alone should not be the criterion for employment of a statistical technique. Simple techniques are preferable insofar as one does not sacrifice other quantities such as precision, accuracy, or sensitivity. Carefully and scrupulously collected observations merit a thorough and efficient statistical analysis. Often one expends considerable time and effort in the collection of data, and the statistical analysis of these data may constitute only a small portion of the total time and effort involved. The savings achieved by employing a short-cut statistical technique may be negligible relative to the total time and effort involved in the investigation. This, of course, is *not* to deny that short-cut methods can be wisely and usefully employed by an investigator as he peruses and explores his data in order to determine what is likely to yield a fruitful analysis.

The fact that nonparametric methods entail fewer assumptions than traditional methods represents another advantage, and undoubtedly their chief one. The paired-sample t test, strictly speaking, requires that the differences emanate from an underlying approximately normally distributed population. This point was not mentioned in discussing this test, primarily because moderate violations of this assumption have little effect on the applicability of the t test. In other words, the t test procedure holds up well even when there are considerable departures from an underlying normal distribution. The signed rank test involves much weaker assumptions. These are that the observations come from a numerically continuous scale of measurement (see p. 17) and that, under the null hypothesis, the distribution of paired differences in the underlying population be symmetric. Thus, within the strictest interpretation, the signed rank test's assumptions are satisfied in considerably more situations than those of the t test.

A similar argument pertains to the independent-samples t test as opposed to the rank sum test. The independent-samples t test also has an assumption of underlying normal distributions in both the treatment and control populations. In addition, implementation of the independent-samples t test required the assumption of equal variability in the two groups. The rank sum test has no such requirements. The sole requirement is that the observations are from underlying continuous scales of measurement. The rank sum test has the null hypothesis that the population distributions in each group are equal.

The test of significance on the product moment correlation necessitated the assumption of an underlying bivariate normal population distribution (p. 211). Spearman's rank correlation test involves no such requirement.

A third advantage of nonparametric methods pertains to the situation in which the basic observations can be expressed only in terms of ranks. Certainly this is the case with the data in Table 2.4 on the evaluation of medical students' performance on an oral examination. The examiners did not quantify the performance of the 12 students; they merely arrayed the students from high to low. This happens in many situations. There may be no device for quantification, but it is still possible to obtain a hierarchy of preferences, i.e., a qualitative ranking of observations. Nonparametric methods are tailor-made for these situations, whereas the classic parametric methods of previous chapters are inapplicable.

Among the disadvantages of nonparametric methods, mention has already been made of the fact that with many observations (say 50 or more) ranking can be more time-consuming than the calculation of sums and sums of squares. However, as was also mentioned, ease or difficulty of calculation should not constitute an important criterion for judging a test.

Critics of nonparametric methods have referred to their predominant concentration on tests of significance. Although methods are available for the determination of nonparametric confidence intervals, these are difficult and somewhat cumbersome to apply. Nonparametric methods do not readily lend themselves to the confidence limit determination as do the more classic methods. Certainly in the medical literature, nonparametric methods deal almost exclusively with tests of significance.

An additional shortcoming with nonparametric methods is the greater difficulty in their application to experimental designs that are more complex than those considered in this text. Classic parametric methods can be easily extended to deal with more complicated experimental arrangements. Although analogous nonparametric procedures have been developed, they do entail considerably more difficulties.

A final comparison of nonparametric with classic methods involves the important question of how nonparametric methods fare when all the assumptions hold to justify employment of classic methods. For example, when the conditions for the paired-sample t test are exactly satisfied, what does one sacrifice, if anything, by employing the signed rank test? The answer is, very little. In terms of the power function (see p. 122), for any alternative to the null hypothesis, the power of the rank tests is approximately 95 percent that of the t test. Another way of stating this is that with fixed types I and II errors, the t test can achieve these specified risks with 95 percent of the observations that are required by the analogous nonparametric rank test. In this sense, nonparametric tests are quite efficient.

Statisticians vary in their enthusiasm for employment of nonparametric techniques. There are a number of elementary statistics texts (for example, [72] and [111]) that emphasize the nonparametric approach and deemphasize the classic t test approach. Others, including this text, Armitage [2], and Snedecor and Cochran [101], emphasize the classic parametric techniques.

For the reader of the medical literature, the discussion may be summarized by stating that when he encounters nonparametric tests, he may view them as quite respectable alternatives to the t tests that pervade the literature. Many investigators employ nonparametric methods only when the t test assumptions suffer gross violations; they are most appropriate in such situations. Even when all the t test assumptions hold, there is little basis for criticism of the investigator who analyzes his data by nonparametric rank methods. The nonparametric methods have high efficiency in this situation and are quite unlikely to result in a conclusion that is materially different from that of the more traditional type of t tests.

EXERCISES

1. Referring back to question 1 for Chapter 6, the following data give the initial weight and weight loss at one year for nine newly diagnosed diabetic patients who received Diabinese for control of their diabetes:

x Initial weight (lb)	y Weight loss at 1 yr (lb)
202 ·	25
177	13
179	41
167	−11
162	−8
150	4
200	0
174	11
163	−4

A. Using the appropriate nonparametric technique, perform tests of significance of the following null hypotheses:

   (1) With DBI treatment, there is no change in weight at one year.

   (2) With Diabinese treatment, there is no change in weight at one year.

   (3) The initial weight is the same among patients receiving DBI therapy as with those receiving Diabinese.

   (4) The weight loss at one year is the same among patients receiving DBI therapy as with those receiving Diabinese.

B. For each test of significance in part A, compare the result with the result of an appropriate t test. (To simplify your calculations, the following sums and sums of squares about the mean pertain to the nine patients on Diabinese therapy: $\Sigma x = 1{,}574$, $\Sigma(x - \bar{x})^2 = 2{,}377$, $\Sigma y = 71$, $\Sigma(y - \bar{y})^2 = 2{,}253$.)

2. Referring back to question 2 for Chapter 6, compute Spearman's rank correlation for each of the product moment correlations previously calculated. How do the two compare?

Chapter 8
Sequential Analysis

Sequential analysis is a technique wherein one conducts a statistical test of significance sequentially over time as the data are collected. After each observation, one analyzes the cumulative data and reaches one of the following three decisions: (1) stop the data collection, reject the null hypothesis, and claim statistical significance, (2) stop the data collection, do not reject the null hypothesis, and claim the results are not statistically significant, or (3) continue the data collection; the cumulated data are inadequate to draw a conclusion.

A sequential test of significance has the same structure as the fixed sample-size tests of Chapters 4 and 5. The investigator specifies a null hypothesis, a significance level, and whether a one- or two-sided test is desired. He further specifies an alternative hypothesis and a type II error. The sequential test of significance results in the same conclusion as before; it either rejects or fails to reject the null hypothesis. The sequential test has the distinct feature that the number of observations required to reach one of these conclusions varies. One may complete the test with few observations, or, with the very same specifications, many observations may be required. Thus, sequential analysis is an alternative technique for conducting the tests of significance discussed in Chapters 4 and 5. There are sequential analogs for a normal distribution test on a mean when the SD is known, for t tests involving a single mean or the comparison of two means, for a test on a single proportion, and for tests involving the comparison of two proportions.

In medicine, one encounters sequential analysis most often in clinical trials (see Chapter 10). Among sequential clinical trials, the comparison of two proportions occurs with greatest frequency. Such tests are illustrated in this section. The reader who is interested in the other forms of sequential tests should refer to Armitage's text, which elaborates the details of the application of sequential methods to clinical trials [3].

A SEQUENTIAL CLINICAL TRIAL

Figure 8.1 depicts a sequential test on a proportion. The data come from a clinical trial of the drug isocarboxazid in the treatment of angina pectoris [46]. Out-patients with angina pectoris were the subjects for the trial. Each participant received isocarboxazid therapy for four weeks and placebo therapy for four weeks. The order of the therapies was randomized (p. 261), and the study was double blind (p. 262). Patients indicated at the conclusion of their treatment regimen whether or not there was improvement in their condition during the course of each drug's administration. The author states, "Only

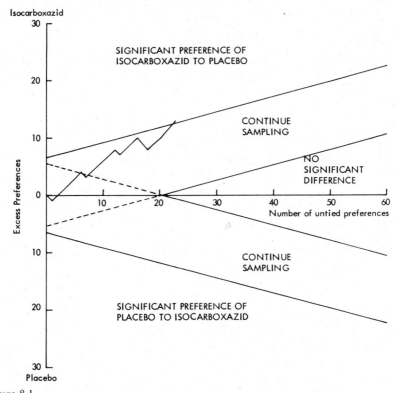

Figure 8.1
An "open" sequential clinical trial: improvement after isocarboxazid versus placebo in the treatment of angina pectoris. (From Grant [46].)

definite statements of marked improvement were accepted as a success." Patients for whom both treatments provided noticeable improvement or for whom neither treatment provided noticeable improvement were discarded from the analysis, analogously to the discarding of the tied pairs in the comparison of proportions in paired samples (p. 172). Only the untied pairs— patients who indicated improvement on one drug and not on the other— entered into the analysis. Thus, each observation in the sequential analysis consisted of either a "success" (an untied pair indicating preference for isocarboxazid) or "failure" (an untied pair indicating preference for the placebo).

The sequential analysis consisted of a plot of excess preferences as the ordinate against the number of untied preferences as the abscissa, and proceeded as follows. A path began at the origin of Figure 8.1. As the patients completed their treatment schedules and their preferences became available, then either of two alternatives pertained: if the patient preferred isocarboxazid, the path went up one unit; if he preferred the placebo, the path went down one unit. (Of course, a preference for both or neither did not affect the path and such observations were discarded.) The two pairs of parallel lines, one pair heading upward, the other downward, represent the boundaries or *stopping rules* for the test. As long as the path remained within the two parallel lines, the investigators continued the data collection and waited for an additional preference. As soon as the path would touch or cross one of the parallel line boundaries, the trial would terminate and the appropriate conclusion would be drawn, depending on which boundary was crossed. The path in Figure 8.1 consists of a plot of the following series of preferences:

$$F, S, S, S, S, S, F, S, S, S, S, S, F, S, S, S, F, F, S, S, S, S, S$$

It may be seen that the path crossed the upper boundary upon the 23rd preference. At this stage, the trial terminated and the investigator concluded that the patients preferred isocarboxazid to the placebo significantly more often in the treatment of angina pectoris ($P < .05$).

In designing the trial, the investigator specified as his null hypothesis that isocarboxazid and the placebo are equally preferable. He indicated his willingness to risk a 5 percent chance of claiming a difference between the two agents when, in fact, they are equally preferred. Further, he stated that should the rate of preference for isocarboxazid be as much as 75 percent, he wished to risk only a 5 percent chance of failing to conclude that isocarboxazid was significantly more preferable. Finally, he indicated that he was as interested in the conclusion that isocarboxazid was preferred significantly more often than the placebo as the conclusion that the placebo was preferred significantly more often than isocarboxazid.

The above specifications, with π denoting the population rate of untied preferences for isocarboxazid, indicate the null hypothesis $\pi_0 = \frac{1}{2}$ with a type I error $\alpha = .05$. The alternative hypothesis was specified as $\pi_1 = .75$ with a type II error $\beta = .05$. These specifications of π_0, π_1, α, and β determine the parallel-line boundaries for the test. The theory of sequential analysis developed by Wald provides the means for obtaining boundaries such that the test achieves the specified error levels [110]. Armitage presents sets of tables and guidelines for choosing the appropriate boundaries for a sequential test [3]. An investigator who plans to perform a test of significance by sequential analysis would profit from reading Armitage's text. The present discussion concerns only the description of sequential tests and their interpretation.

The reader who encounters sequential trials in the medical literature would do well to remember that the boundaries an author employs for his sequential test are derived from the specification of a null and an alternative hypothesis and the corresponding type I and II error levels. It is the author's onus to indicate these values precisely in his published report. Unfortunately, a number of sequential trials have been published in which the investigators have employed one of the designs listed in Armitage's text but have failed to indicate all the above specifications in their published report. With such omission, the results of these trials cannot be interpreted properly.

COMPARISON OF SEQUENTIAL WITH FIXED SAMPLE-SIZE TRIALS

For the trial under consideration in Figure 8.1, the investigator could have employed a fixed sample-size design as described in Chapter 5. In fact, the reader might verify that for the specified error levels and null and alternative hypotheses, the analogous fixed sample-size trial would have entailed $n = 46$ total untied preferences (see the formula on p. 161). The sequential test reached a conclusion after 23 untied preferences. Thus, the sequential test provided a considerable savings in the number of preferences. A conclusion was reached with half the observations that would have been required with the analogous fixed sample-size test. The savings in the number of observations represents the chief advantage and appeal of sequential analysis. This trial produced considerable economy in observations; another sequential trial with these same error levels and boundaries could result in a path that wandered much farther along the "continue sampling" channel. In fact, inspection of Figure 8.1 reveals that it is possible that more than 46 observations might be required before the path crossed a boundary. Thus, it is conceivable that a sequential trial might entail more observations than the analogous fixed sample-size trial.

A question of interest, then, is how many observations *on the average* are required for a path to cross the boundaries of a particular sequential design? To answer this question, one would conceive of many paths with the particular boundaries, and, for each path, one would determine the observation number at which the path first crossed a boundary. One could then calculate the mean number of observations required to cross the boundaries. The average number of observations required to cross the boundaries of a sequential test is called the *average sample number* (ASN). Wald, in his theoretical development of sequential analysis, derived an approximate mathematical expression for the ASN with a particular set of boundaries. The only feature of the expression pertinent to the present discussion is that it depends on π, the population success rate. Application of the ASN expression to the boundaries depicted in Figure 8.1 gives the ASN values of 9 when $\pi = 0$, 31 when $\pi = .50$, and 25 when $\pi = .75$. Further, the maximum value of the ASN is 38 when π is roughly halfway between .50 and .75, i.e., at approximately $\pi = .63$. Since the analogous fixed sample-size test requires 46 observations, the savings in the *average* number of observations with the sequential test are 35 percent when the null hypothesis is true ($\pi = .50$), 46 percent when the alternative hypothesis is true ($\pi = .75$), and 17 percent when $\pi = .63$. Thus, no matter what the true population success rate π may be, sequential analysis offers, on the average, a saving in the number of observations. In some instances, the saving is considerable.

A "RESTRICTED" SEQUENTIAL CLINICAL TRIAL

The design depicted in Figure 8.1 is termed an *open type* sequential design. It is "open" in that a path may wander along the open "continue sampling" channel that is defined by the two parallel line boundaries. Open designs are derived directly from the original development of sequential analysis by Wald. For applications in clinical trials, open designs have the disadvantage that the sample path could proceed rather far along the "continue sampling" channel and thus require a considerable number of observations to reach a conclusion. Even though the chance that this happens may be low, the possibility that it *could* happen represents a somewhat unappealing feature of the use of open designs in clinical trials.

It would seem desirable to curtail a sequential design after a fixed number of observations. In other words, the test proceeds sequentially with the analysis of the cumulative data after each new observation, but the test must reach a conclusion by the time one collects some fixed number of observations. Armitage has developed this modification, and he terms such tests as *restricted* sequential designs [3].

Figure 8.2 illustrates a restricted sequential design for a two-sided test on a proportion. In fact, the null and alternative hypotheses and the α and β error levels are the same as in the previous example, namely, $\pi_0 = .50$ with $\alpha = .05$, against $\pi_1 = .75$ with $\beta = .05$. The test is restricted in that a decision must be reached by the time 62 preferences are recorded. Thus, truncation is at $N = 62$. The sample path proceeds precisely as before. If the path crosses the outer boundaries, the trial terminates and one reaches the conclusion "reject

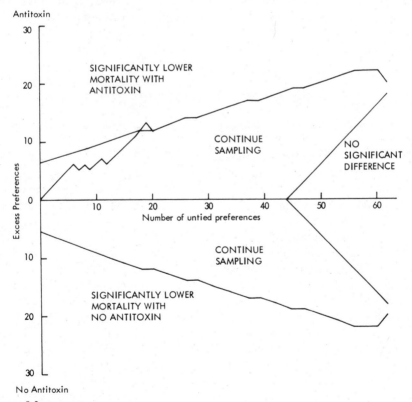

Figure 8.2
A restricted sequential clinical trial: mortality after antitoxin versus no antitoxin in the treatment of clinical tetanus. (From Brown et al. [14].)

233

the null hypothesis; statistically significant." If the path crosses the wedge-shaped inner boundary, the trial terminates and one reaches the conclusion "do not reject null hypothesis; not statistically significant." One of these conclusions must be reached by the 62nd observation.

The path illustrated in Figure 8.2 is for a clinical trial of antitoxin in the treatment of clinical tetanus [14]. Although treatment for tetanus commonly consisted of antitoxin administration, evidence of its value had never been firmly established. The trial was conducted to answer the question: "Does the mortality rate of patients with tetanus who receive a large dose of antitoxin differ from that of those who receive none?" The ethical rationale for conducting the trial and withholding antitoxin from patients with tetanus is discussed in Chapter 10.

With a fixed sample-size approach, the study would have involved the comparison of two independent proportions, namely, the mortality rates in the antitoxin-treated group versus the control group. For sequential analysis, the analog of the comparison of two independent proportions consists of random pairs of patients, each pair consisting of one antitoxin-treated patient and one control patient. The results are analyzed analogously to the comparison of proportions in a paired sample; tied pairs are discarded and analysis is restricted to a test on a single proportion among the untied pairs (p. 172). The authors state:

Successive patients allocated to the two treatments were regarded as paired (i.e., the first patient receiving antitoxin was paired with the first receiving no antitoxin, and so on). The random allocation was so arranged that in each center the numbers allocated to the two groups were balanced after each 10. The pairing was, however, performed in the order in which the record cards were received by the statistician.

If, for any pair, the patient receiving antitoxin survives whereas the patient receiving no antitoxin dies, a "preference" for antitoxin is recorded; when the patient receiving antitoxin dies and the paired patient receiving no antitoxin survives, the preference is for no antitoxin.

The null hypothesis of equal population mortality rates is equivalent to equal preferences among the untied pairs for antitoxin and no antitoxin, or, the probability is ½ that an untied pair is an antitoxin preference. The alternative hypothesis refers to an antitoxin preference rate of $\pi_1 = .75$ among the untied pairs. If the population mortality rate without antitoxin was 75 percent, it may be derived that an antitoxin preference rate of $\pi_1 = .75$ among the untied pairs means a population mortality rate with antitoxin of 50 percent. Thus, the alternative hypothesis corresponds with an alteration in population mortality from 75 percent without antitoxin to 50 percent with antitoxin therapy.

The path depicted in Figure 8.2 crossed the upper boundary at the 18th untied pair. The path continued beyond the point at which it first crossed the boundary because, at the time of crossing, several patients were already under treatment and their results became available subsequently. Even if the path continued farther and crossed back into the "continue sampling" region, the conclusion would not be altered. The conclusion would still consist of a statistically significant difference in mortality rates. The sequential boundaries are theoretically determined according to the first time the path crosses the boundary. It matters not what direction the path takes once it crosses a boundary.

When the sequential trial was terminated, there were 41 antitoxin-treated patients and 38 patients without antitoxin therapy, making up a total of 79 patients. The 18 untied pairs when the boundary was crossed and the two untied pairs that became available later totaled 20 untied pairs and thus accounted for 40 of the patients. This leaves 39 patients to constitute the discarded tied pairs and the few who remained unpaired at the conclusion of the trial. It may be determined that the analogous fixed sample-size trial comparing two independent proportions would have required approximately 168 total patients (half being treated with antitoxin and half with no antitoxin). Hence, in this trial, sequential analysis also produced a considerable saving in the number of observations. The conclusion was reached with less than half the number of patients required by the analogous fixed sample-size trial.

COMPARISON OF THE AVERAGE NUMBER OF OBSERVATIONS WITH "RESTRICTED" AND "OPEN" SEQUENTIAL TRIALS

For the restricted or closed sequential design, one can also determine the ASN values, i.e., the mean number of observations required to terminate the test. Compared with the open design, the restricted design has about the same ASN when the alternative hypothesis is true and a substantially larger ASN when the null hypothesis is true. This may be deduced from the comparison of Figures 8.2 and 8.1. When the alternative hypothesis is true, most sample paths cross the outer boundaries. Since the open and restricted sequential designs have nearly identical outer boundaries in this situation, their ASN functions are therefore similar. Thus, when the alternative hypothesis is true, restricted and open designs offer about the same advantage in savings of observations. Now, when the null hypothesis is true, most sample paths will cross the inner boundaries. By inspection, it may be seen that a path must travel a substantially longer distance to cross the inner boundaries of the restricted design (Figure 8.2) compared with the open design (Figure 8.1). Thus, when the null hypothesis is true, one pays the price of more observations on the average with the restricted design than with the open design. Since the null hypothesis refers to no difference between the two treatments under consideration, it is not as important to economize on sample size here as it is when there is a real difference between the treatments. Thus, the price of an increase in average sample size when the null hypothesis is true is well worth the advantage in truncation that the restricted design affords.

CRITICISM OF THE SEQUENTIAL APPROACH

Much controversy has arisen concerning sequential analysis, particularly its application to clinical trials. The criticism is of two forms: theoretical objections and practical objections.

Anscombe [1] and Cornfield [23] put forth theoretical objections that focus on the underlying structure of a test of significance, namely, the principle of fixed error levels for null and alternative hypotheses. They claim that this is not the appropriate framework for statistical inference in clinical trials. In one sense, their objections also pertain to the classic fixed sample-size methods of inference expounded in Chapters 4 and 5, since these methods also involve fixed error levels. Sequential analysis, however, depends entirely on this substructure; hence, if the framework crumbles, all of sequential analysis crumbles. The fixed sample-size methods, although vulnerable, are not as fragile. From a pragmatic point of view, the alternative substructure for inference that is proposed by these critics and others remains in a developmental stage. The alternative techniques of analysis are not widely available in a useful form for medical investigators. There have been few instances where they have been applied to real data, and there has been virtually no instance of their application in the field of clinical trials. Controversy still rages among theoretical statisticians concerning the fundamental principles of statistical inference. Clearly, the pursuit of sequential clinical trials in its present format will continue to further knowledge of the comparison of two treatment regimens. In the future, however, the collection and analysis of clinical trial data may be within a quite different statistical framework.

Mainland voices the practical objections to sequential clinical trials [69]. There are many instances when sequential analysis is not feasible. For example, if the time between the initiation of treatment and the response is long, then one can gain little by proceeding sequentially. Likewise, if the trial involves several questions and the analysis of a number of different responses, the time of termination for one response will differ from the times of termination for other responses. Such a multi-faceted trial makes sequential analysis inappropriate. Mainland also discusses other practical difficulties.

The sequential trial has been greatly maligned. This author has not occupied a neutral position and has contributed by coming to the defense of the sequential trial against Mainland's criticisms [19]. In essence, I argued that circumstances exist where sequential trials are feasible and where there is benefit to be gained from the potential savings in observation that they offer. By all means, the investigator should not be daunted from employing sequential analysis in such a situation.

Chapter 9
Longitudinal Studies and the Use of the Life Table

The follow-up of chronic diseases can be among the most difficult of medical investigations. One must wait some time, often a very long time, until some event happens. The maintenance of surveillance on patients within the study group can be extremely costly and time-consuming.

The data collected in a longitudinal study are also complex. They do not readily lend themselves to analysis by the methods described in previous chapters. Simple, intuitive approaches to analysis may lead to serious misrepresentation and misinterpretation. Longitudinal data deserve proper analysis. One such method that applies in a wide variety of situations has come to be known as the *life-table* approach.

To illustrate several conceivable approaches with longitudinal data, an investigation will be considered from the medical literature whose goal was the determination of the prognosis among patients with a particular cardiac disorder. The life-table method is developed with these data.

ILLUSTRATION OF A LONGITUDINAL STUDY

An example perhaps best illustrates the difficulties with longitudinal study data. The data presented here are from a published study, but to avoid possible embarrassment to the author concerning the validity of the analysis he presented, his name and the identification of the particular cardiac disease have been deleted. The data, however, are real and are identical with what was presented in the published report.

The study consisted of the identification of all instances of the disease in question in two hospitals during a 10-year period. Strict, generally accepted criteria for diagnosis of the disease were followed, and 164 patients with the disease were identified. The author states:

The clinical records of these patients were obtained and an attempt to trace the patients was made. Only those patients whose present status could be determined were kept in the study. If the patient had died, the date of death was ascertained. If the patient was still alive at the time the study was completed, this fact was established with certainty. A final group of 146 patients remained after these criteria had been met.

Actually, it would have been better if the 18 excluded patients had been retained for some time in the study, at least for that time that they were known to be alive. These patients could have better been withdrawn from the study at the time that they were lost from observation. Their number is small, however, and the data on the remaining 146 patients well illustrate the methods considered in this chapter.

It is clear that patients entered the study at various times during the 10-year period. At time of termination of the study, some patients had died and some were still alive. Also, at study termination, the patients had been observed for varying lengths of time, the maximum possible time being 10 years.

Table 9.1, which was extracted from the published report, describes the duration of survival separately for those patients who were alive at the completion of study and those who had died sometime before completion of the study. The investigator wished to determine the prognosis from these data; in particular, his concern was with mortality. How might he assemble these data to produce a meaningful figure that summarizes mortality experience? The following section considers several intuitively appealing approaches.

Table 9.1. Duration of survival of patients who were living and who were dead at the completion of a study of prognosis for a particular cardiac disorder

Duration of survival (yr)	Patients living at study completion	Patients dead at study completion
<1	3	27
1–2	10	18
2–3	10	21
3–4	3	9
4–5	3	1
5–6	11	2
6–7	5	3
7–8	8	1
8–9	1	2
9–10	6	2
Total	60	86

SOME ESTIMATES OF MORTALITY

Mean Duration of Survival

The author of the report under consideration had chosen to calculate the mean duration of survival among the living and dead patients. The average duration of survival was 4.7 years for the living patients, 2.4 years for the dead patients, and, for all patients, was 3.3 years. These results were compared with results of a previous study conducted some 15 years earlier in another institution. The author notes:

We were surprised to find that in our cases the average duration of survival ... was actually a few months shorter than that reported in the previously mentioned study done 15 years ago. Although no effort was made to match these two studies in terms of the populations studied or methods of case selection, it was expected that the average duration of survival would be longer in the more recent study because of recent advances in the treatment of heart disease.

It turns out that "average duration" does not adequately represent prognosis. The average duration is most affected by the length of the study, namely, 10 years. The point, discussed later (p. 300), is that the average duration has meaning with regard to mortality only when *all* the study members have died. At the time of study termination, 60 of the 146 patients were still alive. In a subsequent 10 years, some of these 60 would have died, and the average survival at that time would, of course, have increased. In fact, as the length of study observation increases, the average survival will increase until the last of the 60 living patients has died. The mean survival of 3.3 years is exceedingly pessimistic if it is viewed as a summary of survival. The 3.3-year average is properly interpreted only as the average length of *observation* of the 146 patients in the study; it has no meaningful interpretation with regard to survival or prognosis.

Mortality Rate

Clearly, one does not want to wait until all 146 patients die before the prognosis can be determined. This would imply the possibility of the investigation outlasting the investigator. However, meaningful information can be obtained by switching from a quantitative to qualitative approach, i.e., by calculating mortality *rates* instead of the average longevity.

Since 86 deaths were observed among the 146 subjects, one might very simply calculate the mortality rate as $(86/146) 100\% = 58.9\%$. This, too, is a relatively meaningless figure and depends greatly on the duration of the study. If one waits long enough, of course, the mortality rate for any longitudinal study is 100 percent. A mortality rate calculated from a longitudinal study has meaning only when a proper account has been taken of the time involved.

Mortality Rate per Person-Years of Observation

One way of taking time into account is to calculate a mortality rate on the basis of *person-years of observation*. Such a mortality rate has as its numerator the observed number of deaths during the study period and as its denominator the total number of years of observation that all patients, living or dead, have contributed to the study. For example, with the data in Table 9.1 and the use of the midpoints for each of the yearly intervals of observation, the 27 patients who died within their first year of the study, together with the three living patients who had been observed for less than one year, each contributed 0.5 person-years of observation. The 18 deaths between the first and second year, along with the 10 living patients who were observed for only between one and two years, each contributed 1.5 person-years of observation. Thus, the total person-years of observation for the study for all 146 patients is $(27 + 3)(0.5) + (18 + 10)(1.5) + \ldots + (2 + 6)(9.5) = 487.0$. With 86 deaths, the mortality rate is calculated as $86/487 = 0.177$ or 17.7 deaths per 100 person-years of observation.

The determination of a rate on the basis of duration of exposure, as illustrated above, suffices in many situations to provide the requisite summary of results from a longitudinal study. For example, this method was used in summarizing the results of a longitudinal study of smoking and lung cancer (see p. 285). In that study, there were two groups of subjects under observation (smokers and nonsmokers), the study lasted some four and a half years, and the outcome of interest was mortality from lung cancer. There were a total of 98,090 person-years of observation among smokers and 15,107 among non-smokers. The resulting death rates per 1,000 person-years in each group permitted the required estimate of a relative risk of 13 for lung cancer mortality of smokers compared with nonsmokers.

There are, however, two distinct disadvantages with rates calculated on the basis of person-years. First, such a rate represents an average over the entire length of the study period. Thus, for the data on the cardiac disorder, the rate of 17.7 per 100 person-years is the average over the entire 10 years. Often interest focuses on more specific rates, such as the mortality experience during the first few years after entry into the study in contrast with that after several years' anniversary of study entry. The 17.7 per 100 person-years figure indicates merely that over the 10-year span, the rate of deaths averaged 18 percent per year; no information is attainable as to whether the mortality rate was high in the first few years and thereafter leveled off. In this sense, a calculation based on person-years of observation is most appropriate when the rate under consideration remains approximately constant over time.

The second difficulty with rates calculated on a person-years basis pertains to statistical inference. It may be seen that in the calculation of the denominator, 100 person-years of observation are treated identically whether they involve 100 persons followed one year, 50 persons followed two years, or 10 persons followed 10 years. The n in the calculation of such a rate is not apparent. It would be entirely fallacious, with the example under consideration, to apply the methods of Chapter 5 and an n of 487. Clearly, the value of n can be no more than the 146 patients who make up the study group. Thus, the rates calculated on a person-years basis are not amenable to standard statistical inferential techniques. Their proper statistical analysis requires the development of special methods.

As a consequence, the rates calculated on a person-years observation basis have limited applicability in summarizing the prognosis from a longitudinal study. They provide only the crudest summary and they suffer from difficulty in statistical manipulation.

Five-Year Mortality Rate

Suppose now that attention focuses on a mortality rate for a particular fixed time period, say, a five-year mortality rate. Using five years as the critical point in Table 9.1, it may be seen that among the 86 patients who died, 76 died within the first five years of their entry into the study and 10 died sometime after their fifth anniversary of entry to the study. Among the 60 living patients, 31 survived beyond their fifth anniversary of entry, while 29 patients who were alive at study termination had not yet been followed for five years. With these data, how might one calculate a five-year mortality rate?

One might consider that the 76 deaths within the first five years, coupled with the total study group of 146, yield a five-year mortality rate of $(76/146) \ 100\% = 52.1\%$. This rate is unduly optimistic. Of the 146 patients, 29 have not yet reached their fifth anniversary of entry into the study. The rate is optimistic in that it assumes all 29 will survive to their fifth anniversary.

To correct for these 29 patients, one might suggest their deletion from the denominator. This results in a five-year mortality rate of $[76/(146 - 29)] \ 100\% = 65.0\%$. This, on the other hand, is an overly pessimistic rate. The 29 patients are removed entirely and are treated as if they never had been in the study. They have survived for part of the five-year interval under consideration, and the calculation entirely disregards this. Somehow, credit for the amount of time they have survived should enter into the calculation.

The *life-table* approach accounts for the survival of these 29 patients and yields a five-year mortality rate of 58.3 percent. This result is derived from the determination of annual mortality rates during *each* of the five years of study observation, from entry until the fifth anniversary of entry. In other words, the basic ingredients for the life-table calculation are estimates of mortality rates during each of the first, second, third, fourth, and fifth years since entry to the study. The following section discusses the basic model and the essential requirements of a life-table determination; then the life-table calculation is illustrated with the data in Table 9.1 on the 146 patients with the cardiac disorder.

REQUIREMENTS FOR LIFE-TABLE CALCULATIONS

The first requirement for the applicability of a life table is a *clear and well-defined starting point*. The dates of the first diagnosis, the initiation of therapy, and the admission to a hospital are frequently used. One might intuitively feel that the date of onset of the first symptoms represents a more desirable starting point for the determination of prognosis. There are two reasons, however, why the date of onset of symptoms makes a poor starting point. The first concerns the obvious difficulty of objective determination of the date of onset. The date of onset of symptoms relies not only on the subject's ability to recall past events, but also on the skill and thoroughness of the physician in taking a history and in interpreting it in making a diagnosis. Levine called attention to the latter in an editorial for the *Journal of the American Medical Association* entitled "Elusive errors in coronary statistics" [66]:

The duration of life from the onset of symptoms to death from angina pectoris will depend on the accuracy of the medical history and the appraisal of symptoms, inasmuch as the diagnosis can be properly determined in no other way. One physician may estimate the duration of life in a particular case as 7 years, whereas another physician having seen the same patient during these years, may estimate the duration of life as 11 years. The latter physician merely learned that the patient had mild symptoms which did not bother him very much four years earlier than the former physician. One man was a poorer historian, not a poorer therapist than the other.

The second difficulty is rather more subtle, or as Levine puts it, more "elusive." This is that the retrospective determination of the date of onset can entail considerable bias in that it excludes all patients who experienced symptoms and who died or reached their endpoint prior to their seeking medical attention and being properly diagnosed. In this way, by dating a patient's starting point back to onset of symptoms, one produces an overly optimistic appraisal of prognosis. Levine, in the same editorial, states:

> There is still one final error that has been frequently made and is still frequently made. It is so elusive that, although attention was called to it in former publications, it is still overlooked. In estimating the average length of life after a first attack of coronary thrombosis (or myocardial infarction), ... those patients can be included in the study who have been actually seen by the investigator *during* the acute attack and who have survived. Often one reads medical journals that the patients referred to were consecutive and the duration of life was estimated from the first attack, but that they were first seen by the physician three months, three years, or ten years after the first attack. Such patients were given a bonus of months or many years, for, had they died soon after the first attack, they would not have lived long enough to be included in such a study. One needs to repeat that in such an analysis *all* consecutive patients who survive an acute attack under the care of a given physician or in a given clinic must be included, whether they are seen thereafter by the investigator or not. Those who are first seen by the investigator months or years after their first attack cannot be included.

Hence, the dates of diagnosis, hospital admission, initiation of treatment, and so forth, although they may not seem as methodologically desirable as starting points, have the advantage of objectivity and avoid the bias discussed above.

Obviously, a second requirement for a life-table calculation is a *clear and well-defined endpoint*. As the labeling of the method implies, death often represents the endpoint, but it need not be death. Statistically, the only requirements are that the endpoint be a dichotomous variable and that each patient have one and only one endpoint. The latter restriction means that the life table does not allow for multiple endpoint episodes for patients. For example, multiple attacks or episodes of disease, multiple periods of remission and exacerbation, multiple occurrences of lesions, or whatever, do not fit within the life-table format. However, the occurrence of the *first* attack, the *first* episode of a disease, the *first* exacerbation of the disease, or the *first* lesion do meet the requirements and can be utilized in a life-table determination. Three examples within this author's experience of dichotomous life-table outcomes other than death are the occurrence of myxedema among patients treated with radioactive iodine, the occurrence of the first episode of hemorrhage among patients with a particular cardiovascular condition, and the occurrence of *either* death *or* reinfarction among patients with myocardial infarction.

The third essential feature of the life-table format is that *patients enter under observation at different times, and, at study termination, have been observed for different lengths of time.* The left-hand portion of Figure 9.1 indicates the observation pattern over calendar time for five sample patients who might number among the 146 in the study under consideration. Patient *A* entered the study at its very start, was alive at the time of study termination, and had been observed for over 10 years. In contrast, patient *C* entered the study during its

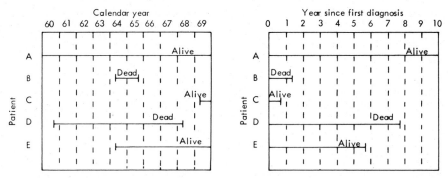

Figure 9.1
Observation patterns for five sample patients in a longitudinal follow-up study of mortality: patterns over calendar time (left) and from time of entry to study (right).

last calendar year, was also alive at the termination date, but had been observed for less than one year. Patient *B* entered the study during its fifth year, died during the study's sixth year, and thereby was observed for less than two years. Patient *D*, on the other hand, entered the study during its first year, died during its ninth year, and was thereby observed for somewhere between seven and eight years.

The fourth distinguishing feature of the life-table format is that *at the time of study termination, the endpoints for some patients are unknown.* This may be for two reasons. First, as illustrated with patients *A*, *C*, and *E* in Figure 9.1, the patients were still under observation and had not yet reached their endpoints at the time of study termination. Second, a patient may be lost to follow-up, e.g., either he moved away, refused to participate any more, or, for one reason or another, could not be traced. Consequently, at study termination the investigator is unaware of whether or not the patient has reached his endpoint. As indicated previously, in the particular study under investigation there were 18 patients who could not be traced and who constitute the losses to follow-up. The investigator chose to exclude them entirely. It would have been preferable to have counted them for the time that they were known to be alive. The losses to follow-up would exhibit an observation pattern similar to that of the deaths (patients *B* and *D*) of Figure 9.1. Instead of labeling their termination in the study as "death," their termination should be labeled "lost to follow-up."

As will be seen later, an assumption is made with regard to those lost to follow-up. As long as the number lost is small, the consequence of the assumption matters little. If, however, there is a considerable number lost to follow-up, then the consequences of the assumption can be important. With a large number lost to follow-up, there is no numerical or mathematical manipulation that can adequately correct for such loss. The results of a life-table determination with large losses to follow-up invite serious questions and may severely misrepresent the situation. For example, if those who are less seriously ill tend to migrate to a more temperate climate, then obviously the determination of the prognosis on the basis of those who remain will result in an overly pessimistic appraisal. On the other hand, if the more seriously ill tend to be referred elsewhere for treatment and thereby become losses to follow-up, then the resulting life-table prognosis on those who stay will be overly optimistic. Good, careful, and complete follow-up represents a prime goal in the conduct of a longitudinal study.

The life table results from the calculation of mortality rates during each of the distinct observation intervals of the study. In the particular example under investigation, the observation intervals were years. Thus, the life table is derived from the calculation of mortality rates during the first year after entry to the trial, between the first and second year after entry, and so on, up to between the ninth and tenth year after entry. Of course, the intervals need not be years, nor need they be equal in width. For example, in an investigation of the prognosis following myocardial infarction, there may be good reason to choose as intervals "under 24 hours," "24 to 48 hours," "48 hours to 1 week," "1 week to 1 month," "1 to 3 months," and so on.

CALCULATION OF LIFE TABLES

As a first step in the preparation of the basic data for entry into the life-table format, the right-hand portion of Figure 9.1 presents the observations on the same five sample patients as in the left-hand portion. The difference between the right and left portions of Figure 9.1 is that the former uses a scale starting at time of entry to the study whereas the latter employs a calendar time scale. In other words, the duration of observation is the same as before (i.e., for each patient, the length of the line in the right-hand portion is identical with that of the left-hand portion), but the observations now commence at the same point, namely, time zero or the date of entry to the study.

Conceptually, the information on each of the 146 patients is obtained in a manner as illustrated in Figure 9.1. The data are then summarized in Table 9.2, which tabulates, for each interval after entry, the number under observation at the beginning of the interval, the number of deaths during the interval, and the number withdrawn alive during the interval. Note that those withdrawn alive comprise two possibilities: those who were withdrawn because the patient was alive and still under observation at termination of study, or those who were withdrawn because the patient was, at that time after entry into the study, lost to follow-up. For example, with the first interval, all 146 patients were, of course, under observation at the time of entry into the study, i.e., at time 0. During the first year, 27 died and 3 were withdrawn alive due to the termination of their observation at study completion. This then leaves $146 - 27 - 3 = 116$ alive and under observation at the beginning of the second interval, namely, the first anniversary of entry to the study. Of these, 18 died and 10 were withdrawn alive sometime between their first and second anniversary dates in the study. This leaves $116 - 18 - 10 = 88$ alive and under observation at their second anniversary of entry to the study. The tabulation proceeds in a similar manner for all 10 years of the study. The

Table 9.2. Rearrangement of data in Table 9.1 to permit calculation of a life table

Year since entry to study x	Alive and under observation at beginning of interval O_x	Deaths during interval d_x	Withdrawn alive during interval w_x
0–1	146	27	3(C)[a]
1–2	116	18(B)[a]	10
2–3	88	21	10
3–4	57	9	3
4–5	45	1	3
5–6	41	2	11(E)[a]
6–7	28	3	5
7–8	20	1(D)[a]	8
8–9	11	2	1
9–10	8	2	6(A)[a]

[a] Letters in parentheses indicate the point at which each of the five sample patients would be counted—see text and Figure 9.1.

letters in parentheses in Table 9.2 indicate where each of the five sample patients in Figure 9.1 would be counted. Note that for the final interval there remain but six patients who were alive and under observation on the 10th anniversary of their entry to the study.

The above summarization lumps patients together regardless of the calendar time in which their observations were obtained. For example, the first-year observations for patients A and E appear together in Table 9.2 despite the fact that, according to the left-hand portion of Figure 9.1, A's first year commenced during the first calendar year of the study whereas E's began during the study's fifth calendar year of operation. Thus, implicit in the life-table determination is the assumption that the rates are independent of calendar time. Patients are grouped together for the calculation of their survival rates regardless of whether their observations were obtained early or late during the time course of the study. In this sense, the life-table method is inappropriate when there have occurred strong secular trends in outcome during the time period the study was in operation.

From Table 9.2, the essence of the calculations is the determination of mortality rates within each of the observation intervals. This would be simple if there were no withdrawals from observation during the interval. One would merely calculate the death rates; the number of deaths during the interval would be the numerator, and the denominator would be the total number alive who were under observation at the start of the interval and at risk of death during the interval. A problem arises, however, with the handling of those who were alive and were withdrawn from the study during the interval. As stated before, an assumption is made concerning them, namely, that they are all withdrawn at precisely the midpoint of the interval of observation, i.e., after half the interval has elapsed. One assumes further that, during the half of the interval that they were not observed, they were subject to half the chance of death for the entire interval. Thus, a death rate is calculated by counting the deaths that actually occurred during the interval and adding an adjustment to them for the deaths expected to occur among those who were withdrawn and for the half of the interval that they were not observed. Thus, for the interval x to $x + 1$, let O_x denote the number under observation at the beginning of the interval, d_x the deaths during the interval, w_x the withdrawals during the interval, and q_x the death rate for the interval. Now, one must add to d_x the expected deaths among the withdrawals for the half of the interval they were not observed, namely, $(w_x)(q_x/2)$. Hence the deaths, with adjustment for withdrawals, are $d_x + (w_x)(q_x/2)$ so that the death rate, q_x, becomes:

$$q_x = \frac{d_x + (w_x)(q_x/2)}{O_x}$$

Solving the above equation for q_x gives

$$q_x = \frac{d_x}{O_x - w_x/2}$$

Thus, for each interval, q_x is determined according to the above formula. The calculations are displayed in Table 9.3.

The q_x values represent the estimated probabilities of death during the intervals. The next column gives their complements, namely, $p_x = 1 - q_x$, or the estimated probabilities of surviving the intervals. It should be noted that these p_x values are interpreted as *conditional* probabilities (see p. 67). Thus, p_x is the estimated chance of surviving the interval x to $x + 1$ provided that the patient has already survived all previous intervals and is alive and under observation at the beginning of the interval.

The cumulative chance of survival is obtained by successive application of the multiplicative law of probability (p. 68). Thus, the chance of surviving one year is $p_x = .8131$. The chance of surviving to the first and then to the second anniversary from entry is $(.8131)(.8378) = .6812$. The chance of then surviving up to the third anniversary is $(.6812)(.7470) = .5089$. This fourth column of Table 9.3, the *cumulative* chance of survival, denoted by P_x, constitutes the life-table function. The cumulative survival to five years is, from the table, $P = .4165$. Thus, the five-year mortality rate previously cited is $1 - .4165 = .5835$.

The survival curve is illustrated by the solid line in Figure 9.2. This graph plots the P_x column as the ordinate against x, the time since entry to study, as the abscissa.

As mentioned before, the author's standard of comparison consisted of a study performed at some other institution about 15 years earlier. The data from the earlier study were also in a format that permitted the calculation of a life table. Furthermore, the earlier study's data were presented with such sufficient detail on age and sex that it was possible to adjust the calculations

Table 9.3. Calculation of the life table and its standard error for the data in Table 9.2

Year since entry to study x	Chance of dying in interval q_x	Chance of surviving interval $p_x = 1 - q_x$	Cumulative chance of surviving P_x	Calculation of standard error of survival curve				
				$O_x - d_x - w_x/2$	$\dfrac{q_x}{O_x - d_x - w_x/2}$	$\sum \dfrac{q_x}{O_x - d_x - w_x/2}$	$\sqrt{\sum \dfrac{q_x}{O_x - d_x - w_x/2}}$	SE(P_x)
0–1	$\dfrac{27}{146 - 3/2} = .1869$	.8131	.8131	117.5	.001591	.001591	.0399	.0324
1–2	$\dfrac{18}{116 - 10/2} = .1622$	.8378	(.8131)(.8378) = .6812	93	.001744	.003335	.0577	.0393
2–3	$\dfrac{21}{88 - 10/2} = .2530$	.7470	(.6812)(.7470) = .5089	62	.004081	.007416	.0861	.0438
3–4	$\dfrac{9}{57 - 3/2} = .1622$	.8378	(.5089)(.8378) = .4263	46.5	.003488	.010904	.1044	.0445
4–5	$\dfrac{1}{45 - 3/2} = .0230$	.9770	(.4263)(.9770) = .4165	42.5	.000541	.011445	.1070	.0446
5–6	$\dfrac{2}{41 - 11/2} = .0563$	.9437	(.4165)(.9437) = .3931	33.5	.001681	.013126	.1146	.0450
6–7	$\dfrac{3}{28 - 5/2} = .1176$	.8824	(.3931)(.8824) = .3468	22.5	.005227	.018353	.1355	.0470
7–8	$\dfrac{1}{20 - 8/2} = .0625$	.9375	(.3468)(.9375) = .3252	15	.004167	.022520	.1501	.0488
8–9	$\dfrac{2}{11 - 1/2} = .1905$	.8095	(.3252)(.8095) = .2632	8.5	.022412	.044932	.2120	.0558
9–10	$\dfrac{2}{8 - 6/2} = .4000$	.6000	(.2632)(.6000) = .1579	3	.133333	.178265	.4222	.0667

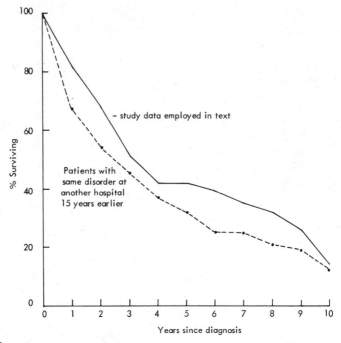

Figure 9.2
Survival curves for prognosis following a particular cardiovascular disorder: results of the life-table calculation in Table 9.3 compared with an analogous life-table determination for patients with the same disorder in another hospital 15 years earlier.

to account for age and sex differentials between the two study groups. The resulting life-table function for this previous study, with adjustment for age and sex, is shown by the broken line in Figure 9.2. It may be seen that the percent survival in the present study is *higher* than that of the previous study at each year following entry to study. This is contrary to the author's conclusion cited on page 238. With the survival rates summarized by an appropriate life-table determination, one can see that the prognosis had definitely improved in the 15-year interval between the two studies, which was what the investigator had initially conjectured.

STATISTICAL INFERENCE WITH LIFE-TABLE VALUES

It should be noted that the P_x values that make up the life table are determinations calculated from a sample of patients. As such, they fall under the concepts of such sample properties as the mean, standard deviation proportion, regression slope, or correlation coefficient, which were discussed in previous chapters. Therefore, the concept of sampling distributions becomes appropriate, and interest may focus on the determination of a standard error on the P_x quantities.

The rationale of the standard error attached to the life-table functions is beyond the scope of this text. An approximate formula for the standard error was proposed by Greenwood [48] and is given as:

$$SE(P_x) = P_x \sqrt{\Sigma \frac{d_x}{(O_x - w_x/2)(O_x - d_x - w_x/2)}} = P_x \sqrt{\Sigma[q_x/(O_x - d_x - w_x/2)]}$$

The last five columns of Table 9.3 illustrate the use of this formula in the calculation of the standard error for the life table. One may consider the P_x values and their respective standard errors as being approximately normally distributed. One can then perform tests of significance or calculate confidence limits on the life-table values. A comparison of two study groups—one that yields a life table with values P_x and the other with corresponding values P'_x— may be achieved by calculating

$$z = \frac{P_x - P'_x}{\sqrt{[SE(P_x)]^2 + [SE(P'_x)]^2}}$$

and referring to the tables of the normal distribution (Appendix Tables A1 and A2). As an example, Harvald et al. presented the results of a clinical trial wherein life tables were calculated and compared for patients with myocardial infarction who were randomly assigned to receive long-term anticoagulant therapy or placebo therapy [54].

Another possibility for analysis of life-table data, especially in studies of prognosis, is the comparison of the life table for a sample of patients with some particular disease with the published mortality tables for the general population. These comparisons are often presented by displaying on a single graph the life table for the study group together with a curve that represents the corresponding survival experience in the general population for a group of individuals who have the same sex and age distribution as the patients. The distance between the two curves (almost invariably, the survival curve for the sample of patients with the disease falls below that for the general population) represents the increase in mortality that can be attributed to the disease. In other words, the distance between the two curves indicates the excess mortality caused by the disease, i.e., that mortality which is above and beyond the natural mortality in the general population. The survival experience of the general population is garnered from population life tables such as those presented in Table 2.18.

EXERCISE

A study of prognosis among patients having cardiac allografts is described elsewhere in the text (p. 302). This study compared the survival patterns of 15 patients having cardiac allografts with 42 potential allograft recipients who could not have a transplant because of the lack of a comparable donor. The table presented here gives the distribution of the months of observation among the survivors and the deaths in the potential recipient and the transplant groups. Of the two sets of data for the transplant patients, one includes and the other excludes the waiting time between the patients' candidacy for transplantation and the time when the transplant was actually performed (see the discussion on p. 302).

Months of observation	42 Potential recipients		15 Transplant patients			
			Including waiting time		Excluding waiting time	
	Survivors	Deaths	Survivors	Deaths	Survivors	Deaths
>1	2	19	–	3	–	5
1–2	1	4	–	2	–	2
2–3	–	2	–	2	–	1
3–4	2	2	–	1	1	–
4–5	1	–	–	1	–	3
5–6	2	–	–	2	–	1
6–7	2	–	1	2	–	1
7–8	4	–	–	–	1	–
8–9	1	–	1	–	–	–
Total	15	27	2	13	2	13

For each of the three sets of data (i.e., potential recipients and transplant patients including and excluding waiting time):

A. Calculate the death rate per person-months of observation. How do the three rates compare?

B. Arrange the observations into a proper tabular format and calculate a life table. Graph the three life tables computed. How do the three survival curves compare?

C. For comparison with the potential recipients, which set of data is more appropriate in the transplant group: with inclusion or with exclusion of waiting time? Why?

D. Before performing and interpreting any tests of significance to compare the prognoses in the two groups, what other factors in the two groups might you want to investigate?

PART III
STATISTICS IN MEDICAL
RESEARCH

Chapter 10
Clinical Trials

Much reference has been made in this text to the evaluation of new drugs or of new medical and surgical procedures. This chapter concerns the principles underlying such experiments. Since these experiments involve human beings as subjects, important ethical questions emerge. Consequently, part of the discussion focuses on aspects of medical ethics. The intent is to elucidate the vital issues, to raise the several pertinent ethical questions, and to cite, from a variety of sources, the views of several experts in the field of clinical trials. By no means is the discussion intended to provide a comprehensive summary of the state of the art of clinical trials or to expound this author's viewpoints. The text, I hope, provides sufficient signposts so that the interested reader can delve further into the literature in this wide and rather controversial field. The methodology and a detailed discussion will be provided for the most common clinical trial format: the comparison of two groups.

EXPLANATION OF THE DIFFERENCE BETWEEN TREATMENT AND CONTROL OBSERVATIONS

The evaluation of a new drug or a new medical or surgical procedure involves the comparison of two series of observations: one series is obtained with the use of the new drug or procedure; the other is a control series that is obtained without its use, though perhaps it may be obtained with the use of some standard therapeutic agent or regimen. For the present discussion, it matters not whether the observations are derived from paired or independent samples or whether they pertain to a nominal or a numerical continuous scale of measurement. Explanations of an observed difference between the treated and control series fall within one or more of the following categories:

1. Sampling variation or chance
2. Inherent differences between the treatment and control groups
3. Differences in the handling and evaluation of the treatment and control groups during the course of the investigation
4. The true effects of the new procedure

Category 1—sampling variation or chance—constitutes the main focus of this book. This is the sole concern of the test of significance. A statistically significant result rules out this category as a likely explanation of the difference. Of course, this process assumes that the correct test was employed and that the arithmetic was without error. All too often data are incorrectly analyzed, for example, when paired data are treated as independent samples. One might be surprised at how frequently, even with employment of the correct test, there is an error in arithmetic in published results. These may seem to be rather trivial points, but they do occur in the medical literature and the reader should be aware that they exist.

Of course, the goal of a comparison is to obtain an explanation in terms of Category 4, i.e., the true effect of the new procedure. With the elimination of sampling variation by the deployment of methods of statistical inference, the problem is how does one eliminate, beyond reasonable doubt, Categories 2 and 3 as explanations? As a first step in solving this problem, it is advantageous to indicate, using examples, precisely what is meant by Categories 2 and 3.

Regarding Category 2—inherent differences between the two groups—consider the following situation for comparing a proposed new surgical treatment as opposed to the traditional medical treatment for a particular disease. The operation is introduced and performed by a number of surgeons. After some experience, an investigator collects observations on the patients who were operated on, along with observations among patients who had received the traditional medical treatment. The investigator then compares statistically the results from surgically versus medically treated patients. With the ad hoc usage of the surgical treatment, however, one might reasonably expect that the better operative risks became candidates for the surgical procedure. The poorer risk patients tended to undergo the traditional medical treatment. Thus, the two groups were inherently different at the start. The operation may offer no improvement whatsoever, but the fact that the surgical patients were initially better risks as compared with the medical patients could explain the statistically significant results that indicated the superiority of surgery.

To illustrate Category 3—the differences in the handling of the groups during the course of an investigation—the following situation is provided. In the test of a new medical procedure, those treated undergo frequent evaluations and are monitored rather carefully in the hospital during treatment in order to avoid possible untoward reactions. Suppose there is no specific control treatment and those patients in the control group are sent home, perhaps with a prescription for extended bed rest, and with some casual follow-up to determine their status at the conclusion of the investigation. Consequently, the group undergoing the new procedure receives much more intensive ancillary medical care than the control group. A statistically significant result favoring the new treatment might be explained entirely by the more intensive, supportive care and attention these patients received as opposed to the control patients.

Note that, in each of these two situations, it was not claimed that the bias definitely existed. The statements were worded to suggest that these biases *could* have occurred. In criticizing a medical report in the literature, the reader or critic need not prove bias. It is sufficient for him to argue persuasively enough to raise serious doubt. It is the onus of the author to design his investigation and to report his results in a manner that accounts for any such doubts.

DEFINITION OF THE CONTROLLED CLINICAL TRIAL AND ITS HISTORY

How, then, does one eliminate Categories 2 and 3, beyond reasonable doubt, as explanations? The answer is found in the use of the *controlled clinical trial.* A scientifically ideal controlled clinical trial is one in which the two series, under simultaneous investigation, are as alike as possible in every respect except that in one series, the patients receive the new drug or procedure, while in the other, they receive the control drug or procedure. The phrase "as alike as possible" means that these conditions are to be maintained both at the outset and during the course of the investigation.

Of course, this scientific ideal is rarely, if ever, achieved. Since clinical trials deal with the medical treatment of human beings, one must often sacrifice what is scientifically ideal for what is possible ethically and what, in the most practical sense, is feasible. The ethics and practical aspects of clinical trials will be discussed at greater length later in this chapter.

Another point to note in the definition is the word "simultaneous." In other words, the clinical trial is based upon concurrent controls. An example of the use of historical controls has already been discussed (see p. 119). Historical controls, i.e., past data on the "old" used as a standard of comparison for present data on the "new," are unsatisfactory. The patients may have changed over time, other factors connected with the treatment may have changed, or even the nature of the disease may have changed.

To those with background and experience in science, the principle of the controlled clinical trial may seem obvious and rather unexciting. Yet, historically, the controlled clinical trial is relatively new to the field of medical research. Atkins [4] states:

Before the last war the controlled clinical trial was virtually unknown. It would of course be absurd not to admit that immense advances in therapeutic knowledge were made before 1945, but if we look at these critically we are bound to observe that the therapeutic measures which have stood the test of time, both medical and surgical, were discovered at infrequent intervals and were in what we might term the Nobel Prize class. I refer to such discoveries as lime-juice in the treatment of scurvy, quinine for malaria, salvarsan for syphilis, Prontosil and the sulphonamide group of drugs, and penicillin. Each of these discoveries led to results so striking and so undeniable that no clinical trial was necessary to establish them firmly as therapeutic agents of the first magnitude. Advances in clinical knowledge, however, cannot afford to wait for these rare mutations in human knowledge. Moreover, if we turn to surgery we find that the impetus for surgical advance up to 1945 came essentially from advances in the contingent fields of bacteriology, anaesthesia, and physiology; advances which were self-evident and led at once to achievements of great importance in surgery itself.

Atkins proceeds to describe a number of what today are deemed horrifying procedures that, in the past, were performed under the guise of surgery and had become established in medical practice on an uncontrolled basis. Atkins continues:

What a chapter of unnecessary misery and occasional tragedy the relation of these matters unfolds. One would like to be able to say that things of this sort no longer occur. Unfortunately, this is not true, but it is true to say that they are becoming less and less common, that the advocacy of a therapeutic measure depends now, not on the force of personality, the standing in the profession, or the "mellifluidity" of the protagonist, but on more soundly based scientific evidence, and the tool for the forging of this evidence is the controlled clinical trial.

There is some controversy as to precisely what study constitutes the first controlled clinical trial. In essence, the general statistical principles of experimental design were first enunciated by the renowned scientist R. A. Fisher [40]. The thrust of Fisher's work, however, pertained to research in agriculture and the biological laboratory. With regard to medicine, the British Medical Research Council (MRC) trial of streptomycin in the treatment of tuberculosis [76] is recognized by many as an important milestone in the development of the controlled clinical trial. (The data shown in Table 2.3 came from this study.) It certainly was the one study that produced wide recognition for the controlled clinical trial as a device for the sound, scientific investigation of the therapeutic effect of a new agent. It has been argued [26] that prior to the MRC trial of streptomycin for tuberculosis there were several published investigations that met all the requirements for what today has become known as the controlled clinical trial. However, these studies have not received widespread recognition.

OTHER UNSATISFACTORY COMPARISONS

In setting up the treatment and control series, some intuitively appealing procedures consist of the comparison of volunteers for treatment with those who do not volunteer or the comparison of patients of physicians (or in hospitals) that employ the new treatment with patients on whom the treatment has not been employed. With regard to volunteers versus nonvolunteers, Hill has stated the case against this type of comparison rather eloquently [56]:

Another very frequent source of error in the assessment of a vaccine lies in the comparison of persons who volunteer, or choose, to be inoculated (or volunteer on behalf of their children) with those who do not volunteer or choose. The volunteers may tend to come from a different age group and thus, on the average, to be older or younger; they may tend to include more—or fewer—males than females; they may tend to be drawn more from one social class than another. Thus, in the early days of vaccination against poliomyelitis one survey in the U.S.A. showed that the vaccinated children came more from the white families, more from mothers with a high standard of education behind them, and more from fathers in the "white collar" and relatively well-paid occupations. Given adequate records these, and similar easily defined characteristics, can be identified. The comparisons of the inoculated and uninoculated can then be made within like categories. But far more subtle and undetectable differences may well be involved. The volunteers for inoculation may be persons more careful of their health, more aware of the presence of an epidemic in the community. They may on such occasions take other steps to avoid infection, e.g. the avoidance of crowded transport or cinemas. It may (as in the example quoted above) be the more intelligent mothers who bring their children to be inoculated; and more intelligent mothers may also endeavour to protect their children from infection in other ways. They may too, perhaps, have small families so that the inoculated child is automatically less exposed to infection from siblings. Thus in one pioneer trial of vaccines against whooping cough it was found that 47 per cent. of the inoculated children were only children, i.e. with no sibs, compared with only 20 per cent. of the control children.

Lastly, with diseases that do not have a uniform incidence and do not themselves confer a lasting immunity, e.g. influenza and the common cold, there may well be in the act of volunteering a grave element of self-selection. Persons who rarely suffer from such minor illnesses are unlikely to volunteer, those who are constantly troubled by them may well seek relief through inoculation. In other words, self-selection may tend to bring the susceptibles in the inoculated class and leave the resistants as "controls." The comparison is, then, valueless. We are not comparing like with like. Such dangers are not imaginary; they have been demonstrated often in carefully documented trials.

Similar arguments pertain to the comparisons of patients in different hospitals or of different physicians. The types of patients may differ, the supportive and ancillary care may differ, and the quality of the hospital or the skills of the physician may differ. These all tend to throw serious doubts on comparisons made on this basis.

RANDOMIZATION

In dealing with Category 2, "randomization" represents the one-word answer for the question of ensuring that the control and treated groups are alike at the start of the investigation. *Randomization* means that patients are allocated to the treatment and control groups by chance.

It is worthwhile to point out that one should not confuse randomization or random assignment with haphazard assignment. Random assignment follows a predetermined plan that is usually devised with the aid of a table of random numbers. The pattern of assignment to treatment may appear to be haphazard, but this arises from the haphazard nature with which digits appear in a table of random numbers, and not the haphazard whim of the investigator in allocating patients.

Randomization ensures that the personal judgment and prejudices of the investigator and of the patient do not influence treatment allocation. In the instance cited earlier of evaluation of a new surgical treatment, randomization tends to protect against the surgical group being overloaded with the good operative risks.

Note that the effects of randomization were cautiously worded with the qualification "tends to." Randomization achieves a balance in the long run. However, with a small series of patients, randomization may not always produce groups that are alike in every respect. In any randomized clinical trial, it is wise to compare the relevant characteristics of the treatment and control groups subsequent to randomization in order to ascertain that balance was achieved. In fact, as a general rule, a report of a clinical trial should include among its first tables one in which the treatment and control groups are compared on the several important characteristics relating to the disease under study. With virtually every disease, such a tabulation should involve, at the very least, a comparison of the sex and age distribution.

As an example, Brown et al. reported the results of a clinical trial of antitoxin versus no antitoxin in the treatment of clinical tetanus [14] (see also p. 234). Table 10.1, taken from this report, indicates the comparison of treatment and control groups with regard to the factors relevant to the disease. Note that the treatment and control patients differed slightly in their severity on admission. The analysis of the data took this discrepancy into account, and appropriate adjustments were made to correct for the severity differential. The major point, however, is that Table 10.1 enables the reader to judge for himself the comparability of the groups.

This text does not detail the procedures one would employ in using a table of random numbers to achieve a random assignment scheme to treatment and control groups. One should note, however, that the use of tables of random

Table 10.1. Comparison of characteristics of treatment group (antitoxin) and control group (no antitoxin) in a controlled clinical trial of treatment for clinical tetanus

Characteristic	Antitoxin group	No antitoxin group
Total cases	41	38
Locality and race:		
Nigeria; Black	35	32
West Indies		
Black	5	3
Others	1	3
Sex:		
Male	23	21
Female	18	17
Mean values:		
Age (yr)	24.8	27.1
Incubation period (days)	10.1 (26 cases)	9.7 (29 cases)
Period of onset (days)	3.0 (33 cases)	3.2 (34 cases)
Intercurrent disease or complications:		
None	18	15
Pulmonary infection	5	10
Hyperpyrexia	6	7
Laryngospasm	1	2
Postpartum	6	5
Miscellaneous	12	6
Severity on admission:		
Local	0	2
General		
Mild	9	4
Moderate	12	9
Severe	10	23
Site of wound:		
Limbs	22	22
Head and neck	1	1
Trunk	1	1
Genital tract	6	5
Not known	11	9
Sepsis (excluding postpartum cases):		
Present	10	8
Absent	25	25

Data from Brown et al. [14].

numbers entails a certain degree of care and attention. It is well worth the effort to take such care and ensure that the tables are used properly and efficiently. Most often, the investigator will wish to achieve randomization with *balance*. That is, after so many allocations (for example, every four), there are equal numbers assigned to each group (for example, two to treatment and two to the control). The interested reader may consult Armitage's text [2] for the details of methods of random assignment.

There are several intuitively appealing alternatives to the use of random numbers. These appear simple and, on the surface, seem to simulate random assignment. Experience has shown, however, that they are fraught with dangers of bias. One such assignment method is the use of alternate cases. As individuals become eligible for inclusion in a trial, one is assigned to the treatment group, the next to the control group, and so on, in a strictly alternate fashion. In many circumstances, the "alternate case" method will simulate random assignment. It does, however, allow for personal bias and selection to enter. The resulting shadow of a doubt can cripple and destroy the credibility of a clinical trial.

For example, one of the early trials of anticoagulants in the treatment of myocardial infarction employed a slight variation on the alternate case method. Patients who were admitted to hospital on odd days of the month received anticoagulants, and those who were admitted on even days were assigned to the control group, which received no anticoagulants. The assignment scheme resulted in a gross imbalance in the numbers of patients in each group with many more in the anticoagulant group, more so than could be accounted for by the fact that several months have more odd than even days. This led to the suspicion that random assignment was not being achieved. It appeared that some physicians preferred the anticoagulant treatment for their patients. If he knew of the alternate-day assignment scheme, a physician could arrange for the admission of his patient to the trial on a day on which the patient would receive assignment to the treatment group the physician preferred for him. The tendency was for admission on days that placed patients in the anticoagulant-treatment group. Thus, the physician, not chance, influenced assignment to treatment group, so serious doubt arose concerning the comparability of the two groups of patients and consequently the validity of the results.

As another example, Mahon and Daniels refer to a clinical trial of the antiinflammatory effect of the drug oxyphenbutazone among postoperative obstetrical and gynecological patients [68]. Rather than using strict random assignment, the scheme called for the use of the drug among patients on one side of a ward, while the control group consisted of patients on the other side. The results revealed that there were 148 patients in the drug-treated group and 87 in the control group. If strict randomization had been followed, one would have expected half of the total of 235 patients to be in the drug-treated group. The assignment to groups clearly falls short of being random and here, too, the results of the study become suspect.

Another example is the clinical trial of propranolol in the treatment of the acute phase of myocardial infarction as reported by Snow [102] and used previously in this text to illustrate the comparison of two independent proportions (Example 5.8). Snow used alternate assignment to the propranolol-treated and control groups. Hamilton, in a letter to the editor of *The Lancet*, stated [51]:

Since Dr. Snow knew what treatment his patients were going to receive, bias may have occurred in the selection of cases for inclusion in the trial; and it is also possible, though not so likely, that bias may have arisen in rejecting them for the trial after investigation.

Snow and Clarke, on the defensive, replied [103]:

We are well aware of the need to avoid the bias which Professor Hamilton suggests may have arisen in the admission of patients to the trial because it was known what treatment they would receive. We do not agree that this knowledge could have influenced selection, since it is quite impossible to regulate the inflow of good-risk or bad-risk patients; all were admitted as urgencies and not from the waiting list. A difficulty might have arisen in the unlikely event of two patients being admitted simultaneously, but in fact this never happened. Moreover, the admission of patients was made by the medical officer on duty, who had no other connection with the trial.

Finally, in another letter to *The Lancet* editor, Rossiter stated [93]:

Had Dr. Snow allocated his patients at random to the two groups, the only possible explanation would have been an effect of propranolol in reducing mortality. But Dr. Snow allocated alternate patients to the two groups; so another explanation is that the alternate patients differed consistently. If the allocation was strictly controlled, as Dr. Snow emphasizes, and if there was no possibility, for example, of an assistant or nurse altering the order for any reason, then it is hard to imagine how this particular allocation could have had more than a slight effect on the difference found between the death rates. This is not to say that alternate allocation can take the place of randomization. Had randomization been used, then this doubt about Dr. Snow's results would not exist.

Clearly, randomization could have been employed in this trial without difficulty, and its use would have prevented the above criticisms. The investigator would not have needed to rally to the defense of his allocation procedure. (Further aspects of Snow's study are discussed later in this section.)

Other suggested possibilities for the random assignment to groups include the tossing of a coin or the drawing of a slip of paper from a hat or bowl. Aside from the effect such procedures might have on the doctor-patient relationship, they open up many possibilities for the physician to exercise personal bias and judgment in his assignment of patients to groups.

If one is going to randomize, one should do so correctly. Randomization is not that difficult to achieve. Without proper randomization, the investigator is immediately on the defensive and increases his vulnerability to the critical onslaught of his peers. One method that has been proved effective is the use of sealed, serially numbered opaque envelopes. As patients meet the appropriate criteria and and become eligible for entry into the trial, the next in a pile of sealed, serially numbered opaque envelopes is opened. Inside is a card that indicates whether the patient is assigned to the treatment or control group. The ordering of the cards within the envelopes is determined from a table of random numbers.

In drug trials, hospital pharmacies often aid in the conduct of randomized clinical trials. Provided with a master list of study numbers and random number assignments, the pharmacy will prepare and store numbered packets of the indicated drugs. As patients enter the trial and receive medication, the pharmacy takes the next numbered packet in the series. When additional medication is needed, an appropriate mechanism is established to ascertain that the patient receives his same medication.

The above discussion refers to the independent-samples situation. What does randomization entail with paired samples? For a self-pairing situation, randomization applies to the order in which patients receive the drugs under study. With two drugs, *A* and *B*, it means random assignment to receive the drugs in the order *AB* or *BA*. As indicated before (p. 136), such an experimental plan is called a *cross-over design*.

When the investigator forms matched pairs of subjects, randomization means the assignment of the two members of the pair at random to each of the treatment and control procedures under study.

A situation intermediate between paired and independent samples involves *stratified randomization*. In this situation, strata or groups are formed and randomization occurs separately for the subjects in each stratum. As patients become eligible for inclusion in the trial, their appropriate stratum is determined and they receive the next random-number assignment within that stratum. Cooperative clinical trials that involve the joint participation of several institutions in different localities usually involve some form of stratified randomization when they employ separate randomization plans with balanced numbers at each institution; in other words, the localities are the strata. McKissock et al. reported a clinical trial of posterior communicating aneurysms that utilized stratified randomization [75]. Patients, as they entered the trial, were classified according to their hypertensive status (hypertensive or normotensive), age (50 and under or over 50), and operative risk (good or poor), yielding a total of eight strata. Within each stratum, patients were randomly assigned with their numbers balanced to the two treatments under study.

Stratified randomization has the advantage of assuring balance between the two groups, at least on the characteristics that determine the strata. In the aneurysm trial described, the investigator had assurance that the two groups of patients were balanced with respect to hypertensive status, age, and operative risk. Had stratification not been employed, he would have run the risk that chance might produce imbalance with regard to these important factors, especially if the number of subjects in the trial was small. The disadvantage with stratified randomization is that it is administratively difficult and cumbersome to execute. In many cases, the extra assurance of balance with stratified randomization is simply not worth the effort.

In this discussion of randomization, it is worth mentioning that a confusion often exists in the use of the phrases "random assignment" and "random selection." Strictly speaking, this section deals with random assignment, namely, the process by which subjects are assigned to treatment groups in an experiment. Random selection pertains more to surveys and refers to the process whereby a sample of subjects is selected at random from a larger population. Clinical trials rarely entail random selection; the investigator takes the patients available to him for study, provided they meet the criteria for entry into the trial. Random assignment, however, as this section has emphasized, constitutes a fundamental principle on which the controlled clinical trial is based.

A further advantage of random assignment or allocation in an experiment is that the process of statistical inference (e.g., the conduct of a test of significance or the determination of confidence limits) need no longer depend on the supposition that one simulates random selection from some larger underlying population. Consider, for example, the comparison of two groups in independent samples where there are n_T sample observations in one group and n_C in the other and where the assignment to each group was strictly on a random basis. Conceptually, one may view the particular two samples at hand as being one of the many possible outcomes resulting from the random assignment of a total of $n_T + n_C$ observations into one group of n_T and another of n_C.

For instance, with the random assignment of 20 observations into two groups of 10 each, one views the result as one outcome from the 184,754 possible ways of splitting 20 observations into two groups of 10 each. The total of 184,754 possible outcomes then becomes the underlying population. For a test of significance in comparing the means or proportions in the two groups, one asks, under the null hypothesis, how often among the 184,754 possible outcomes would one find a difference as large as or larger than that observed? As before, if this probability is less than the predetermined significance level, the conclusion is that observed results are unlikely to be explained by chance. Thus, the fact that one group received treatment while the other served as a control would appear to make a difference. In other words, what was observed could not be explained as a chance event that resulted from the random assignment of 20 into two groups of 10. Note that the inference in this situation pertains only to the particular experiment at hand.

According to such reasoning, it is not necessary to assume that each group of 10 simulated a random sample from some larger treatment and control populations. In essence, random assignment alone provides a sufficient rationale to conduct and interpret a test of significance in a comparative experiment.

However, any interpretation that involves referring the findings to a larger target population involves issues of representativeness, bias, and simulation of random selection as discussed on pages 4 to 7 and 119 to 120.

BLIND TECHNIQUES AND PLACEBOS

Blind techniques and placebos provide the means for eliminating factors unintentionally associated with treatment (Category 3). In a *single-blind trial,* the patient is unaware of whether he is in the treatment or control group; in a *double-blind trial,* both the patient and the physician are unaware of who is assigned to each group.

Obviously, the intent of blind procedures is to eliminate the biases and prejudices of the patient or of both the patient and the physician. With regard to the physician, this means not only protection against his favoritism for the drug, but protection against his providing a more favorable assessment in the control group. A physician, in trying to be fair in his assessment of a new drug or procedure in which he himself has some interest, may bend over backward and tend to give more of the benefit of a doubt to patients in the control group. The double-blind study protects against his being overly prejudicial in either a positive or negative fashion. With regard to the patient, the blind study protects against his saying what he believes will please—or, in this day and age, what will displease—the physician.

When there is no standard drug to be used in a blind or double-blind manner for comparison with the new drug, placebos are employed. Translated literally from Latin, *placebo* means "I will please." It is interesting to note how the dictionary definition of *placebo* has changed over time. In 1947, *Dorland's Illustrated Medical Dictionary* [32] defined it as: "A make-believe medicine given to please or gratify the patient." The 1965 edition [31] defined it as: "An inactive substance or preparation, formerly given to please or gratify a patient, now also used in controlled studies to determine the efficacy of medicinal substances." Some might consider this definition to be rather narrow. There need be no restriction to "medicinal substances."* One might consider placebo medical procedures or even placebo surgery. Initially, the possibility of placebo or sham surgery on human subjects may sound horrifying to many individuals, yet such studies are conducted. This point is later discussed in the section dealing with ethical issues, where the ethical rationale for placebo surgery is set forth.

As an example of an extensive and somewhat complex placebo procedure, Ruffin et al. present the results of a double-blind clinical trial of gastric freezing of ulcers [94]. Patients in the "freeze" and control groups were prepared in an identical manner. They were both intubated. The authors state:

An attempt was made to have every aspect of the sham gastric "freeze" identical to the true "freeze" with the one exception of the temperature of the coolant circulating in the balloon. Thus, the exact procedure as described for gastric "freezing"—preparation of patient, volume of coolant in gastric balloon, duration of procedure and monitoring—was followed.

To accomplish the sham "freeze", a tube assembly was constructed to look exactly like the one used in the true "freeze". However, the assembly used in the sham procedure had a shunt proximal to the gastric balloon at 30 cm from the incisors, so that the coolant from the refrigerating unit was circulated only in the proximal part of the tube. Thus, in both procedures, the tube became frosted, and the patient felt a cold tube in the mouth, pharynx and upper esophagus. In the sham procedure, two small auxiliary tubes permitted the balloon to be filled and circulated with tap water at 37° by an auxiliary pump and filling apparatus mounted permanently on the Swenko hypothermia machine.

It is interesting to note that this study also employed the "sealed envelope" technique. When the patient was prepared for the procedure, the next numbered envelope was opened and the card inside indicated whether he would receive a true ($-10°C$) or sham ($37°C$) "freeze." Of course, the physician who administered the "freeze" knew whether it was real or sham. The study was double-blind in that another physician, unaware of which procedure had been employed, performed the follow-up evaluation of patients.

Clearly, not all clinical trials can be double-blind. Obviously, with many procedures, such as a radical mastectomy, double-blind trials are impossible. In other situations, although a double-blind trial may be theoretically possible,

* The recently published 1974 edition [31a] adds "Also a procedure with no intrinsic therapeutic value, performed for such purposes."

it is not feasible to plan a trial with this degree of control. The need for a double-blind trial depends on the nature of the response used to assess the results. The more subjective the outcome may be, the greater is the rationale for a double-blind trial. For example, if one deals with extremely subjective responses—such as the relief of angina symptoms, an effect on tension, anxiety, or mental status, headache relief, the relief of pain, or the arrest of hayfever or allergic symptoms—then the tighter control of the double-blind study can become extremely important. When the outcome of a trial is more objective—for example, life or death, or perhaps the level of some substance in the blood or urine—then there is less call for the exactitude of the double-blind trial. However, even with as objective an outcome as life or death, some might argue that failure to perform a double-blind trial may suggest the possibility of bias. Clearly, the argument is not as cogent as it is when dealing with subjective phenomena such as those mentioned above.

In today's world of medical research, the randomized, double-blind, controlled clinical trial maintains a secure and respected position. If two investigators each perform a controlled clinical trial testing the same drug in a similar manner except that one employs a double-blind experimental design whereas the other does not, and if they arrive at opposite conclusions, greater credence attaches to the results of the investigator who employs the double-blind technique.

Snow's previously mentioned trial of propranolol treatment in myocardial infarction may serve as a case in point [102]. Mention has already been made of the trial's lack of random assignment to the propranolol-treated and control groups. In addition, the trial was not double-blind. There were three subsequent trials of propranolol treatment in myocardial infarction, all of which employed random assignment to treatment groups [5, 17, 105]. Furthermore, two of these additional trials employed double-blind techniques as well. In none of the three subsequent trials could a difference in mortality rates be detected. Also, the doses used were not the same as Snow's. The editor of *The Lancet* commented on the comparison of Balcon's and Clausen's results with those of Snow [34]:

The discrepancy between these results and Snow's is hard to explain. Balcon et al. suggest that the design of the trials was responsible, since Snow did not use random allocation or double-blind administration of tablets. Moreover, the doses of propranolol were different. But Clausen et al. did not apparently use a double-blind method, and their dose of propranolol was lower than that of Snow, while that used by Balcon et al. was higher; so it is difficult to explain the discrepancy on this basis.

In the light of the information now available on the action of propranolol on the myocardium and coronary circulation and the results of these two trials, there seems to be no indication for its routine use in acute myocardial infarction.

Thus, the lack of a double-blind technique represents another vulnerable facet of Snow's study when compared with these other experiments.

ETHICAL ISSUES

Several key ethical issues arise within the context of the clinical trial as an experiment on human beings. This section purports to list these questions and their answers, thereby providing the rationale for the controlled clinical trial.

1. *Is it ethical to have a control group? Can a potentially beneficial drug or treatment be withheld from a patient who might derive some value from its use?*

Clinical investigators answer with a qualified "yes." Their rationale is that if the state of scientific knowledge is such that the investigator does not know whether the drug or treatment is of value, then it is ethical for him to perform a controlled trial and to allocate patients at random to the treatment and control groups. If he believes that the treatment *is* of value, then it is unethical for him to participate in a controlled trial. Of course, this is often not a clear-cut matter. Atkins, who deals largely with advanced cases of breast cancer, states [4]:

The fact that randomization is essential for the prosecution of such trials introduces serious ethical problems. In the first place a trial of this nature cannot be instigated unless the investigator is genuinely completely uncertain in his own mind regarding the relative merits of two methods of treatment to be contrasted. At the Breast Clinic at Guy's Hospital we have a very simple rule about this. If we would allow a member of our own family to enter the trial it is ethical; if not, it is not ethical. A further safeguard is that this decision has been made unanimously by our whole group.

The proponents of clinical trials argue further that if a physician can honestly state, "I do not know whether this treatment is of value," then his proper ethical stance is to propose a clinical trial to obtain an answer once and for all. It may be quite unethical to continue to use an unproved treatment without its having been subjected to proper assessment.

Hill cites several examples where, in retrospect, the ethical course of action would have been to conduct a controlled clinical trial [57]. One of his examples concerns a clinical trial of antibiotics used prophylactically among surgical ward patients who ran a risk of postoperative chest infection or who had chronic chest disease. The initial question was whether it was ethical to withhold the potentially beneficial antibiotic and to allow some patients to receive a placebo. The trial resulted in no difference between use of the antibiotic and placebo therapy. In retrospect, the question was whether it would have been ethical *not* to do the trial and to administer routinely a powerful antibiotic.

Another example that Hill cites concerns a trial of long-term anticoagulant therapy in the treatment of cerebrovascular disease. It seemed to be a good idea to administer anticoagulants to patients thus afflicted. The initial question was whether it was ethical to withhold the potentially beneficial anticoagulant. A controlled trial was started and had to be stopped before completion because of an untoward number of cerebral hemorrhages in the anticoagulant group. Here, too, in retrospect, the conduct of a controlled trial and the identification of the risk of hemorrhage was clearly the ethical procedure, rather than the routine employment of the potentially dangerous anticoagulant.

Another point worth mentioning is that the time to conduct a controlled trial is early in the development of a new treatment or drug. If one waits too long, the treatment may become so well ingrained in medical practice that the conduct of a proper controlled trial becomes difficult or nearly impossible. Chalmers, in a letter to the editor of *The Lancet* concerning the anticoagulant effect of a purified fraction of Malayan pit viper venom (arvin), states [16]:

How early in the development of new drugs should the process of randomization be introduced into the therapeutic trial? I am firmly convinced that the first patient to receive a new agent should be randomized. . . .

There are far more potent ethical reasons for randomizing from the beginning patients treated by a new drug. When the first patient with a thromboembolic problem received arvin, there was absolutely no knowledge of its relative efficacy or toxicity. If the drug eventually turns out to be less effective or more toxic than heparin, that patient would have been lucky to have landed in the control group. If the converse eventually is true then the initial patients assigned to arvin by chance would be the lucky ones. Randomization is most ethical when there is no knowledge about relative efficacy and toxicity, and this state exists in its purest form at the time the first patient is to be treated.

The standard argument against early randomization is that an improper trial would result if the drug has not previously been explored in selected patients to determine the proper dose and to decide whether or not a randomized trial is ethical. Is it proper for patients to be selected arbitrarily for earliest trials of a new agent when it is even more likely at that time that they might do better if they received standard therapy?

Finally, it is apparent that most existing treatments have been either accepted or rejected without a proper therapeutic trial because conclusions were reached as a result of uncontrolled studies which, for assumed ethical reasons, could not be challenged by proper studies.

The conclusion is inescapable that randomization should begin with the first patient.

Of course, there are many procedures and treatments that concurrently constitute "good" medical practice and whose effectiveness remain unproved. These procedures may so be ingrained in practice that it is virtually impossible to conduct a proper clinical trial at the present time. Some examples are salicylates in the treatment of rheumatoid arthritis and digitalis in the treatment of congestive heart failure.

An additional merit to the early initiation of a clinical trial is that, when a new drug or technique is in short supply, random allocation represents the fairest way of drug distribution. Hill indicates that this situation prevailed with the trial of streptomycin in tuberculosis shortly after World War II and also with the cooperative United Kingdom–United States trial of corticosteroids in rheumatic fever in the early 1950s [57]. Both of these trials commenced shortly after the respective drugs were developed. At the times of the trials, it was impossible to secure sufficient drug supplies to treat all patients. Thus, a randomized, controlled clinical trial not only assessed the new drug properly, but it also served to ensure its fair distribution.

In certain instances, it may not be feasible to conduct a trial in one geographical area, but it is feasible to do so elsewhere. For example, consider the trial of tetanus antitoxin in the treatment of clinical tetanus that was cited previously (p. 257). In the United Kingdom, such a trial was not feasible because treatment with antitoxin was "orthodox practice despite the lack of evidence that it is beneficial." However, the trial was feasible elsewhere since "there are hospitals in India and in Africa, where tetanus is common, in which tetanus anti-toxin is not used in all cases, both because the worth of this remedy is considered unproved and because money for supplies is not always to be had" [14].

Similarly, in the design of a trial there may be several types of patients the investigator will want to exclude, purely on an ethical basis. For example, the thalidomide tragedy has clearly demonstrated the wisdom of excluding pregnant women from therapeutic trials for conditions unrelated to pregnancy. Likewise, there are often valid ethical reasons for excluding the very young and the very old.

The design of a clinical trial requires careful determination of precisely what patients may ethically be recruited to participate.

2. How far can one go with placebos and dummy treatments? Can placebo or sham surgery be justified?

Beecher has argued the rationale for placebo surgery most persuasively [7]:

Some responsible physicians with the highest motives have said *they* could never carry out a sham procedure in any of *their* patients. Of course this can be done only with the full consent of the individuals involved, who must express a willingness not to know whether or not they were subjected to the full procedure until after the study is completed. The position of the high-minded physician or surgeon who says that he never could be a party to such a "sham procedure," however, is worthy of some consideration. He introduces a new treatment or operation and carries out scores to hundreds of these, and with his colleagues and followers some thousands of procedures are done. As with most major undertakings some risk is involved: major surgery is always associated with a death rate. Then an equally high-minded investigator comes along who, *with the consent of his patients*, carries out a properly designed study which might in many cases consist of no more than 25 sham operations and 25 full procedures, for a total of 50 individuals. This investigator finds that the procedure has no more power than a placebo, transient at best. What then is the position of the high-minded physician or surgeon who refused to make such a clear-headed study? Those who have been subjected to his new procedure have lost a great deal of money and time. They have experienced discomfort and suffering, and several are dead. How, then, is the high-minded practitioner to face up to his failure to carry out a properly designed study? It does indeed seem at times that we are more considerate of our laboratory animals and their welfare than we are of the welfare and lives of our patients when we deny them an adequate test, when we subject them to the continuing risks of inadequately designed major therapeutic procedures.

He proceeds to relate a case in point, namely, the ligation of the internal mammary arteries in the treatment of angina pectoris. The operation, originating in Italy in 1939, spread quickly to the United States where, on an uncontrolled basis, it became rather popular. The enthusiasts had the first round in the literature and published summary results of case reports that touted the benefits of the operations and stressed the relief of symptoms and palliation of the disease that were achieved. Beecher notes that among these reports one can detect an occasional deleterious operative effect, such as a death on the way to the operating room or on the operating table. The skeptics had the second round in the literature. They described the immediate beneficial postoperative effects of the procedure and then went on to indicate how these soon wore off and how, within not too long a time, the disease syndrome had resumed its preoperative course. Finally, a controlled clinical trial was conducted with a small number of patients. The procedure was done under local anesthesia and only at the time of operation was the surgeon informed whether he should ligate the arteries or merely make a skin incision.

The physician who evaluated the patient afterward was unaware of whether the patient had received the full or sham operative procedure. The results of evaluation revealed no difference in the course of the disease among patients receiving the sham operation as compared with the full procedure. The operation was quickly discredited.

The double-blind clinical trial of the gastric freezing of ulcers referred to previously (p. 263) represents another instance in which the results of a carefully designed, rigorous, therapeutic trial dealt the final blow to an unproved procedure. With both ulcers and angina, the assessment of the course of the disease is a highly subjective matter, so the advantages to be gained by a double-blind trial become substantial. Whether a particular controlled trial should or should not be double-blind often remains a most controversial issue. Today, the double-blind trial is analogous to the Good Housekeeping seal of approval. Some feel that the pendulum has swung too far in the double-blind direction and that many medical investigators are afflicted with "placebomania." In this connection, Hill states [57]:

I believe a useful question to ask oneself is "to what extent is an exact control essential?" The answer certainly is not that one of the group must *always* be a mirror-image of the other. The ethical problem may sometimes, I believe, be met in realizing that and in not making the best the enemy of the good. . . .

The doctor will also wish to consider the doctor/patient relationship. Harm may be done if the public comes to believe that doctors are constantly using them as guinea-pigs. In exhibiting new treatments they are, it is my belief, doing that willy-nilly, but the public does not realize it. But they need not go out of their way to make it obvious by an *unnecessary* use of dummy pills.

As with drugs and medical procedures, there are many surgical procedures today that are part and parcel of "good" surgical care, but whose benefit has never been adequately established; they may, in fact, be no better (or perhaps worse) than sham surgery. One often looks with scorn at what was done in the past under the guise of standard medical practice. Who knows which of today's standard medical and surgical procedures will become tomorrow's objects of ridicule?

3. *Must the investigator obtain the patient's consent to participate in the trial? Should the patient be told the nature of the two (or more) treatment possibilities?*

At the time of this writing, the legal answers to both questions in the United States are "yes." Informed consent is the requirement for all clinical studies. Beecher states the case rather emphatically [6]:

All so-called codes are based on the bland assumption that meaningful or informed consent is readily available for the asking. . . . This is very often not the case. Consent in any full informed sense may not be obtainable. Nevertheless, except possibly, in the most trivial situations, it remains a goal toward which one must strive for sociologic, ethical and clear-cut legal reasons. There is no choice in the matter.

Informed consent, however, is not always a clear-cut issue. Not all agree with Beecher, with perhaps the greatest dissent coming from Great Britain. For example, Hill states [57]:

Having made up your mind that you are not in any way subjecting either patient to a recognized and unjustifiable danger, pain or discomfort, can anything be gained by endeavoring to explain to them your own state of ignorance and to describe the attempts you are making to remove it? ... Once you have decided that either treatment *for all you know* may be equally well exhibited to the patient's benefit, and without detriment, is there any real basis for seeking consent or refusal?

In a similar manner, Atkins argues [4]:

From the point of view of ethics the problem arises of whether patients should be informed that they are taking part in a trial. Often this is desirable, and may in many instances be helpful and encourage the patient to attend for the frequent examinations that may be demanded in the interests of the trial rather than the patient. Nevertheless, it is not always desirable, and at a meeting of the Medical Research Council which was attended by the Treasury Solicitors, and where the legal and ethical aspects of this matter were considered, it was decided that there was no obligation on the part of an investigator to inform a patient that he was participating in a trial. Particularly is this so in the trial of methods of treatment for desperate cases or advanced disease. If the trial is ethical by the criteria outlined [see p. 265], and if therefore the choice of treatment is really being made by the "toss of a coin", it is not considered to be the best part of doctoring to inform a patient so gravely ill that we do not know how to treat her, and that the choice of treatment is being so determined.

For a more detailed discussion of the ethical questions in controlled clinical trials, the reader is referred to the previously cited paper by Hill [57] and the issue of *Daedalus* [47] that is devoted exclusively to this subject.

DESIGN OF CLINICAL TRIALS

Although the underlying principles may appear simple, the design of a controlled clinical trial can often be a complex endeavor. However simple the study may appear, it is worthwhile to plan it carefully and to attempt to account for all possible exigencies. This text will not cover the details of clinical trial design; several good texts are available [53, 58, 70, 109, 118].

The final citation in this chapter is from an editorial in the *New England Journal of Medicine* entitled "Bias, the Achilles heel of the therapeutic trial" and serves to indicate the scope of what is needed in the design of a trial [35]:

The major difference between medicine as it is practiced today and that of half a century ago is the more widespread and vigorous application of scientific principles in research and practice. These standards as they apply to practice are also generally championed in the more specific field of therapeutics, in which the clinical evaluation of drugs is among the most complex and difficult to carry out of all medical endeavors. Even when the investigator thinks he knows the type of patient that may benefit from the drug under consideration and has a suitable number of such patients available, is aware of the general dose to use and the therapeutic effects to look for and has at hand also a reasonable (although not infallible) set of measurements with which to quantitate these effects, he has taken only the preliminary steps to organizing his study. Yet to be considered are further plans, including the allocation of subjects into control or treatment groups, proper recording technics, statistical evaluation, assignment of confidence limits and others. In setting these standards, moreover, the almost ineradicable factor of *bias* crops up as an everpresent hazard.

For the physician reading the literature, it is wise for him to be ever vigilant to uncover bias as a possible explanation for the results encountered. Remember, it is the author's onus to demonstrate that bias did not occur or was unlikely to have arisen.

Chapter 11
Medical Surveys

In contrast with the experimental nature of clinical trials in which the investigator can manipulate the allocation of patients to study groups, *medical surveys* deal with observational studies on humans where such manipulation is impossible. The ensuing discussion focuses on how observational studies provide evidence of a statistical relationship or association between some factor, termed the *risk factor*, and a disease. Familiar examples are smoking and lung cancer, oral contraceptives and thromboembolic disease, and elevated serum cholesterol level and coronary heart disease. The primary purposes of this chapter are to delineate the various methods by which these relationships are established and to indicate each method's merits and disadvantages.

In the discussion of these study methods, one immediately encounters the classic problem over the distinction between association and causation (or disease etiology). This is still a controversial and somewhat philosophical issue. The reader is referred to Hill's text for a more complete discussion of the distinction [56]. To avoid the problem, one would best view the methods discussed in this section as providing links, and usually, most important ones, in a chain of evidence that can culminate in the verdict "causation."

CASE REPORTS AND CLINICAL OBSERVATIONS

Strictly speaking, case reports and clinical observations do not fall within the framework of statistical studies. They refer to observations by the clinician of unusual occurrences of a disease, of the coexistence of diseases, or of clusters of hitherto rarely occurring diseases. Often these observations may concern merely a handful of patients and may be entirely devoid of numerical material. They do serve, however, as excellent sources for ideas, hunches, and hypotheses that may, in turn, lead to a whole host of statistically based studies. In other words, clinical observations often form the first link in what may become a chain of evidence that leads to the firm establishment of a relationship. As such, they deserve some mention.

It is hard to find a more suitable example than the following excerpt from the clinical observations of Gregg, a practicing ophthalmologist, and contained in a paper that he presented to the Ophthalmological Society of Australia [49]:

In the first half of the year, 1941, an unusual number of cases of congenital cataract made their appearance in Sydney. Cases of similar type which appeared during the same period, have since been reported from widely separated parts of Australia. Their frequency, unusual characteristics and wide distribution warranted closer investigation, and this report is an attempt to bring to notice some of the more important features of what might almost be regarded as a mild epidemic. . . .

Although one was struck with the unusual appearance of the cataracts in the first few cases, it was only when other similar cases continued to appear that serious thought was given to their causation.

The remarkable similarity of the opacities in the lens, the frequency of an accompanying affection of the heart and the widespread geographical incidence of the cases suggested that there was some common factor in the production of the diseased condition, and suggested it was the result of some constitutional condition of toxic or infective nature rather than of a purely development defect.

The question arose whether this factor could have been some disease or infection occurring in the mother during pregnancy which had then interfered with the developing cells of the lens. By a calculation from the date of birth of the baby it was estimated that the early period of pregnancy corresponded with the period of maximum intensity of the very widespread and severe epidemic in 1940 of the so-called German measles.

Special attention was accordingly paid to the history of the health of the mothers during pregnancy, and in each new case it was found that the mother had suffered from that disease early in her pregnancy, most frequently in the first or second month.

Thus, Gregg's clinical observations launched the numerous investigations that have today established beyond doubt the association between rubella during the first trimester of pregnancy and congenital defects.

VITAL STATISTICS

Vital statistics data often serve as the first clue in establishing an association. National vital statistics data are under constant scrutiny. In particular, examination of time trends in mortality and morbidity rates according to cause provides a fertile source for hypotheses concerning association. The appearance of a perturbation in death rates leads to speculation regarding possible explanations, and a whole host of statistical studies may follow. For example, the Surgeon General's report, "Smoking and health" [92], notes that as early as 1900 an increase in lung cancer death rates had been noted, and it was suggested then that the parallel increase in cigarette smoking might somehow be implicated.

Sometimes, vital statistics data can be used effectively in establishing evidence of an association by the comparison of vital rates in different geographical regions, i.e., those regions where the factor under question is absent versus regions in which it is present. As an example, Colton and Buxbaum investigated the association between motor vehicle inspection and motor vehicle accident mortality [20]. This study is described in some detail in order to illustrate the merits and disadvantages of the use of vital statistics.

The investigation was based on Ralph Nader's allegation that mechanical failure contributed to the occurrence of motor vehicle accidents [80]. Following this reasoning, it would seem that an attempt to identify and correct mechanical defects should have a demonstrable effect on the occurrence of motor vehicle accidents and their sequelae. Motor vehicle inspection clearly represents such an attempt. The fact that some states had compulsory motor vehicle inspection, while simultaneously others did not, made a vital statistics study feasible. Thus, the study asked the question: Is there any difference in motor vehicle accident mortality rates in the states with inspection as compared with noninspection states?

Table 11.1 summarizes the results for the designated study year, 1960. At that time there were 17 states classified as having motor vehicle inspection and 34 as not having inspection. The motor vehicle accident mortality rates shown are age-adjusted by the direct method (see p. 47) for the total United States population from 15 to 64 years old (roughly, the driving age population).

Table 11.1. Age-adjusted[a] motor vehicle accident mortality rates by sex and race in inspection versus noninspection states, U.S. (including District of Columbia), 1960, ages 15 to 64 years (rates per 100,000 population)

Race-sex group	17 Inspection states	34 Noninspection states	Ratio[b]
White males	30.0	44.0	1.47
Nonwhite males	36.1	54.6	1.51
White females	9.1	13.5	1.49
Nonwhite females	9.0	13.1	1.45
Total population	20.0	29.1	1.45

[a] Adjusted to total U.S. population by age, 1960.
[b] Rate in noninspection states divided by rate in inspection states.
Data from Colton and Buxbaum [20].

Table 11.1 presents rates separately by race and sex groups. The last column of Table 11.1 indicates that noninspection states had approximately one-and-a-half times the age-adjusted mortality rates as inspection states. The differences in rates are highly statistically significant ($P < .001$) and, therefore, are unexplainable by chance variation. (The method for testing the difference is beyond the scope of this book.) A more detailed inspection of the age-specific rates (see p. 45) by five-year intervals for each of the four race and sex groups indicated nearly uniformly higher mortality rates in the noninspection states.

It might be mentioned that 1960 was chosen as the study year because of its coincidence with the decennial census. To derive the age-adjusted rates displayed in Table 11.1, it was necessary to secure data on the number of motor vehicle accident deaths and on the total United States population, each set of which was classified according to state, age, sex, and race. These data were available in such detail only for the census year.

An immediate question about any statistical comparison emanating from an observational study such as that presented in Table 11.1 is, "Has like been compared with like?" The inspection states were self-selected and not randomly allocated. Hence, are those states that chose to inspect motor vehicles similar to those not inspecting them, at least for the crucial variables that are known to bear upon motor vehicle accident mortality rates? With this question in mind, one's immediate response to Table 11.1 might be, "Show me which are the inspection and which the noninspection states." Figure 11.1 presents such a display.

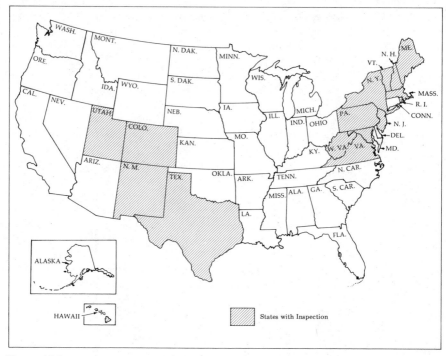

Figure 11.1
Motor vehicle inspection states, United States, 1960. (From Colton and Buxbaum [20].)

In 1960 the self-selected inspection states clustered in the Northeast and Southwest. Thus, the possibility arises that characteristics other than inspection might contribute to, or possibly explain, the differences exhibited in Table 11.1. For example, one such possibility is population density. It is well known that fatal accidents occur more frequently in rural areas as opposed to populous areas. This results in an exceedingly strong inverse relationship between motor vehicle accident mortality rate and population density. Since inspection states tend to be more densely populated, they will, of course, exhibit lower accident mortality rates, apart from any effect of inspection. The same argument applies to other characteristics of inspection versus noninspection states.

There are statistical techniques available that remove or adjust for the effects of uncontrolled, disturbing variables such as population density. With the data at hand, *covariance adjustment* was employed. The methodology underlying this technique is beyond the scope of this text and can be found in more advanced texts [2, 12, 101]. The results of its application, however, are of interest. The male mortality rates in Table 11.1 were adjusted by covariance to remove the effects of three disturbing variables: population density, per capita income, and mortality rates from other accidents. The rationale for the adjustment for the latter variable was that inspection states might tend to be

274

Table 11.2. Statistical comparison in inspection versus noninspection states of age-adjusted motor vehicle accident mortality rates before and after adjustments for population density, per capita income, and the mortality rate from other accidents, U.S. 1960, white and nonwhite males 15 to 64 years old (rates per 100,000 population)

Comparison	Age-adjusted rates		Ratio	Difference	SE of difference	P value
	Inspection states	Noninspection states				
White males:						
Before covariance adjustment	30.0	44.0	1.47	14.0	3.70	<.001
After covariance adjustment[a]	35.5	42.3	1.19	6.8	2.10	<.001
Nonwhite males:						
Before covariance adjustment	36.1	54.6	1.51	18.5	6.53	<.01
After covariance adjustment[a]	42.0	53.0	1.26	11.0	3.90	<.01

[a] Adjustment made simultaneously for population density, per capita income, and the mortality rate from other accidents. Data from Colton and Buxbaum [20].

more safety conscious and would therefore have lower rates from other accidents.

Table 11.2 summarizes the results of the covariance adjustment, the adjustment being made simultaneously for all three disturbing variables. The basic rates in Table 11.2 have, of course, already been adjusted for age by use of the direct method (p. 47). One interprets the covariance-adjusted rates in Table 11.2 as the rates that would prevail if the aggregate of inspection and noninspection states had identical population density, per capita income, and mortality rates from other accidents. Note that the magnitude of the difference in rates is considerably reduced following the covariance adjustment; for white males there is a difference of 14.0 before adjustment to 6.8 after, and for nonwhite males there is a difference of 18.5 before adjustment to 11.0 after. Thus, the disturbing variables account for a goodly portion of the initially observed difference, namely 51 percent $(100\%[14.0 - 6.8]/14.0)$ for white males and 41 percent $(100\%[18.5 - 11.0]/18.5)$ for nonwhite males. In other words, roughly half of the initially observed differences in motor vehicle accident mortality rates between inspection and noninspection states could be attributed to the difference in these two groups of states with respect to population density, per capita income, and mortality rates from other accidents. With covariance adjustment, however, note too that the standard error of the difference also decreases. The important point is that after the covariance adjustment the application of an appropriate test of significance reveals that inspection states maintain a significantly lower mortality rate compared with noninspection states. In other words, with the removal of the effects of differences between the groups with respect to population density, per capita income, and the mortality rates from other accidents, the resulting difference in motor vehicle accident mortality rates remains unexplainable by chance variation. Of course, the possibility remains that there are other disturbing variables, as yet unaccounted for, that could contribute to and possibly explain the difference in mortality rates. The possibility of unaccounted disturbing variables lingers as a chronic problem in all forms of observational studies.

Other aspects of this study deserve mention in order to illustrate some of the difficulties encountered with this form of vital statistics study. One important aspect concerns a suitable definition for the factor under study, in this case, motor vehicle inspection. Readers who have had experience with automobile inspection in more than one state can attest to the considerable variation among states in inspection procedures. These range from the most cursory check to a quite thorough examination. Further, some states inspect once a year and others twice a year. Some use state-owned and state-run inspection sites; others use private service stations franchised by the state. The data were deemed insufficient to analyze separately for each of these characteristics. Hence, the category "inspection states" represents a considerable range of inspection possibilities. An additional difficulty with the definition of inspection was that one state inspected only those vehicles four or more years old (it was classified as an inspection state), another required inspection only of used cars purchased out of state and of state cars 10 or more years old (it was classified as a noninspection state), while still others maintained inspection programs only in a few municipalities (they were classified as noninspection states). Thus, the grouping of the 17 inspection states is a crude classification that covered many situations and, in some cases, involved rather arbitrary decisions. These are characteristic of the problems encountered with observational studies: classifications must often be crude, and in many instances arbitrary decisions are necessary. The author of a report on an observational study has the obligation to inform the reader specifically of the definitions he has established for the factor under study and the rules for classification of the observational units. This can be a most arduous task.

An obvious difficulty with vital statistics studies concerns the pertinence of the response variable, which most often consists of mortality rates. Mortality may not be the variable of chief interest. It may, however, be the only variable for which data are available. For example, it might be more appropriate with the automobile inspection study to consider the rates at which motor vehicle accidents occur or the per capita costs of motor vehicle accidents rather than the motor vehicle accident mortality. Mortality represents only a portion of the consequences of a motor vehicle accident. Although accident rates and cost data may be more meaningful, they simply are not readily available in sufficient detail to conduct any meaningful analysis. The mortality data, however, are readily secured.

One might also quibble with the denominator in the mortality rate. The rates employ population in the denominator (i.e., mortality per 100,000 persons), whereas some feel that a rate in terms of the risk of exposure to motor vehicle accidents is more meaningful. Motor vehicle accident morbidity and mortality rates often employ in the denominator "million miles driven." Such data are available by state and are derived by multiplying the total amount of gasoline sold in the state (such data are published by the Petroleum Institute) by a constant average miles-per-gallon figure. However, the "million miles driven" denominator cannot be broken down according to sex, race, and age, which form the crucial variables in comparison of rates. The rates employed in the study used population as denominators, not because they most accurately reflect risk of accident mortality, but because they are the only denominator data available in sufficient detail to present the comparisons of Table 11.1 and 11.2.

Another point concerns the validity of the vital statistics data. The census data, for the most part, are quite accurate. There are occasional abberrations that cause concern among demographic experts, but these are rare and, considering the magnitudes of the numbers involved, these generally will have little effect on vital statistics rates. With regard to the numerator, there is a virtually universal reporting of deaths. Errors in reporting demographic information such as age, sex, and race are known to occur, but these, too, for the most part, have little impact on mortality rates. It is the accuracy of the recording of the cause of death that causes the main controversy between the proponents and opponents of vital statistics studies. In the study under consideration, there would be little controversy concerning the accuracy of the reporting of motor vehicle accident. For vital statistics studies involving other causes, such as pneumonia, influenza, heart disease, cirrhosis of the liver, and so forth, the controversy may be considerable.

With all these difficulties, what then are the chief advantages of vital statistics studies such as that described? Very simply, vital statistics studies are exceedingly economical and easy to perform. The data collection usually involves no more than obtaining the official government publications that provide the tabulations of the deaths for the numerators (issued by the National Center of Health Statistics) and of the populations for the denominator (issued by the United States Bureau of the Census). As a coinvestigator in the motor vehicle inspection study, this author had to travel no further than the university's medical library to secure the necessary data for calculation of the mortality rates. A phone call to the American Automobile Association prompted the receipt of a list of the inspection procedures in each state during 1960.

Thus, vital statistics studies, in spite of all their inadequacies and inaccuracies, provide an exceedingly quick and economical means for establishing one link in the chain of evidence for an association.

CROSS-SECTIONAL SURVEYS

A *cross-sectional survey*, as distinct from the retrospective and prospective studies described later, does not involve time. A cross-sectional survey provides a snapshot view of a relationship at an instant of time. Such surveys usually apply to the association of two diseases.

As an illustration, Table 11.3 abstracts data from a survey that concerned, in part, an association between bacteriuria and hypertension [78]. In this

Table 11.3. Bacteriuria and hypertension among females 30 to 59 years old, field survey, Jamaica, West Indies

| | Diastolic blood pressure | | | |
	110 mm Hg or more	Less than 110 mm Hg	Total	Percent hypertensive
Bacteriuria				
Yes	18	31	49	36.7
No	103	874	977	10.5
Total	121	905	1026	
Percent bacteriuria	14.9	3.4		

Data from Miall et al. [78].

study, the investigators went from house to house in the community, measured the dwellers' blood pressure, and secured urine samples. Note that the results are expressed in the format of the fourfold table (see p. 175). The figures in the bottom row summarize the percent of bacteriuric cases among normotensives (diastolic blood pressure less than 110 mg Hg) compared with hypertensives (diastolic blood pressure of 110 mm Hg or more). Alternatively, the figures in the last column summarize the percentage that are hypertensive of the nonbacteriuric women compared with the bacteriuric women. One might apply the methods of Chapter 5 (see Table 5.2) to compare the proportions of those who are bacteriuric or, alternatively, to compare the proportions of those who are hypertensive. It may be seen that the results of critical ratio or chi-square tests comparing the proportions of bacteriuric cases are identical with those comparing the proportions of hypertensive cases. Thus, with the fourfold table, it matters not whether one compares row or column percentages; the respective tests of significance yield identical results.

Since the cross-sectional survey does not involve time, one cannot say which disease occurred first. Clearly, both hypertension and bacteriuria involve a substantial asymptomatic component. One cannot say whether bacteriuric women are more likely to develop hypertension or whether hypertensive women are more likely to develop bacteriuria. All that may be concluded from the data is that bacteriuria and hypertension tend to be associated.

RETROSPECTIVE STUDIES

As the term implies, *retrospective studies* involve going back in time. A retrospective study starts with cases of the disease in question. The investigator identifies, as a standard of comparison, a control group without the disease. Then for each case and each control, the investigator goes back in time and obtains a history to indicate the presence or absence or the level of the risk factor under study. The question is whether the risk factor is present more frequently or occurs at a higher average level among cases of the disease as compared with controls. If there is sufficient evidence that it is, the investigator will conclude there is an association between the risk factor and the disease.

Although "retrospective" is the commonly applied label, many epidemiologists prefer the more accurate designation, *case-control study*.

Sartwell's study of oral contraceptives and thromboembolism [97], which was used previously to illustrate the comparison of matched proportions (Example 5.11), serves as an example. As has been noted, the study identified cases of thromboembolism during a three-year period among married women, 15 to 44 years of age, who had been discharged from several teaching hospitals in a number of large northeastern cities. The controls consisted of women who were discharged from these same hospitals with diagnoses other than thromboembolic disease. The controls were individually matched to cases within each hospital so that each case-control match had discharge dates within six months of one another, were in the same five-year age group, and had identical marital status, city of residence, race, parity, and hospital pay status. The investigator then secured contraceptive histories for the resulting 175 case-control pairs of women. Analysis of these results (p. 174) revealed a significantly higher proportion of the cases with a history of oral contraceptive usage prior to hospitalization than controls. Thus, the study provides evidence of an association between oral contraceptive usage and the occurrence of thromboemobic disease.

Three critical aspects of retrospective studies deserve attention: (1) the criteria employed for definition of cases and identification of the factor under study, (2) the selection of controls and their comparability with the cases, and (3) the accuracy of the histories of exposure to the risk factors.

First, with regard to the definition of cases, care must be exercised to ascertain that those designated as cases actually have the disease in question. In the study under consideration, Sartwell states [97]:

> The term "idiopathic thromboembolism" is used in this report to refer to diseases in women who, at the time they developed thromboembolism, did not have any medical, surgical or traumatic condition that is associated with this disease. . . .

> Reasonable medical evidence to support the diagnosis of thromboembolism was required. . . . Only cases in which the hospital diagnosis was unequivocal were accepted and the records were reviewed independently by two physicians, one a board-qualified internist, who rejected those cases which they considered doubtful. . . .

Thus, the criterion for the definition of the disease had as its goal the exclusion of cases that might have been attributed to known predisposing or precipitating thromboembolic factors. The list of exclusions from the study included such possibilities as recent surgery, trauma, or pregnancy, a history of thromboembolic disease, varicose veins, diabetes, hypertension, and so forth. Of importance, the list of exclusions applied equally to candidates for the case group and the control group.

Reliance on the information contained in records represents a characteristic feature of retrospective studies. In fact, some such studies rely entirely on records. It is an obvious but important point that a study can be only as good as the records on which it is based. The validity and reliability of the information in records often represent the Achilles heel of retrospective investigations.

For the study being considered, the identification of cases and controls relied on the information in the hospital record. Thus, accuracy in the diagnosis of thromboembolic disease and diligence in its recording become important. Clearly, physicians may differ in the criteria they apply and in their skills for diagnosing various diseases. In addition, the criteria for diagnosis of a disease may change over time. A retrospective inquiry may yield a spurious association if physicians tend to diagnose the disease more often when the risk factor is present than when it is absent. In the present example, this would imply that physicians were more likely to seek, and consequently record, thromboembolic disease as the discharge diagnosis among oral contraceptive users than among nonusers. If this selective factor prevailed, one would, of course, find more oral contraceptive users in the case group, quite apart from any increased risk with the use of oral contraceptives.

Another point with regard to the use of records in the study at hand is that the cited diagnostic criteria indicate care was taken to eliminate what may be called *false positive diagnoses*, i.e., discharge diagnoses of thromboembolic disease when, in reality, the patient had no such disease. Little can be done, however, to pick out *false negative diagnoses*, i.e., discharge diagnoses that failed to indicate thromboembolic disease when, in fact, the patient had such disease.

The definition of the factor's presence consisted of the use of oral contraceptives within two years of hospital admission. The authors noted that several oral contraceptive users had employed other contraceptive methods as well during the two-year period. In addition, the duration of oral contraceptive use ranged from the date of hospital admission to more than a year before hospital admission. Thus, the dichotomy of oral contraceptive use or nonuse comprises a variety of possibilities. However, the authors do present data to indicate that the ranges of possibilities for oral contraceptive use were distributed similarly among cases and controls.

The second major area of importance concerns the selection of the controls and their comparability with the cases. The goal of the retrospective study is to obtain controls as similar as possible to the cases in all important respects except for their not having the disease in question. Matched pairs is the technique commonly employed in retrospective studies as an attempt to achieve this goal. The oral contraceptive study employed one-to-one matching (the matching factors have already been listed). Even with matching on these several variables, the question remains as to how similar the cases and controls were with regard to other variables which were not employed in the matching procedure but which are possibly related to the phenomena under study. Sartwell presents data on the comparison of cases and controls by family income, religion, education, smoking history, past weight, and the occupations of the patient and husband. Significant differences were detected in education, in the proportion who had been working just prior to hospitalization, and in the proportion whose occupation or whose husband's occupation was in a medically related field. The full analysis of the data took these discrepancies into account. However, as with the vital statistics study previously described, there remains the possibility that other presently unidentified characteristics may differ among cases and controls and contribute to or partially explain the observed difference.

The third factor of great importance in retrospective studies is the means for securing the history concerning presence of the risk factor. In the thromboembolism study, personal interviews with each identified case and matched control provided the required data on contraceptive usage. Sartwell states:

Both groups were interviewed to ascertain whether they had used oral contraceptives before hospitalization ....

The plan was to have the interviewers deal with other topics including medications of various types taken before the hospitalization in question (e.g., analgesics, tranquilizers and sedatives, drugs for weight control), the respondent's previous health and the medical and reproductive history of her husband and herself. The interview was designed to avoid concentrating the respondent's attention on a possible drug-thromboembolism relationship and thereby possibly obtain biased answers.

Thus, care was taken to ensure that the history of risk factor exposure was sought similarly among cases and controls. Many retrospective studies fail to consider the comparability of cases with controls in the manner in which the history is sought. When the form of inquiry differs for cases and controls, the possibility arises that more intensive interviewing and probing into the history of the cases may produce a spuriously high prevalence of the presence of the risk factor.

The above possibility pertains particularly to retrospective studies where the information regarding the presence or absence of the risk factor is derived entirely from records. A record that does not mention the risk factor does not necessarily entail the absence of the risk factor. There may be no mention of the factor merely because whoever completed the record failed to ask the question. Thus, the risk factor can artificially occur more frequently among cases than among controls merely because it was looked for and recorded more frequently among cases than among controls. As an example, suppose the thromboembolism study had relied entirely on the hospital records for the indication of oral contraceptive use. It seems quite plausible that the women discharged with thromboembolism would, during their hospital stay, have been more likely to have had their contraceptive histories queried and noted in their hospital records than would control women. Hence, a record's failure to mention oral contraceptive use does not imply the patient's lack of use of oral contraceptives. "No mention" may mean merely "neglect to inquire." And, it is most plausible that the neglect to inquire occurred more frequently among controls than among cases. Thus, the cases could spuriously demonstrate a higher frequency of oral contraceptive use as compared with controls.

Even with personal interviews conducted in an identical manner, there is the possibility of different responses being elicited in the case and control groups. For example, had the interviewer suggested to the subject that the study concerned a contraceptive-thromboembolism association, one might expect more ready recall and more indication of contraceptive use among the thromboembolic cases than among the controls. Precautions were taken to couch the key oral contraceptive question within a general inquiry on reproductive and contraceptive history. Even with this safeguard, there remains the possibility that thromboembolic women may have better recall or may be more prone to reveal to the questioner their contraceptive history. Vessey and Doll, who had previously conducted retrospective studies on this association in Great Britain, state [108]:

A woman's ability and willingness to recall details of her contraceptive history may be affected by whether she has suffered an illness which might be associated in her mind with the type of contraceptive she had used.

There is another possibility for bias that applies particularly to retrospective studies. This concerns the interplay of admission rates to the treatment and control groups, and is called *Berkson's fallacy* (thus named not for Berkson having committed it, but for his having been the first to elucidate its nature). The fallacy is rather subtle and is elaborated in the following chapter (p. 305).

For the present, it may be summarized verbally by saying that spurious associations may arise in a study sample when there are differing rates of admission from the underlying population to the sample group. Persons who have both the disease and risk factor under investigation may be more likely to be included in the study sample than persons who have either the disease alone or the risk factor alone. The result is a spuriously high frequency of the risk factor among the study's cases. In the present example, this would mean that women who actually have thromboembolic disease and who have used oral contraceptives are more likely to be hospitalized and to have thromboembolism recognized and recorded than those women who had thromboembolism alone. Sartwell considers this possibility and presents evidence to indicate that its occurrence in his study was highly unlikely.

With the establishment of a statistical association between a risk factor and a disease, one often wishes to obtain some indication of the increase in disease risk brought about by the factor's presence. The retrospective study has the disadvantage that the magnitude of the increased risk cannot be estimated directly. An indirect estimate, however, is possible. This estimate is based on the assumptions that the disease is of low incidence in the population and that the cases and controls in the study constitute a random sample of the underlying populations. The latter assumption is rarely true, but in practice its violation does not seem to alter the results appreciably. In a retrospective study that employs matched pairs, the increased risk of the disease, called the *relative risk*, is estimated as the ratio of the numbers of untied pairs. The numerator of this ratio is the number of pairs for which the case member exhibits the risk factor while the control member does not; the denominator is the number of pairs for which the control member exhibits the risk factor while the case member does not. Thus, for the oral contraceptive-thromboembolism study, relative risk is estimated as $57/13 = 4.4$. This means that based on the sample results, users of oral contraceptives have approximately 4.4 times the risk of thromboembolic disease as nonusers.

Had the contraceptive-thromboembolism study involved independent samples rather than matched pairs, as is summarized in the following fourfold table, then one would estimate the relative risk as $(ad)/(bc)$.

		Cases	Controls
Risk	Present	a	b
Factor	Absent	c	d
	Total	$a + c$	$b + d$

The above discussion has focused on the weaknesses of the retrospective study. What then are its advantages? Without doubt, the advantages are its economy, the relative speed with which the study can be completed, and the fact that there is usually little or no difficulty in finding a suitable number of cases. Further, another advantageous feature of the retrospective study is that these rather simply collected observations often serve as a spur to the more thorough study of a problem with additional statistical type studies as well as with considerable subsequent laboratory and clinical investigation.

PROSPECTIVE STUDIES

In contrast with a retrospective study, a *prospective study* goes forward in time. One identifies a group of persons who have the risk factor and a suitable control group without the risk factor. The study proceeds forward in time in that both groups are followed to determine new cases of the disease in question. One calculates the rates of disease occurrence or incidence and compares this incidence among those with and without the risk factor.

It is possible to conduct a prospective study entirely with retrospective material. For example, records obtained many years ago, when coupled with records of more recent vintage, may provide sufficient material to calculate and compare disease incidence rates. To avoid the confusion of words, epidemiologists prefer the term *cohort studies* for these forward-in-time investigations. However, "prospective study" is the more commonly used designation among the medical community.

A classic among prospective studies is that of Doll and Hill on smoking and lung cancer [30]. Although by 1950 several retrospective investigations had already been completed, the Doll and Hill study was the first large-scale prospective investigation of this association. On October 31, 1951 the investigators sent a simple questionnaire to all members of the medical profession in the United Kingdom (approximately 60,000 individuals). The questionnaire asked for information on whether or not the respondent smoked, on what, if anything, he smoked (cigarettes, pipes, or cigars), and on how much he smoked. More than two-thirds of the physicians, some 41,000, replied in sufficient detail for their results to be included in the study.

The responses to the questionnaire enabled the investigators to classify each subject as a smoker or nonsmoker. One should note that, as in the other studies cited, such a definition encompasses a wide variety of possibilities. For example, smokers might range from those who smoke a minimal amount to those who consume several packs a day, and from those who may have recently adopted the habit to those who are veterans of many years of smoking. The category of smokers might include those who smoke cigarettes with those who smoke cigars or pipes. Likewise, the group of nonsmokers may include individuals who presently abstain but who have an extensive history of cigarette smoking. Again, it is the author's onus to indicate clearly to the reader the criteria he employed for defining the risk factor. In this investigation, the authors state:

A non-smoker is defined as a person who has never consistently smoked as much as 1 g. of tobacco a day for as long as one year (1 cigarette is equivalent to 1 g. of tobacco).

The first follow-up occurred some four and a half years later. The Registrar-General and the medical associations provided the investigators with death certificate information for every medically qualified decedent during the intervening time. Of course, some deaths occurred abroad; in such instances the requisite information had to be secured from the appropriate authorities in other countries.

Restricting attention to males over 35 years old, there was a total of 1,714 deaths among all study participants during the four-and-one-half year period; 82 of these deaths were attributed to lung cancer. In addition, for three other deaths, lung cancer appeared on the death certificate as a contributory but not primary cause. This gave a total of 85 deaths associated with lung cancer.

In order to confirm the diagnosis for each of the 85 deaths, the investigators wrote to the physician who had certified the death and, when necessary, to the hospital or consultant to whom the patient had been referred. As a result, one case was rejected because histological examination of the operative specimen failed to confirm carcinoma.

Table 11.4. Lung cancer mortality rates of cigarette smokers versus nonsmokers, British physicians age 35 years or older during a 4½ year follow-up period

	Nonsmokers	Smokers
Man-years of exposure	15,107	98,090
Lung cancer deaths	1	83
Death rate per 1,000 man-years of exposure:		
Crude	0.07	0.85
Age-adjusted	0.07	0.90

Data from Doll and Hill [30].

The results are presented in Table 11.4. With this longitudinal study, the investigators chose to employ man-years of exposure (p. 239) as the denominator for the calculation of lung cancer mortality rates. As discussed in Chapter 9, such a technique was necessary because the participants varied in their length of observation in the study. In addition, in order to correct for any possible age discrepancy between smokers and nonsmokers, the authors employed age-adjusted rates (p. 47). The results in Table 11.4 clearly indicate an association between smoking and lung cancer. It may be seen that smokers, compared with nonsmokers, have $0.90/0.07 = 13$ times the risk of lung cancer mortality.

Although the Doll and Hill study was the first large-scale prospective investigation, it may be interesting to note that the subsequent United States' Surgeon General's report on smoking and health reviewed their data along with data from six other large-scale prospective studies and 29 retrospective studies, each of which provided confirming evidence of an association [92].

The Doll and Hill prospective study employed routinely collected records, namely, the death certificates. Rather than rely solely on the death certificate statement of cause, however, the investigators sought confirmation from the original sources that provided the diagnostic information. As with the retrospective study, the quality of a prospective study that relies entirely upon information in medical records is, of course, only as good as the quality of the record. No information in the record may, as before, indicate merely that information on the characteristic in question was not sought.

Prospective studies that proceed from present to future time do have the distinct advantage of permitting uniformity in observation both for the present identification of the risk factor and for future recognition of new instances of the disease. Often, the investigator can examine the subjects at the start of a prospective investigation, establish rigorous criteria for determining the risk factor's presence, and ascertain that those who already have the disease are excluded. Careful and complete follow-up at frequent intervals along with the application of uniform and rigorous criteria for disease identification represent the ideal for a prospective study.

Another advantage of the prospective study is that the investigator can determine the comparability of the two groups at the start of the investigation. He can identify variables for which an adjustment will be necessary in the analysis, and he can begin to make plans for performing such adjustments.

Furthermore, in a prospective study the investigator usually has considerably more leeway in what he can measure and how he will measure it; most often, he will not have to rely predominantly on information contained in records.

A further advantage of the prospective study is that one obtains a direct estimate of the magnitude of increased risk. The 13-fold increase in lung cancer mortality with smoking represents such an estimate.

Another example of a prospective investigation, one which is community-based and which involves repeated medical examination of participants, is the Framingham Heart Study [27]. This study commenced in 1950 with the recruitment of approximately 5,000 men and women residents of Framingham, Massachusetts, who were between 30 and 59 years of age. This represented a random sample of two-thirds of the town's population. Rather than focusing on a single association, the goal of the Framingham study was to identify the host of risk factors associated with heart disease. Initially, the participating subjects underwent a thorough medical examination that emphasized cardiovascular evaluation. The cohort was examined biennially, and, at this writing, the 12th examination cycle is underway on the approximately 4,000 remaining members of the cohort. In addition to the biennial examinations, there are also records of hospitalization, obituary notices, and other sources of information that are continuously monitored to provide data on the occurrence of new cardiovascular disease episodes. From this prospective inquiry, there has streamed a wealth of information identifying the association between risk factors and heart disease (the earliest was the report of Dawber et al. [28] and, at this writing, the latest is that of Kannel et al. [62]).

In the prospective study, as in the other types of studies described, there is the question of the comparability of the two groups, i.e., those with and without the risk factor. There may remain the possibility of an as yet unidentified crucial variable distinguishing the two groups and explaining the association. Prospective studies usually involve some aspect of cooperation on the part of the subject and his willingness to participate. Not all subjects eligible for study will agree to participate. This can then raise questions of differential selection among those with and without the risk factor and the possibility of bias. Thus, for example, in the study of smoking and lung cancer, Doll and Hill considered the suggestion that smokers in good health were less likely to respond to the initial questionnaire than were corresponding non-smokers in good health. This might come about because smokers would tend to have more difficulty in completing the questionnaire than nonsmokers. In particular, a healthy smoker would have been more inclined not to respond than a healthy nonsmoker. The result would be an over-representation of the healthy among the nonsmokers, thereby yielding artificially lower mortality rates among nonsmokers. Doll and Hill went to considerable effort to investi-gate whether such a bias was likely to be present, and they reached the con-clusion that it was highly improbable.

The examples cited demonstrate the major difficulty in executing prospec-tive studies. Prospective studies are large, time-consuming, and expensive. The rarer the disease in question, the larger is the number required under observation in order to obtain a suitable number of cases. Likewise, extremely long periods of follow-up may be required before sufficient numbers of cases develop. The smoking and lung cancer study indicates that the acquisition of data on 80 or more lung cancer deaths required nearly five years of observation on some 40,000 subjects. The Framingham study with its biennial examinations requires considerable effort and expense.

The reader may well appreciate that good follow-up presents a major difficulty in the execution of a prospective study. As has been indicated in Chapter 9, subjects may move away or refuse to participate. The possibilities that the termination of follow-up occurs at differential rates among the groups under observation and that the termination of follow-up may be related to development of the disease can raise serious questions pertaining to the validity of the study's results. Sometimes, poor follow-up is not always attributable to the subject's disinclination to participate. Over time, the enthusiasm of the investigator or his collaborators may wane, and the diligence with which they seek out and track subjects may diminish, thereby causing extreme difficulty in the maintenance of appropriate follow-up.

Whatever the difficulties of the prospective study, it does have the capability of providing, among all the various observational studies, the most firmly based evidence of association.

PROSPECTIVE EXPERIMENTS

One step beyond the prospective survey is the *prospective experiment* that would entail the investigator's manipulation of the risk factor among the study participants. In many situations, this is impossible; for example, the associa-tion between smoking and lung cancer could not be feasibly made the subject of experiment. Sometimes, however, an experiment is feasible. For example, the association between cholesterol level and heart disease initiated a prospective experiment in which subjects were randomly assigned to receive various cholesterol-lowering agents. Thus, as a consequence of the association between elevated cholesterol level and heart disease, this experiment asks the question whether the reduction of cholesterol level reduces the incidence of heart disease. Within the framework of Chapter 10, the prospective experiment falls under the classification of a clinical trial, and the principles enunciated in that chapter are therefore relevant.

Chapter 12
Fallacies in Numerical Reasoning

The art of statistics involves the assembling of numerical material in a meaningful way. There are traps and pitfalls that beset the inexperienced investigator as he proceeds to collect and interpret numerical data. Several of the more common fallacies in numerical reasoning that lurk to ensnare the unwary investigator form the contents of this chapter. Of more consequence is the fact that these gaffes often escape notice by editors and referees of medical journals and thus lurk to ensnare the unwary reader as well. No doubt some of the ensuing fallacies are quite obvious; others, however, are hopefully somewhat more subtle. Insofar as possible, the examples employ real data from published medical investigations. The goal is to use these examples to assist the reader in identifying these errors in logic; *by no means* is the intent to impugn the motives or integrity of the investigator or to deride the quality of what appears in the medical literature. These errors do occasionally occur in the present literature, and by perusing these examples, the reader will hopefully learn to recognize similar cases when they appear.

DENOMINATORS

Much numerical evidence centers on the determination of rates, risks, or chances. It is important to remember that a rate consists of both a numerator and a denominator. In medicine it is a relatively simple task to obtain the numerator. Obtaining the proper denominator, however, is quite another matter. One is often tempted to interpret the numerator data as if they were a rate.

Example 12.1.　Table 12.1 gives the age distribution of "patients aged 15–45 who were fully investigated for carotid stroke in the neurosurgical unit in the ten years 1956–1965. Of the 65 women in the series, 23 were pregnant or puerperal at the time of their stroke" [59]. From these data on the age and pregnancy status of female stroke patients, the author concluded: "When the quinquennial incidence for 15–45 is considered it becomes clear that nonpregnant women do, indeed, become more prone to strokes at a later age than pregnant women."

If one takes age 35 as a reference point, then the data do indicate more than three-quarters of the nonpregnant stroke patients were 35 to 45 years of age, compared with less than one-eighth of the pregnant women. But these are numerator data. The author's concern is with risk or the *rates* at which patients with stroke occur among pregnant and nonpregnant women. His missing ingredients are the denominators. The proper denominators are the numbers of pregnant and nonpregnant women in the population served by this hospital and at risk of stroke during this time period. To calculate the appropriate quinquennial incidence rates, he would need these denominator data classified by age.

Table 12.1. Age distribution of nonpregnant and pregnant women investigated for carotid strokes

| Age (yr) | Number of female patients investigated for carotid stroke | |
	Nonpregnant	Pregnant
15–19	1	—
20–24	2	7
25–29	4	6
30–34	4	7
35–39	10	3
40–44	21	—
Total	42	23

Data from Jennett and Cross [59].

It seems that the more apparent explanation for the small number of pregnant stroke patients between the ages of 35 and 45 is simply that there are relatively few pregnant women in this age group. In fact, it seems likely that the magnitude of the denominators would reveal that, among women over 35 years old, considerably more were nonpregnant than pregnant, so much so that if the investigator calculated the *rates* at which stroke cases occurred, the rate would be higher for pregnant women. The reader may verify that if roughly only one-tenth or less of the women at risk between age 35 and 45 were pregnant, then their rate of strokes would be higher than that for the nonpregnant women. Certainly, the finding of fewer than 1 in 10 pregnant women among all women over 35 years old appears most plausible. The data, as they appear in the table, say nothing of incidence because they entirely lack denominators.

Sometimes, in search of denominator data, one is tempted to employ an inappropriate denominator. The resulting proportions or percentages are then misinterpreted as rates.

Example 12.2.　　Analysis of the admissions to a large municipal hospital in a northeastern city over a five-year period revealed that, among white patients, hemorrhage from gastric and duodenal ulcers occurred at a rate of 4.8 per 1,000 admissions, whereas among nonwhites this occurred at a rate of 1.6 per 1,000 admissions [13]. The conclusion was drawn that hemorrhage from ulcers is more prevalent in white than in nonwhite persons.

　　The concern with prevalence indicates that the appropriate denominators are the total numbers of whites and nonwhites in the population served by the hospital (presuming one could adequately define such a population, which is extremely difficult in a large metropolitan area). The quantities the investigator calculated represent the proportions of total admissions to the hospital for whites and nonwhites. If, in the population served by the hospital, the nonwhites are hospitalized more often than whites for all other conditions, then, of course, the proportion of total nonwhite admissions for bleeding ulcers will be smaller than that for whites. In other words, the prevalence of bleeding ulcers might actually be the same for whites and nonwhites, but the more frequent hospitalization of nonwhites for all other conditions might explain the figures presented.

　　It may be of interest to the hospital staff to know that bleeding ulcers accounted for a greater percentage of their white patients compared with their nonwhite admissions. However, it is entirely fallacious on the basis of these data to draw any conclusion concerning the frequency of the disease outside the particular hospital since the proper denominator data are lacking.

Example 12.3.　　As another illustration of the temptation of improper denominators, consider the following data by race on total infant deaths, infant deaths due to congenital malformations and birth injuries, and total live births in the United States for 1965:*

	White	Nonwhite
Infant deaths from all causes	67,198	25,668
Infant deaths from congenital malformations and birth injuries	34,370	8,291
Total live births	3,123,860	636,498

* Data from the U.S. Public Health Service [91].

One might calculate that (34,370/67,198) 100% = 51.1% of the white infant deaths and (8,291/25,668) 100% = 32.3% of the nonwhite infant deaths were due to congenital malformations and birth injuries. One might then attempt to conclude that white infants are at greater risk of mortality from congenital malformations and birth injuries than nonwhite infants. These percentages, however, say nothing about the *risk* of death from this cause; they indicate merely that proportionately more white than nonwhite infant deaths are attributable to this cause. To calculate the *risk* of death from congenital malformations, the figure for "total live births" represents the proper denominator for those at risk. The death *rates* for congenital malformations and birth injuries are 34,370/3,123,860 = 0.0110, or 11.0 per 1,000, for whites and 8,291/636,498 = 0.0130, or 13.0 per 1,000, for nonwhites. Thus, nonwhite infants have a slightly higher mortality risk from congenital malformations and birth injuries than white infants.

Finally, one common cause of denominator difficulty pertains to reports on the characteristics of an accumulation of patients with some particular disease. The patients may represent what a particular physician has seen in his own practice or may represent all cases admitted to a hospital over a particular time period. Among the first tables one is likely to encounter in such a report is the age distribution of the cases.

Example 12.4.   Table 12.2 presents the age distribution of 553 coronary heart disease patients seen by an investigator (a cardiologist) over a 10-year period [74]. The text summarizes this tabular result with the statement, "The peak age incidence is 46–55 years." Strictly speaking, this statement claims that the data reveal persons 46 to 55 years old are at greater risk of coronary heart disease than persons of other ages.

Table 12.2. Age distribution of coronary heart disease patients seen by a cardiologist during a 10-year period

Age (yr)	Number of patients	Percent of patients
35 and below	37	6.7
36–45	99	17.9
46–55	214	38.7
56–65	140	25.3
65 and over	63	11.4
Total	553	100.0

Data from Mathur [74].

Clearly, the data permit no such conclusion. The denominator—the population, by age, at risk of coronary heart disease—is missing. All that the investigator may conclude is that in *his* practice during this time he has seen relatively more patients in this age group than in any other. Another cardiologist, practicing in some other area, could likely produce an entirely different age distribution for his coronary heart disease patients. For instance, a cardiologist practicing in the center city is likely to encounter a very different age distribution for his coronary heart disease patients compared with a cardiologist practicing in the outer suburbs. To calculate the age incidence, one needs the denominators for the population at risk by age.

COMPARISON GROUPS

Much of medicine is comparative. This is especially so with regard to retrospective methods of inquiry. When one identifies a group of patients with a disease and inquires about their symptoms, their past history, or their previous exposure to some agent, the interpretation of the results usually requires a corresponding determination among a group of controls without the disease.

Example 12.5.　A medical news report with the headline, "Even at home, drinkers run risk of getting smashed," stated [38]:

> A man's home may be his castle, but it's really not much safer than a highway when drinking is involved. Of the roughly 8.5 million persons who are injured at home each year according to a . . . survey, one-quarter have been drinking at the time. . . .

> Based on interviews and Breathalyser tests or venous blood samples of over 8,000 patients admitted to . . . Hospital's emergency service, . . . 22% of persons involved in home accidents had been drinking.

There may well be such an association between drinking and home accidents but these data are meaningless without a comparison figure for the drinking habits of a group of controls *not* involved in a home accident. For all one knows, among the population served by this hospital, one-quarter or more of all individuals may have been drinking on any given night.

Another example is provided by a book review of a treatise on marijuana.

Example 12.6.　The reviewer takes the book's author to task for his statement on the "stepping stone" hypothesis, which claims that marijuana use leads to heroin use. The reviewer states [87]:

> . . . in my view the weakest part of the book is the chapter on addiction and the "stepping stone" hypothesis—that is, the hypothesis that marijuana

use leads one to try hallucinogens and heroin. Is there really a relation between marijuana and other drug use? All available evidence shows that there is though the author is skeptical of this fact and fails to cite some of the evidence supporting it. That a large number of heroin addicts have tried marijuana is dismissed with the comment, "doubtless they all drank milk, ate food, read comic books, wore clothes and rode bicycles before they used either cannabis or heroin, yet, so far as I know, no one has maintained that any of these activities lead to . . . heroin use." This is a frequent but incorrect argument.

To demonstrate his point, the reviewer cites data on 14 students who had used LSD. Of these, 13 had used marijuana; all 14 had, in addition, experience with alcohol. These data on their own shed little light on an association between LSD and marijuana. However, the key to the reviewer's point concerns a control group of 233 students who had never used LSD. The data on marijuana and alcohol usage for both LSD users and controls are as follows:

	14 students who used LSD	233 students who never used LSD	Difference in percent
Percent having used marijuana	92.8	33.0	59.8
Percent having used alcohol	100.0	94.4	5.6

Thus, it is when the reviewer presents the control data for the 233 not having used LSD that one sees a striking difference (59.8 percent) in the percentages having used marijuana compared with almost no difference (5.6 percent) in the percentages having used alcohol. Thus, the control data point to an association between LSD and marijuana and no association between LSD and alcohol. The reviewer states:

The proportion of alcohol users (or milk drinkers, comic book readers, etc.) in the population is so high that just by chance, most hard drug users will be included. All the data now available show that marijuana use is not related to alcohol but is related to LSD and heroin use.

AGE

There is hardly a disease one can think of in which age does not play an important role in morbidity and certainly in mortality. Of any investigation that deals with morbidity or mortality, the reader would do well to ask, "Has age been properly taken into account?" Sometimes the answer is "no."

Example 12.7.   The following excerpt pertains to one portion of a paper that dealt with emotional factors and neoplastic disease, in this particular example, cancer mortality and marital status [64]:

> One part of the life-history that has been tested is the hypothesis that the cancer patients underwent the loss of a crucial cathexis* before the first signs of the neoplasm were noted. . . . Our prediction is that cancer mortality rates should vary in different classes. . . .
>
> The marital group with the highest cancer mortality rate should be 'widowed'. The loss of a spouse due to illness or accident will frequently mean the loss of a major and intense relationship.
>
> The next highest cancer mortality rate should be the 'divorced'. Lower than the 'widowed' because, a priori, we would say that a lower proportion of the divorced made their marriage a major focus of their relationship and energies, although the rates should be higher than for either of the two remaining classes. . . .
>
> The lowest cancer mortality rate should be found in the 'single' group. We would predict that this group would have least often established and lost a major cathexis in the marital area. . . .
>
> So far as marital groups then, we would believe that the pattern of relationships we are looking for would be found statistically in descending order as follows: 'widowed', 'divorced', 'married', 'single'. We predict that cancer mortality rates follow the same order.

To document this hypothesis, consider the data in Table 12.3 on cancer mortality and marital status for American females from 1929 to 1931. If one looks merely at the mortality rates for all cancers, their progression by marital status seems to fall in line with the crucial cathexis prediction. It may seem rather surprising, however, that from single to widowed women there is as much as a ninefold difference in mortality!

Table 12.3. Cancer mortality rates by site and marital status, U.S. females, 1929–31 (rates per 100,000 population)

Marital status	Site					
	Breast	Uterus	Ovary and fallopian tubes	Vulva and vagina	Other	Total
Single	15.0	9.0	3.3	0.5	33.4	61.2
Married	24.5	35.0	4.7	0.8	71.8	136.8
Divorced	29.3	57.2	6.0	1.5	81.8	175.8
Widowed	74.4	94.4	9.6	4.3	344.4	527.1

Data from LeShan [64].

* *Cathexis:* "Concentration of mental or emotional energy upon an idea or object" [31].

The rates are calculated correctly with appropriate numerators and denominators. There is, however, a much more plausible alternative explanation to crucial cathexis for the differences in rates: the simple explanation is the difference in age. The data in Table 12.3 are *crude* death rates. Cancer is one disease whose mortality is related strongly to age. Thus, it is not at all surprising to find that among single women—who are considerably younger than married women who, in turn, are younger than divorcees who, in turn, are younger than widows—the cancer mortality rates are as different as those shown in Table 12.3. Age has been entirely neglected in the comparison of mortality by marital status.

The commonly employed technique to account for age is the calculation of age-adjusted rates as described previously (p. 47). For the data in Table 12.3, the original sources of information that the author had cited [55] yielded the required distribution of both the cancer deaths and the female U.S. population by age and by marital status. Using as a standard the age distribution of the total American female population in 1930, age-adjusted cancer mortality rates were calculated by the direct method (Table 2.16) and are presented in Table 12.4. One interprets these rates as the

Table 12.4. Age-adjusted[a] cancer mortality rates by site and marital status, U.S. females, 1929–31 (rates per 100,000 population)

Marital status	Site					
	Breast	Uterus	Ovary and fallopian tubes	Vulva and vagina	Other	Total
Single	43.7	25.4	8.2	1.3	97.4	176.0
Married	25.0	34.3	4.4	1.0	85.9	150.7
Divorced	35.7	60.8	6.1	1.5	128.0	232.2
Widowed	28.3	45.9	5.4	1.4	105.1	186.3

[a] Adjusted to total U.S. female population by age in 1930.
Calculated from data presented by Herring [55].

mortality rates that would prevail if each of the four marital status groups had the same age distribution as the total American female population. The age-adjusted rates tell quite a different story. First, the order of magnitude of the differences between the rates is considerably lower than the ninefold difference among the crude rates of Table 12.3.

Second, the rates are not in line with what was anticipated with the crucial cathexis hypothesis. Third, and parenthetically, they reflect some of the well-known facts of cancer epidemiology. Marriage has some advantages and disadvantages with regard to cancer mortality; the married woman as compared with the single woman has less risk of mortality from breast cancer, but a higher risk of mortality from cancer of the uterus.

The average age at death represents another common misuse of age data. Since age data are usually fairly easy to obtain for a group of deaths, one is tempted to summarize mortality experience by using the average age at death.

Example 12.8.   When the hazards of radiation became known, there was speculation that radiologists, because of their long-continued exposure to low dosages of ionizing radiation, would experience reduced longevity compared with other physicians. To compare the mortality experience of radiologists with other physicians, an investigator collected data on the age at death of all American physicians who died during the period from 1930 to 1954. The investigator classified physicians by their specialties, and the figures below give the average age at death for five medical specialty categories [112]:

Category	Average age at death (years)
Radiologists	60.5
Dermatologists	62.3
Pathologists	62.4
Specialists with some radiation exposure (gastroenterologists, urologists, etc.)	63.7
Other physicians with no exposure to radiation	65.7

Comparison of the top and bottom averages indicated that "radiologists die five years earlier on the average than physicians having no known contact with radiation."

One cannot conclude from these data, however, that radiologists have a poorer mortality experience than other physicians with no exposure to radiation. The key variable that remains unaccounted for is the age distribution of *all* radiologists and *all* other physicians. Since radiology is a relatively new specialty, few entered the field in its early stages. Thus radiology, when compared with other more established specialties, will have a deficit of elderly physicians. If among the population of living physicians, there are more elderly "other" physicians than elderly radiologists, then, even if the two groups died at the same age-specific rates, the other physicians would reveal a higher average age at death than radiologists.

Consideration of some extreme examples may aid in understanding this point. The average age at death of full professors will be higher than that of assistant professors; the average age at death of generals will be higher than that of lieutenants; and the average age at death of presidents will be higher than that of congressmen. This is because, respectively, there are more older full professors than assistant professors, generals than lieutenants, and presidents than congressmen.

Table 12.5. Hypothetical data to illustrate fallacy of "average age at death": Mortality of radiologists versus other physicians

Age group (yr)	Mid-point (yr)	Radiologists			Other physicians		
		Number in population	Death rate	Number of deaths	Number in population	Death rate	Number of deaths
25–44	35	390	.003	1	470	.003	1
45–64	55	540	.024	13	390	.024	9
65–84	75	70	.100	7	140	.100	14
Total		1,000		21	1,000		24

Identical age-specific death rates

Average Age at Death:

$$\text{For radiologists:} \quad \frac{(1)(35) + (13)(55) + (7)(75)}{21} = 61 \text{ yr}$$

$$\text{For other physicians:} \quad \frac{(1)(35) + (9)(55) + (14)(75)}{24} = 66 \text{ yr}$$

To illustrate how the fallacy operates, Table 12.5 presents mortality data for hypothetical populations of 1,000 radiologists and 1,000 other physicians. For simplification, the table employs three age groups. Within each age group, the radiologists and the other physicians die at identical death rates. One obtains the numbers of deaths in each age group (the product of the number in the population and the death rate), and, using the midpoint of the age range, one calculates the average age at death, shown at the foot of the table. The resulting five-year difference in average age at death cannot be attributed to differential mortality experience; it is attributed solely to the different age compositions of the two populations, mainly the fact that there are considerably more elderly persons (i.e., age 65 to 84 years) among the "other" physicians than among radiologists. Thus, when dying at the same rates, the larger number of elderly "other" physicians yields more elderly deaths compared with radiologists. This is what most affects the average-age-at-death calculations.

The moral is, beware of average-age-at-death figures. They are not a helpful summary of mortality and can be seriously misleading. The proper analysis of mortality would involve the determination of age-specific mortality rates. This requires, of course, denominator data on the age distribution of the population. Seltzer and Sartwell performed such an analysis for radiologists compared with those in other specialties [100]. Interestingly, they concluded that radiologists had a somewhat less favorable mortality experience, although it was by no means as poor as that suggested by the difference in the average-age-at-death data.

FOLLOW-UP

The complexities of longitudinal studies have already been discussed. As was noted in Chapter 9, the difficulty in assembling longevity data is that, by the time the investigator wants to draw his conclusions, some of his patients have died, some are alive, and some have been lost to follow-up. In addition, within each of these three groups, patients have been observed for differing lengths of time. The mean observation time of the deceased makes an intuitively appealing summary mortality figure.

Example 12.9. Consider the following excerpt from a study whose aim was to determine prognosis following blindness due to diabetic retinopathy [8]:

> Review of a series of 180 blind diabetic patients who had received guide dogs ... over a 17-year period (1947–1964) included 85 deceased and 95 living diabetic patients (as of November 1, 1964) .... Of the 85 deceased diabetics in this series, the average lifespan after the onset of severe blindness due to diabetic retinopathy was 5.8 years. This suggests that the life expectancy of a diabetic is very poor after the onset of blindness due to severe retinopathy.

The prognosis may be poor, but not as poor as these data

seem to indicate. The calculation is based only on the deaths within the 17 years of the study. The longest possible survival time, therefore, is 17 years, presuming that the patient was recruited at the start of the study in 1947 and died at the end of the study in 1964. The possible survival time for any patient starting in the study after 1947 is, of course, less than 17 years. For example, a patient entering on November 1, 1963 and dying in 1964 could contribute at most one year's survival to the calculation. The most important factor is that the author's calculation entirely neglects the 95 patients who were alive in November 1964 when the study was terminated.

One might suggest that the investigator should include the survival times of the 95 living patients, that is, their survival up until the date of study termination. This, however, would not help. As noted in Chapter 9 (p. 239), the mean "survival" of all 190 patients as of November 1964 would represent merely the average duration of observation of all 190 patients and would fail to present any meaningful summary of the duration of life.

The point is that mean survival cannot be calculated until *all* 180 patients under observation have died. By averaging the survival time only among those deaths that occurred in the 17-year study period, the investigator is drastically selecting for early death. No wonder the prognosis seems so poor!

The fact that the calculation of mean survival time must await the death of all subjects under investigation does not imply the impossibility of an investigator's making a meaningful statement of mortality. The raw data on diabetic retinopathy in the example above would fit within a life-table format and thereby would permit the calculation of a survival curve (see p. 244). Alternatively, calculation of a death rate per person-years of exposure would also provide an appropriate mortality summary (see p. 239).

Example 12.10. This example represents a hybrid of the average age and incomplete follow-up difficulties. It concerns a report on a familial relationship in cancer of the breast [83]:

As are most clinicians who deal with carcinoma of the breast we have long since been convinced that it is a familial disease. Among our patients there are many who have an impressive family history of mammary carcinoma.

One aspect of the familial pattern as revealed in our data which we wish to present in more detail is the age at which the disease appears. . . .

In our data there were a total of 182 pairs of mothers and daughters with mammary carcinoma developing at a known age. . . . The mean age of the mothers was 59.7 years; that of the daughters 47.5 years.

> This difference of 12.2 years is convincing evidence that mothers with mammary carcinoma pass on to their daughters a likelihood of developing the disease at an earlier age than they themselves get it. No matter how statisticians may interpret these data they are all too real to be ignored.

Apart from any changes that may have occurred because of the ability to diagnose breast cancer at an earlier stage and the possibly keener surveillance among daughters of women with breast cancer, there are other shortcomings to this conclusion. The study involves the "incomplete follow-up difficulty" in that, among the investigator's patients, no doubt there are many mother-daughter pairs for which at the time of the study the mother has breast cancer and the daughter does not, but the daughter will develop the disease in the future. In other words, at the time of the investigation, many daughters fated to acquire breast cancer have not yet lived long enough to develop it and be counted in the study. Thus, the investigator's requirement of the occurrence of breast cancer in both mother and daughter is deliberately selective for those instances in which the daughters develop breast cancer at an early age.

The "average-age difficulty" is involved in the sense that the mothers with breast cancer come from a population having a high proportion of older women, whereas the daughters with breast cancer come from a population with very few older women. One must consider the age distributions in the underlying populations of mothers and daughters. Breast cancer is strongly related to age, and the age distributions of mothers and daughters differ substantially. In other words, breast cancer at an older age can pertain to the mother member and not to the daughter member of the study pair.

This argument does not imply the absence of a familial component in breast cancer. There well may be a relationship, but it clearly cannot be demonstrated with the data presented.

COMPARISON OF LIKE WITH LIKE

The essence of statistical comparisons in medicine is that one compares like with like. The discussions of clinical trials and medical surveys in Chapters 10 and 11 emphasized this point. "Like with like" means that what are compared are alike in important characteristics at the start of an investigation, handled alike during the course of the investigation, and treated alike in the analysis of results. In this discussion of fallacies, it is worth remembering this important concept.

Example 12.11. The following example illustrates an instance where a question arose concerning whether the investigator compared like with like in the analysis of his results. In addition, this study involved the incomplete follow-up fallacy. The report stated [77]:

> The aim of the analysis described here is to answer the question: Does cardiac transplantation at the present stage of development prolong the life of patients with advanced, therapy-resistant heart disease?

> Sixteen cardiac allografts have been done in 15 patients.... All patients had end-stage heart disease which was resistant to further medical treatment.

> [During this same time period] 42 other patients were considered as possible and acceptable recipients for cardiac allografts.... The group of potential recipients comprised patients considered for heart transplantation which could not be performed for lack of a comparable donor.

> To compare the survival times of the potential recipients with those of the transplant patients, we added the waiting time of the transplant patients from the moment they were considered as recipients to the post-operative survival time.

Apart from the overall comparability of the transplant and potential transplant patients, it was the last sentence in the above excerpt that came under considerable criticism. This pertained to the investigator's supplementation in the transplant group of their average waiting period (it came to 22 days) with no corresponding adjustment for the potential recipients. One letter to the editor of the journal stated [65]:

> Firstly, the 22-day average waiting time cannot be directly added to the postoperative survival time, for any patient dying while awaiting operation would automatically be allocated to the control group who did not receive operations, thus unfairly loading that group with short survivals.

Another claimed [52]:

> Of necessity transplant patients had to live until they were operated on; the comparison group was under no compulsion to survive a comparable period.

The investigators became ensnared in the incomplete follow-up fallacy when they later stated:

> The mean survival time for the 15 transplanted patients up to March 1, 1969 was 111 days compared with a mean survival of 74 days for the 42 potential recipients.

The letters to the editor focused considerable attention on the incomplete follow-up and one letter, using the data the author had presented, contained a life-table calculation. The result was that, if one discounts the first month's survival (which roughly corresponds with the 22-day bonus survival time of the transplant group), the remaining survival patterns of the transplant and comparison groups are quite similar. The numbers involved, of course, are quite small.

The following three fallacies do not concern errors in numerical logic. They pertain to the misapplication of statistical techniques. Since these occur somewhat frequently, they are worthy of mention in this section.

INAPPROPRIATE SAMPLE UNITS

Reference has already been made to the difficulty involved when multiple measurements are obtained on sample units (p. 41). It is indeed tempting to treat the total number of observations as the sample size in subsequent statistical determinations. This can be quite misleading, as was indicated with the 800 blood pressure measurements on 10 hypertensive patients (p. 42).

In a similar manner, the use of person-years of exposure might suggest the inappropriate use of the number of person-years as n for the calculation of tests of significance. For example, with the smoking and lung cancer data of Table 11.4, it would be most inappropriate to use ns of 15,107 and 98,090. This is clearly demonstrated by considering what would happen if, alternatively, the results had been expressed in person-months or person-weeks of observation. The data would remain unchanged, but the presumed n would increase 12-fold or 52-fold, respectively, which cannot be right. The point is that rates calculated on the basis of person-time exposure do not readily lend themselves to application of the common statistical methods of inference in this text. Techniques beyond those covered here are required.

NORMAL LIMITS

Another common error in the application of the methods of statistics is the routine determination of "normal limits" by the calculation of a mean ± 2 SDs for some quantity measured among a group of healthy subjects. These normal limits are interpreted as including the values for 95 percent of the healthy individuals. It must be remembered that the property of 95 percent of a distribution being contained within the mean ± 2 SDs applies only to a *normal* distribution. Many distributions of medical quantities do not follow or even approximate the normal distribution. Before one can calculate "normal limits" as the mean ± 2 SDs, one must have convincing evidence that the distribution closely resembles the normal. Normal limits are best obtained from careful, large-scale investigations of healthy individuals in which the percentage distribution of the characteristic can be empirically determined. For further information, the interested reader should refer to the intriguingly titled paper, "Health, normality and the ghost of Gauss" [37].

MULTIPLE SIGNIFICANCE TESTING

Many current studies involve a considerable number of different measurements on each subject. The methods of statistical tests of significance are easy to apply, and, with the advent of computers, P values can be spewed forth almost ceaselessly. As an extreme possibility, there is the danger that an investigator may be tempted to allow his statistical analysis to generate his hypotheses. The philosophy underlying this approach is to measure everything, test the results for each measurement by computer, and then pick out all those items that achieve statistical significance.

To illustrate this "needle-in-the-haystack" research approach, consider the following hypothetical example concerning a psychological test comprising 550 items.

Example 12.12.   An investigator studying psychological factors in prematurity administers the Minnesota Multiphasic Personality Inventory (MMPI) to women attending a prenatal clinic. The MMPI consists of 550 statements, and for each statement the subject answers whether the statement is true or false about herself. (Sample statements are, "I loved my mother," "I dream frequently," "I believe there is a God," and "Sexual things disgust me.") After the women are delivered, they are classified as having delivered a normal or a premature infant. For each of the 550 items on the MMPI test, the investigator will construct a fourfold table, the column headings being "Normal Delivery" and "Premature" and the row labels being "Item Answered True" and "Item Answered False." He might plan to calculate chi-square for each fourfold table and test the difference in the percentage answering "true" among women having delivered normal babies compared with women having delivered premature babies. He may then propose to select from the resulting 550 tests of significance those items that achieve significance at the 5 percent level. He might then claim that these items represent the personality discriminants between the two groups of women.

The point is that with multiple testing, when each test is at the 5 percent level, one must consider the long-range interpretation of the 5 percent significance level. If all the 550 null hypotheses tested were actually true, then by chance alone the investigator would expect 5 percent, or $(550)(0.05) = 28$ items, to achieve statistical significance. Thus, it should come as no surprise to him if he were to find, say, 30 items significant at the 5 percent level. If he found considerably more, he would certainly be convinced that there were some differences in the responses of the two groups of women. Of course, it would be impossible for him to pick out which differences were real and which reflected merely the expected 5 percent from repeated applications of the test of significance.

BERKSON'S FALLACY

Berkson's fallacy deals with the possibility of spurious associations between diseases or between a disease and a risk factor. The essence of the fallacy is that the interplay of differential admission rates from an underlying population to a select study group, such as a series of hospital admissions or a set of necropsy protocols, can lead to the observation of an artificial association in the study group.

Example 12.13.   An investigation of a possible association between tuberculosis and cancer began with identification of 816 instances of cancer among the necropsy protocols at a large metropolitan teaching hospital during a particular time period [84]. For controls, 816 necropsy protocols were obtained during the same time period for patients dying from a wide variety of causes except any cancer. For both cancer patients and controls, the records were reviewed to determine whether or not the patients had had tuberculosis. The results are summarized in the following fourfold table:

		Cancer	Control
	Present	54	133
Tuberculosis	Absent	762	683
	Total	816	816
	Percent with tuberculosis	6.6%	16.3%

Chi-square (1 df) = 36.75, $P < .001$

The difference in the proportions with tuberculosis, according to the chi-square test (p. 175), is highly statistically significant. Note that there is a *negative* association between tuberculosis and cancer; the frequency of tuberculosis is *less* among cancer patients than among controls. As a matter of fact, on the basis of the above observed negative association and its suggestion of tuberculosis-cancer antagonism, an investigation commenced whereby human malignancies were treated with tuberculin [85].

To illustrate the nature of Berkson's fallacy, assume that ideal study conditions prevail, that the diseases involved are uniformly and objectively defined according to strict diagnostic criteria, and that, further, the cases and controls are alike in all relevant aspects so that differences in age, sex, and other clinical characteristics can be neglected as explanations of the observed difference in rates.

Before considering the cancer and tuberculosis data from the example above, consider the following hypothetical situation concerning a possible association between two diseases, A and X. A control disease B is identified (B may refer to all diseases other than A or it may be a particular "control" disease that is known to bear no relation whatsoever to X). The study will consist of determining the relative frequency of X among the cases of A compared with the cases of B.

The following hypothetical data (in round numbers) show the nature of the fallacy. The argument is developed by considering an underlying population in which there is *no* association between A and X, i.e., X occurs *equally* frequently among the patients with diseases A and B. Then, by allowing members of the underlying population to enter the study group at differing admission rates, the spurious study association will be demonstrated.

Assume there are population counts of 1,000 persons each with disease A and B. Assume further that 100 in each group have disease X. Thus X occurs among 10 percent of the cases of A and 10 percent of the cases of B in the underlying population. Hence, there is no association between diseases A and X. The data for the population are:

		Population	
		Disease A	Disease B
	Present	100	100
Disease X	Absent	900	900
	Total	1,000	1,000
	Percent with X	10%	10%

Now presume the following rates of admission to the study group:

If Disease	Probability of entering study group
A	.20
B	.80
X	.50

In other words, only a portion of the population wend their way into the study group, and further, with differing diseases, the proportion who enter the study group differ. With the study group defined as the cases in a particular hospital or among a set of necropsy protocols, these differential study entry rates with different diseases seem perfectly reasonable.

Now consider persons with two diseases, namely, those with A and X and those with B and X. Such patients may enter the study group because of either disease. As a first-order approximation, assume that with two diseases the forces causing a patient to be admitted to the study group operate independently. A patient with diseases A and X may enter the study in two mutually exclusive ways: either having A causes him to be admitted, or having A does not cause him to be admitted but having X does. Using the additive law of probability (p. 64),

Pr(Either A or X causes admission) $=$

PR(A causes admission) $+$

Pr(A does not cause admission but X causes admission)

With the forces causing admission operating independently, application of the multiplicative law of probability (p. 67) above to the last term gives the desired result:

Pr(Either A or X causes admission) $=$

Pr(A causes admission) $+$

Pr(A does not cause admission) Pr(X causes admission)

With the figures given, it may be seen that the following chances of admission to the study group prevail:

1. Patients with both diseases A and X: $.2 + (1 - .2)(.5) = .6$
2. Patients with both diseases B and X: $.8 + (1 - .8)(.5) = .9$
3. Patients with disease A alone: $.2$
4. Patients with disease B alone: $.8$

Thus, 60 percent of those with A and X, 90 percent of those with B and X, 20 percent of those with A alone, and 80 percent of those with B alone enter the study from the population.

Application of these admission rates to the general population figures gives for the study group:

		Study group	
		Disease A	Disease B
Disease X	Present	$(100)(.6) = 60$	$(100)(.9) = 90$
	Absent	$(900)(.2) = 180$	$(900)(.8) = 720$
	Total	240	810
	Percent with X	25%	11%

Thus, in the study group, disease X occurs more than twice as frequently with A as with B, i.e., 25 percent among the cases of A and only 11 percent among the cases of B. Application of the chi-square test yields $\chi_c^2(1 \text{ df}) = 28.03$, $P < .001$. Thus, the difference is highly statistically significant and not explainable by chance variation. The result, however, is entirely explainable by the differential admission rates to the study group.

Now consider the following somewhat more complex set of data. In contrast with the preceding example, the numbers are not rounded off and in the general population the total with disease A is not the same as the total with disease B.

		Population	
		Disease A	Disease B
Disease X	Present	79	409
	Absent	1,318	6,830
	Total	1,397	7,239
	Percent with X	5.6%	5.6%

As before, there is no association between A and X in the population, i.e., X occurs among 5.6 percent of the cases of A and with the same frequency among the cases of B.

Next, assume that there are the following admission rates to the study group:

If Disease	Probability of entering study group
A	.578
B	.100
X	.250

As before, the same assumptions apply concerning the admission to the study group of patients with two diseases. This then gives the following chances for entry to the study:

1. Patients with both diseases A and X: $.578 + (1 - .578)(.250) = .684$
2. Patients with both diseases B and X: $.100 + (1 - .100)(.250) = .325$
3. Patients with disease A alone: $.578$
4. Patients with disease B alone: $.100$

Application of these rates to the population figures yields for the study group:

		Study group	
		Disease A	Disease B
Disease X	Present	$(79)(.684) = 54$	$(409)(.325) = 133$
	Absent	$(1,318)(.578) = 762$	$(6,830)(.100) = 683$
	Total	816	816
	Percent with X	6.6%	16.3%

It remains now to define disease A as cancer, disease B as all other diseases excluding cancer, disease X as tuberculosis, and the study group as the necropsy cases at a particular hospital over some particular period of time. The data are precisely those cited at the outset. Thus, the association observed in the study group may be spurious. There may be no association between cancer and tuberculosis in the underlying general population, but differential admission rates to the necropsy study group produce the observed association.

The attribution of Berkson's fallacy hangs on the argument of differential study admission rates. The data cited to illustrate the fallacy were hypothetical. Thus, the above argument has not *proved* the spuriousness of the observed association. It has merely raised a shadow of a doubt by indicating that the association *might* be spurious. From the data reported, one has no idea of the relationship between cancer and tuberculosis in the underlying population nor does one have any indication of the actual rates of admission from the population to the study group. The issue is the plausibility of the existence of differential study admission rates. In any study that purports to establish an association and where it appears likely that differential rates of admission apply, then at least some portion of the observed association should be suspect as being attributable to Berkson's fallacy. In dealing with highly select study groups, such as a necropsy series or a collection of hospital records, the selective factors are so varied and widespread (see the discussion on p. 6) that differential admission rates become immediately suspect. It is the onus of the investigator to establish beyond reasonable doubt that selective factors did not operate to the extent of permitting a substantial differential in admission rates from the underlying population to the study group.

The interested reader will find further details of Berkson's fallacy discussed by Berkson [9, 10] and Mainland [70, 71].

EXERCISES

Comment critically on the following statements, pointing out in which way the statement may be fallacious or misleading. Indicate what alternative approach or additional data, if any, are needed to answer the question posed in each statement.

1. A report of acute leukemia concerned all patients over 13 years old who were admitted to a particular university hospital over a 15-year period. The following table gives the age distribution of patients for each five-year interval in the 15 years:

Age (yr)	Five-year time interval		
	First	Second	Third
14–29	41	50	51
30 and over	49	76	109
Total	90	126	160

From these data the authors concluded that the incidence rate of acute leukemia had risen and that the increasing incidence was largely restricted to persons over 30 years old.

2. The following data give the sex and race distribution of 158 cases of abdominal aortic aneurysms that were found by autopsy at a number of metropolitan hospitals in a large southern city over a 10-year period:

Sex and race	Number of autopsies with abdominal aneurysms
White males	93
Black males	30
White females	22
Black females	13
Total	158

The authors concluded from these data that the incidence of abdominal aneurysms was almost three times more frequent in white than in black persons and at least three times more frequent in men than in women. In this study, the authors also speculated regarding the incidence of abdominal aortic aneurysms in the total United States. The 158 autopsies with aneurysms were derived from a review of 26,500 autopsies (amounting to 0.6 percent of such autopsies). Since there was a total of approximately 1.6 million deaths in the total United States during the year, the authors speculated that there are approximately $1.6 \times 10^6 \times .006 = 9,600$ abdominal aortic aneurysms annually among all deaths in the United States.

3. A study involved the observation of 102 children under 5 years old with untreated hemangioma simplex. Spontaneous involution occurred in 52

cases; of those, there were 36 for which the size of the lesion was known. Of these 36, 30 were 1 cm or less in diameter and 6 had a diameter of 1 to 3 cm. The authors recommended on the basis of these results that one should immediately treat hemangiomas measuring 1 cm or more since hemangiomas of larger size have a poor chance of spontaneous involution.

4. A review of a clinic's records of diabetic patients revealed approximately 3,000 cases for which data on maximum weight were available. It was found that approximately two-thirds of the patients had been, at some time, 11 percent or more overweight. This provides evidence of an association between obesity and diabetes.

5. Among 110 patients diagnosed with myelofibrosis, there were 85 for whom a complete follow-up was obtained. Among these 85, 55 had died and 30 were still alive at the time the investigator completed his study. For the 55 dead patients, the investigator computed their mean survival time as 2 years and 3 months. He concluded that this observed short duration of life subsequent to diagnosis emphasizes the seriousness of this disease.

6. The obituary columns of an issue of the *Journal of the Americal Medical Association* revealed that the average age at death of 10 board-certified physicians was 60.0 years compared with 73.3 years for 26 physicians who were not board certified. This difference in means was statistically significant ($P < .01$) and therefore provides support to the argument that specialty practice is more stressful and life-shortening than general practice.

7. Data on 123 consecutive unselected female patients with hyperparathyroidism at a university hospital revealed that 36 were under 45 years old and 87 were 45 years old and older. This led the author to conclude that, in women, hyperparathyroidism was more common in the menopausal and postmenopausal age groups.

8. Consecutive patients attending a diabetes clinic were interviewed concerning the age at death of their parents. The analysis included only patients whose parents, both father and mother, had died. The author's rationale for this restriction was to avoid a possible bias due to the fact that wives are usually younger than their husbands. Comparison of the mean age at death revealed that fathers of diabetic patients lived significantly longer than mothers ($P < .001$).

9. An investigation of coronary heart disease in chronic schizophrenic patients consisted of 1,275 autopsy protocols of white males over 40 years old who died of any cause at some 30 hospitals during a five-year period.

Of the 1,275 patients, 394 or 31 percent died from coronary heart disease. In comparison, the investigator cited vital statistics for the United States which indicated that during this time interval, there were approximately 4 million deaths in the total United States among white males 40 years old or older and that only 25 percent died from coronary heart disease. This result provides evidence of an excessive mortality risk from coronary heart disease among chronic schizophrenic patients.

10. Among hospital records of 1,000 varicose-vein patients, 4.7 percent indicated a history of rheumatic fever. As controls, the records of 1,000 patients treated for inguinal hernias revealed only 0.3 percent with a history of rheumatic fever. The two groups of patients were comparable in age and social class. The difference in the rates for a history of rheumatic fever was statistically significant, $P < .001$. Thus, these data provide evidence of an association between varicose veins and rheumatic fever.

11. A review of hospital records of 271 patients with carcinoma of the stomach revealed that 40 had a previous history of fractures of the upper limb, clavicle, scapula ribs, or sternum. Records of 271 patients without stomach cancer, matched for sex and age and admitted to the hospital during the same period, served as controls. Among the controls, a history of fractures at similar sites was discovered in only 18. The difference in the rates for a history of previous fractures was statistically significant, $P < .01$. Thus, these data provide evidence for an association between fractures and gastric cancer.

12. Although the layman generally associates heart attacks with overexertion, they are far more likely to occur during periods of rest. More than one-half the victims of heart attacks are stricken while sleeping or resting and less than 2 percent are afflicted while engaged in strenuous activity such as sports, running, lifting, or moving a heavy load.

13. Among general hospitals in a certain geographical area, the mean length of stay of patients undergoing appendectomy was 11 days, but for patients undergoing gastrectomy the mean length of stay was 27 days. Thus, in terms of the utilizaton of hospital resources, gastrectomy is a more important operation than appendectomy.

14. That Alaska is a more healthy environment than Massachusetts is supported by the fact that in 1968 the mortality rate for Massachusetts was 10.9 deaths per 1,000 population while in Alaska it was 4.9 deaths per 1,000 population, more than a twofold difference.

15. Among 182 guests attending a luau, 38 persons had an acute onset of abdominal cramps and diarrhea within 6 to 50 hours after the meal. The

table below gives for each food served at the luau the percentage of the 38 gastroenteritis cases who indicated that they had consumed that food:

Food	Percent of 38 cases eating food	Food	Percent of 38 cases eating food
Kalua pig	100	Liver	50
Chicken long rice	97	Poi	89
Squid luau	95	Sweet potato	89
Lomi salmon	95	Haupia	74
Poki aku (raw fish)	89	Cake	82
Crab	82	Kulolo	79
Opihi	89		

Since, among the 38 gastroenteritis cases, kalua pig was the food consumed with greatest frequency and it was the only food consumed by everyone who became ill, it clearly becomes suspect as the possible vehicle for transmission of a foodborne infectious agent.

Chapter 13
Critical Reading of the Medical Literature

The approach of this book, like other statistics texts, has in some ways been fragmentary. The text enunciated the principles and commonly employed methods of statistics by proceeding from one topic to another in a hopefully logical, but necessarily disjointed, manner with excerpts from published studies serving as illustrations. The previous three chapters, which dealt with more subjective and quasi-statistical issues, have also employed a fragmentary approach by citing portions of studies to illustrate particular aspects of clinical trials and medical surveys or to identify a particular fallacy in numerical reasoning. The theme of this final chapter is a plea for an integrated approach to the critical reading of the medical literature. Obviously, knowledge of the principles and basic methods of statistics is but one of the several skills involved in the critical evaluation of published numerical evidence in a medical report. Whatever statistical understanding the student may have gained from taking courses in statistics or from the mastery of texts such as this, his statistical understanding needs to be synthesized with his medical expertise and logical skills in order for him to achieve an effective critical approach to the medical literature.

TEACHING EXERCISE IN THE CRITICAL APPRAISAL OF A MEDICAL REPORT

To provide training in such a comprehensive approach to the appraisal of published medical reports, this author has employed, as an integral portion of his course in biostatistics for medical students, exercises in the critical reading of the medical literature. The exercise consists of selecting a paper from the current literature, which is distributed to each student in the class along with a copy of the "Outline for Critique of a Medical Report":

Outline for Critique of a Medical Report*

   I.   Object or hypothesis
       A.   What are the objectives of the study or the questions to be answered?
       B.   What is the population to which the investigators intend to refer their findings?

  II.   Design of the investigation
       A.   Was the study an experiment, planned observations, or an analysis of records?

---

*Credit for the outline goes to Dr. David D. Rutstein who developed it, implemented it in the teaching program, and guided this author in its use as an instructional device.

315

B. How was the sample selected? Are there possible sources of selection which would make the sample atypical or nonrepresentative? If so, what provision was made to deal with this bias?

C. What is the nature of the control group or standard of comparison?

III. Observations

A. Are there clear definitions of the terms used, including diagnostic criteria, measurements made, and criteria of outcome?

B. Was the method of classification or of measurement consistent for all the subjects and relevant to the objectives of the investigation? Are there possible biases in measurement and, if so, what provisions were made to deal with them?

C. Are the observations reliable and reproducible?

IV. Presentation of findings

A. Are the findings presented clearly, objectively, and in sufficient detail to enable the reader to judge them for himself?

B. Are the findings internally consistent, i.e., do the numbers add up properly, can the different tables be reconciled, etc.?

V. Analysis

A. Are the data worthy of statistical analysis? If so, are the methods of statistical analysis appropriate to the source and nature of the data and is the analysis correctly performed and interpreted?

B. Is there sufficient analysis to determine whether "significant differences" may in fact be due to lack of comparability of the groups in sex or age distribution, in clinical characteristics, or in other relevant variables?

VI. Conclusions

Which conclusions are justified by the findings? Which are not? Are the conclusions relevant to the questions posed by the investigators?

VII. Constructive suggestions

Assume you are planning an investigation to answer the questions put in this study. If they have not been clearly put by the authors, frame them in an appropriate manner. Suggest a practical design, criteria for observations, and type of analysis that would provide reliable and valid information relevant to the questions under study.

The students are instructed to read the paper and prepare a written critique following the outline. The students' critiques are read, corrected, commented upon, and then discussed with them in small group-conference sessions. The discussion leaders for each session consist of a physician and a biostatistician.

This is to ensure that salient medical points as well as statistical features emerge in the discussion with the students of the paper at hand. During the course, at least two papers are chosen for critiques: one representing a medical survey, the other representing a clinical trial. By no means is the choice restricted to papers with major defects in either design, execution, or analysis. Much can be learned from the critical dissection of a well-conceived, well-executed, and well-reported study.

Before reviewing the major points on the outline, one should first note that it is impossible to devise a set of questions that apply universally to *all* medical reports. The questions on the outline must, of necessity, be exceedingly general. Even so, not every question applies to every medical report. For a particular report, several questions in the outline become more important than others. Also, many other important and relevant questions that are not on the outline will emerge. The point is that the application of the outline guides the student to a systematic and logical appraisal and places him in the proper position for asking the remaining crucial questions that apply only to the particular report in hand.

STUDY OBJECTIVES

The reader should have a clear understanding of the objectives of the study. Sometimes he gains such understanding merely by reading the title of the paper. In many situations, the author states his objective or the question to be answered at the beginning of his report. There are situations, however, in which the author does not do so explicitly and the reader must glean the objective from the conclusions or summary or from a reading of the entire report. Nevertheless, effective critical appraisal hinges on the reader's initial understanding of the aim of the investigation.

With a view toward the inferences to be drawn from the study, it is well for the reader to identify the author's target population. More often than not, an author fails to indicate specifically the population group to which he intends to refer his findings. The reader will thus have to identify the target population by implication. Undoubtedly, the author will describe the particular group that participated in the study. If he had intended to confine his results solely to the group he studied, there clearly would be no point in publishing his paper. Publication of an inferential study indicates an intent to apply the results to some larger group. The reader needs to determine as best he can the nature of this larger group. With such identification, the reader can assess whether selective factors or bias could, beyond reasonable doubt, materially have affected the results so as to hinder conclusions regarding the target population. The discussion in Chapter 1 concerning target populations and the population sampled is particularly relevant.

DESIGN

Careful reading of the "Materials and Methods" section of a paper permits the reader to assess the adequacy of the study design. First, he should have a clear understanding of the type of study. Is it an experiment, a planned observation study, or the analysis of records? These are hierarchical, but not mutually exclusive, categories. Experiments involve both planned observations and the analysis of records. Planned observations, in turn, involve the analysis of records. However, not all analyses of records involve planned observations, and, correspondingly, not all planned observations are obtained from an experiment. It is worthwhile to note that the chief distinction between an experiment and planned observations is that in an experiment, the investigator manipulates the factor under study. It is he who determines which experimental units (be they patients, laboratory animals, cells, or bacteria) receive which treatments (be they drugs, tests, or laboratory procedures). In planned observations, the investigator does not allocate the factor under investigation; he may have different groups of individuals that vary according to some factor, but these groups result from circumstances beyond the investigator's control. For one reason or another, those in one group may have received one treatment while those in another group received some other.

Some disagree with this distinction between planned observations and an experiment. They argue that, each time a physician administers a drug or performs some test or procedure on a patient, he is interfering with the natural course of events. They would label such interference as an experiment. For example, consider a study that compares those who volunteered with those who failed to volunteer for some treatment. This author would term such a study as one of planned observations. Others would claim that since, in the volunteer group, the investigator interfered with the natural course of events when he administered the treatment, he therefore performed an experiment. The distinction is semantic. This author prefers to label as *experiments* solely those situations in which the investigator presumably could affect the allocation to a particular group, and this is the sense with which the word has been used in this book.

To illustrate the three types of studies, the study of association between cancer and tuberculosis (p. 305) represents a clear-cut example of the analysis of records. The data were derived entirely from routinely collected records of necropsy protocols maintained at the investigator's hospital. The study was, of course, planned. However, the observations were obtained entirely from the available records and were independent of the investigator's plan to conduct a study. The survey of physicians in the examination of the relationship between smoking and lung cancer (p. 284) illustrates a case of planned observations. The investigators planned to collect the basic data that enabled them to classify physicians by smoking status. Obviously, the investigators could exercise no choice as to the allocation of who did and did not smoke. Routine records, which were available regardless of the conduct of the study, also entered into the picture. These, of course, were the death certificates, autopsy protocols, and other hospital records that enabled the investigators to identify the deaths from lung cancer during the study period. The study of propranolol treatment in myocardial infarction (p. 11) illustrates an experiment. The investigator determined the allocation of propranolol or no propranolol to the study patients with myocardial infarctions. His critics raised some doubts about his method of allocation and suggested the possibilities of bias (p. 260). The possibility that his allocation scheme may have been defective matters not in classifying the study as an experiment. The important point is that the investigator could choose who, in the study, would and who would not receive the factor under investigation: the drug propranolol.

The methods employed by the investigator for selecting subjects for his study need clear specification. The reader should be attuned immediately to the identification of possible sources of selection or bias that might hinder conclusions regarding the target population, as identified in the preceding section of the outline (section I.B).

If the essence of the study is comparison, the nature of the control group or the standard of comparison needs clear delineation. Here, the important question is the comparability of the treatment and control groups. Has the investigator sufficiently demonstrated their comparability? Might the two groups possibly differ appreciably with regard to characteristics which are not considered by the investigator and which might materially affect the results? If the groups are not comparable in some important aspect, then the analysis should account for such a discrepancy. In essence, has the author provided the reader with evidence beyond reasonable doubt that he is comparing like with like?

OBSERVATIONS

The usefulness and applicability to other patients of the results presented in a medical report depend on there being clear definitions of the terms involved. First, if the study deals with a disease, the reader must know precisely what constitutes the disease. The investigator is obliged to provide the reader with suitable diagnostic criteria that can be employed in selecting study patients. Gifford and Feinstein, in their critical review of 32 reports of studies on anticoagulant therapy for acute myocardial infarction, state [44]: "The first scientific requirement in any investigation of therapy is a clear, precise statement of diagnostic criteria for the disease under study." For example, it is insufficient to state merely that the study concerned patients with acute myocardial infarctions. Acute myocardial infarction to one physician, in one type of practice and in one locality, may encompass quite a different spectrum of disease from that of another physician in some other type of practice and in another locality. It behooves the investigator to indicate precisely his criteria for acute myocardial infarction among the patients in his study. Of course, simple reference to widely employed criteria that are available elsewhere in published form serves as an entirely acceptable substitute and can conserve valuable space in a printed report. The reader is also entitled to a listing of exclusions from the study group along with the rationale for such exclusions.

In addition to diagnostic criteria, and especially so for clinical trials, it is the author's onus to define carefully the nature of the treatment or procedure as well as the nature of the control regimen. If the study involves follow-up, then this, too, needs clear description. Finally, similar attention must also be devoted to the clear definition of criteria determining the outcome.

In his assessment of the methods of observation, the reader should attune himself to the identification of possible bias and selective factors that could tend to produce inconsistencies in the handling and evaluation of patients among the different groups during the course of the investigation. The essential question with any inconsistency in observation or evaluation is whether it is of such sufficient impact that it could influence materially the results of the study. Here, too, it is the author's onus to demonstrate beyond reasonable doubt that his methods of observation were sufficiently consistent or to argue persuasively that any inconsistencies could not possibly alter his conclusions.

The last question in this section of the outline concerns reliability and reproducibility, which are two of the most difficult items to assess in a report. Often the reader can do no more than to give his impression. The question, however, is of utmost importance in terms of the usefulness of the results. Frequently, there are some clues in a paper that, at the least, inform the reader of the author's concern with and awareness of reproducibility and reliability. When a subjective element enters into an assessment, an author will often refer to, and sometimes provide data on, the results of evaluations by independent observers and their degree of agreement. Also, when the study involves considerable laboratory work, an author may devote some attention to data concerning measurement or laboratory error (see p. 39 for discussion). It is well for the reader to be suspicious of results from a study that remains entirely devoid of any concern with reproducibility and reliability, especially when the study involves some subjective element either in diagnosis, observation, or the assessment of outcome.

PRESENTATION OF FINDINGS

This section pertains more directly to the material covered in this book. An author must walk the fine line of clear and concise data presentation, but must still detour into enough necessary detail for the reader to judge the importance of the data by himself. Important findings require proper documentation For example, if an important result is that males fared better than females, that statement alone is insufficient. The reader is entitled to see the figures or the summary statistics so he may judge for himself that males did indeed do better than females.

It is surprising how often there are numerical inconsistencies contained within papers published in even the most reputable medical journals. Perhaps this is due in part to the many drafts and revisions most papers undergo between the completion of an investigation and final publication. Furthermore, in comparison with textual proofreading, computational and tabular proofreading requires considerably more concentration and is considerably more tedious. The following represent some quick checks the reader might employ for detection of numerical inconsistencies: (1) A column should add to the indicated totals at its foot, and likewise for rows; (2) Percentages, if mutually exclusive categories, should add to 100 percent; (3) Numbers in tables and figures should reconcile with those in the text; and (4) The totals of various tables should agree unless the author has specifically indicated additions or deletions to the basic study group or unless he has noted a restriction to some particular subgroup. Perhaps the astute reader will be able to identify numerical inconsistencies in this text.

ANALYSIS

This text has focused on the statistical analysis of medical data. The first question in this section of the outline, however, is most important as a preamble to the consideration of an analysis. Do the design and methods of observation for the study permit the statistical analysis of the results? A major defect in design or some extreme bias in the method of observation can render any assessment of an analysis irrelevant. When a statistical test of significance was first employed in this text, it carried the warning that some reasonable simulation of random sampling from an underlying population is presupposed (p. 118). The citation from the *New England Journal of Medicine* editorial in the same discussion warned that *any* set of numbers can be submitted to a statistical analysis. The point is whether the investigator has sufficient justification to perform these computations in order to draw the corresponding inferences concerning his underlying population.

If successful, this book will serve as a guide to the reader for evaluating the appropriateness of a statistical analysis and interpreting its results. The methods contained in this book pertain to the commonly employed statistical techniques in the medical literature. No doubt, the reader will encounter methods in the literature that are beyond the scope of this text. The more advanced statistical texts mentioned in previous chapters may serve as useful references for the reader who wishes to delve farther into more complex statistical methods. The employment of less common statistical methods requires proper documentation by the author, although the medical reader who pursues such references may find them beyond his interest and mathematical capabilities. Often, advice may have to be sought from one's statistical colleagues. An important point, however, is that the structure and interpretation of many complex statistical methods are still within the same framework as the more simple methods described in this text. Although the reader may find the arithmetical calculations and the statistical quantities far removed from what appear in this text, the interpretations of the resulting P values or confidence limit statements are identical.

It is important to note that the thorough analysis of medical data entails taking into proper account those variables that are strongly related to the phenomenon under study. Mention has already been made of the importance of age in virtually all diseases. Many of the fallacies discussed in the preceding section depended on the lack of an adequate accounting for age. Sex is often an additional crucial variable, and the question of its proper treatment in an analysis is worth attention. The reader's background, knowledge, and experience in the particular field under study will enable him to ascertain which other important variables deserve attention in a particular analysis.

CONCLUSION

The logical and orderly analysis of a paper according to the preceding sections of the outline will lead the reader to a virtually automatic verdict regarding the author's conclusions. The critical appraisal is essentially completed with the reader's ascertainment of whether the investigator's conclusions tie in with the stated or implicit study objectives as delineated in the first section of the outline.

CONSTRUCTIVE SUGGESTIONS

To offset the rather negative and destructively critical approach suggested by the preceding sections, the final section of the outline urges the student to temper his criticism with some constructive suggestions. If he has found fault with what the investigator has done, then he should suggest a better way of doing it, but one that is within reason. Upon reflection, the reader might conclude that there is no feasible alternative study. He may often come to the realization that the somewhat imperfect study conducted by the investigator leaves little room for improvement. He then has to grapple with a choice between the alternatives of no study whatsoever and the imperfect study at hand. A further advantage to this final section of the outline is that it hopefully encourages a constructive attitude among the potential referees for tomorrow's medical journals.

Answers to Exercises

Chapter 2

1. A. There appear to be more readings ending in 0 and 8 than one might expect. This phenomenon is called "digit preference."
   B. Reader provides.
   C. If, for example, the lowest class was 90 to 98 mm Hg, then the true limits are 89 to 99 mm Hg and the midpoint is 94 mm Hg.
   D. They are not compatible with the raw data. The interval 95 to 99 permits only two possible raw data readings (96 and 98), whereas 100 to 104 permits three (100, 102, and 104). Thus, these intervals are unequal in width when one considers the raw data.
   E. Using the raw data, the median is 121 mm Hg, the mean is 122.5 mm Hg, the SD is 12.5 mm Hg, and the CV is 10.2 percent. With use of a frequency distribution as the basis for these calculations, the results should be very similar.
   F. One might consider factors associated with the instrument (e.g., calibration, dirty tube, or cuff width) and the observer (e.g., the rate of inflation and deflation of the cuff, interpretation of sounds, hearing acuity, or his ability to read a moving column).
   G. (1) Yes, the results should be generally compatible. The range of 105 to 140 mm Hg encompasses 51 or 85 percent of the 60 observations.
      (2) There are several reasons for disagreement such as the lack of uniform conditions for measuring blood pressure, the inexperience of medical students in determining measurements, and the preselection of medical students as healthy persons.

2. A. First, the class intervals are not mutually exclusive; second, the working units are incorrectly assigned (they did not take account of unequal widths of class intervals); and third, the fv^2 column was incorrectly calculated as $(fv)^2$.
   B. Use of case records of a university hospital constitutes one selective factor; these hospitals tend to get the more serious and complicated cases. A study based on hospitalized patients is another selective factor, since many patients with angina pectoris are not hospitalized.
   C. Since angina pectoris is a very subjective type of disease, it would be difficult to pinpoint precisely when its symptoms began. One must also rely on the ability of the subject to recall and report

dates and events that may have occurred many years ago. In addition, much depends on the skill and diligence of the examining physician in taking the patient's history.

3. A. median
    B. (1) mean and median   (2) mean
    C. mean, median, mode
    D. median, modal, mean
    E. mean, mean, mean
    F. mean
    G. mode, mean

4. A. The variances are (1)1,147 (mg percent)^2 and (2)1,206 (mg percent)^2.
    B. Reader provides.
    C. The mean of six variances is 93 (mg percent)^2.
    D. (1) The appropriate variance is that calculated in part C.
        (2) The appropriate variance is that calculated in part A(2).
    E. To determine the unbiasedness use the technique on standard specimens with a known triglyceride level. To determine the precision, run replicate measurements on several specimens. One would also want to consider the cost, the amount of time involved, the personnel and equipment needed, and perhaps any possible added discomfort or inconvenience to the subjects.

5. A. The crude cancer mortality rate for widows is 529.8 deaths per 100,000 population.
    B. The age-adjusted cancer mortality rate for widows, when calculated by the direct method, is 187.6 deaths per 100,000 population.
    C. The age-adjusted cancer mortality rate for widows, when calculated by the indirect method, is 170.8 deaths per 100,000 population. (The expected cancer deaths were 19,396.1 and the standard mortality ratio was 106.2 percent.)

6. A. and B. The computations and rates for prevalence and incidence are shown in this table.

Sex and age (yr)	CHD prevalence rate		Fourteen-year CHD incidence rate	
	Calculation	Rate per 1,000	Calculation	Rate per 1,000
M: 35–44	7/865	8.1	86/(865 − 7)	100.2
45–54	26/731	35.6	135/(731 − 26)	191.5
55–64	18/348	51.7	83/(348 − 18)	251.5
F: 35–44	4/1,095	3.7	15/(1,095 − 4)	13.7
45–54	13/883	14.7	76/(883 − 13)	87.4
55–64	11/437	25.2	72/(437 − 11)	169.0

C. No. One needs to know how many died so that they can be excluded from denominator. Also, one must change the age categories over the fourteen years.

Chapter 3

1. $1 - .98^{45} = .597$
2. $1 - (.8 \times .7 \times .5) = .72$
3. A. Both die: $\pi_T \pi_C$
   Both survive: $(1 - \pi_T)(1 - \pi_C)$
   Treatment member survives, control member dies: $(1 - \pi_T)\pi_C$
   Control member survives, treatment member dies: $\pi_T(1 - \pi_C)$
   B. Untied pairs: $(1 - \pi_T)\pi_C + \pi_T(1 - \pi_C)$
   C. $(1 - \pi_T)\pi_C/[(1 - \pi_T)\pi_C + \pi_T(1 - \pi_C)]$
   D. Reader provides.
   E. Reader provides.
4. The drug passes the screen if there is at least one remission. When $\pi = .20$, $\Pr(\text{Pass}) = 1 - .8^6 = .74$; when $\pi = .30$, $\Pr(\text{Pass}) = 1 - .7^6 = .88$.
5. A. Wife is a living widow: $\Pr(\text{H dies, W lives}) = .1864 \times .9035 = .1684$
   Husband is a living widower: $\Pr(\text{H lives, W dies}) = .8136 \times .0965 = .0785$
   Relative probability: $.1684/.0785 = 2.15$
   B. The probability that a person age 65 survives to age 75 is, from Table 2.18, the number alive at age 75 divided by the number alive at age 65 (i.e., in the l_x column):
   White male: $38,749/65,440 = .5921$
   White female: $61,894/81,114 = .7630$
   The probability that both survive 10 years is $.5921 \times .7630 = .4518$.
6. The chance that someone with a positive test has cancer is computed as follows:

Event	Notation	Probability
Cancer	A_1	.02
No cancer	A_2	.98
Positive test for cancer patient	$B\|A_1$	.80
Positive test for noncancer patient	$B\|A_2$	.05
Patient with positive test has cancer	$A_1\|B$	?

By Bayes' formula,

$$\Pr(A_1 \mid B) = .02 \times .80/(.02 \times .80 + .98 \times .05) = .246$$

The chance that someone with a negative test has cancer is computed similarly:

Event	Notation	Probability
Negative test for cancer patient	$C|A_1$	.20
Negative test for noncancer patient	$C|A_2$	.95
Patient with negative test has cancer	$A_1|C$	?

By Bayes' formula,

$$\Pr(A_1|C) = .02 \times .20/(.02 \times .20 + .98 \times .95) = .004$$

Regarding nonstatistical issues, one would also consider the cost, the consequences of a false positive result (i.e., what is the impact of telling a subject that he has shown a positive test result for cancer when he is actually healthy?), and what can be done medically with those who are discovered to be positive.

7. To answer these questions, first set up the following notation:

C = patient with Cushing's syndrome
Not C = patient without Cushing's syndrome
O = osteoporosis on initial examination
Not O = no osteoporosis on initial examination

From the specifications, one can determine that:

$\Pr(C) = .75$, $\Pr(\text{Not } C) = .25$, $\Pr(O|C) = .65$, and $\Pr(O|\text{Not } C) = .03$

A. The question asks for $\Pr(C|O)$, which, by Bayes' formula, is

$$.65 \times .75/(.65 \times .75 + .03 \times .25) = .985$$

B. False positive rate: $\Pr(O|\text{Not } C) = .03$
False negative rate: $\Pr(\text{Not } O|C) = 1 - \Pr(O|C) = 1 - .65 = .35$

C. (1) $\Pr(O \text{ and } C) = \Pr(O|C)\Pr(C) = .65 \times .75 = .4875$
(2) $\Pr(\text{Not } O \text{ and Not } C) = \Pr(\text{Not } O|\text{ Not } C)\Pr(\text{Not } C)$
$= [1 - \Pr(O|\text{ Not } C)]\Pr(\text{Not } C)$
$= (1 - .03)(.25) = .97 \times .25 = .2425$

D. $1 - (\pi_1 + \pi_2)''$

8. A. Reader provides.
B. Probability of at least one ill: $1 - 81/256 = 175/256$
Probability of at least one ill and one healthy: $1 - 81/256 - 1/256 = 174/256$
C. Reader provides.

9. $\Pr(0, 1, \text{ or } 2 \text{ successes out of } 5) = (1 + 20 + 160)/3125 = .0608$

10. A. $z = 2.00$; Appendix Table A1 gives 2.3 percent.
B. Appendix Table A1 gives $z = 1.28$; $1.28 = (x - 500)/100$, so $x = 628$.

    C. $z_U = 2.00$, $z_L = 1.00$; thus the percentage is $100(1 - .023 - .159) = 81.8$ percent.

    D. New system: $z = 1.7$; old system: $z = 1.8$. Hence, 89 in the old system is a better score; it cuts off a smaller percentage in the upper tail of the normal distribution.

11. Mean: 260 mg per 100 ml
     SD: 60 mg per 100 ml

12. 0.9 percent

13. A. $z_L = -1.4$, $z_U = 1.6$; thus the chance of a value outside the range is $.081 + .055 = .136$.

    B. Pr(one inside) $= 1 - .136 = .864$; Pr(all four inside) $= .864^4$; therefore Pr(at least one of four outside) $= 1 - .864^4 = .443$.

    C. $1 - .864^n = .95$; $n = (\log .05)/(\log .864) = 11$ men.

14. A. Pr(false positive) $= .212$; Pr(false negative) $= .629$.

    B. Not very useful; there is too much overlap between the two distributions.

    C. The correct answer is (5).

Chapter 4

1. A. $z = \dfrac{525 - 500}{100/\sqrt{100}} = 2.50$

The chance, from the one-tailed normal table (Appendix Table A1), is .006. Although such a mean score for the school falls somewhat beyond chance expectation, there may not be too much cause for celebration if the school has a past history of even better National Board performance.

    B. $z = 2.50 = \dfrac{x - 80}{5/\sqrt{64}}$; $x = 81.5625$

    C. From Appendix Table A1, $z = 1.65$. Hence,

$$1.65 = \frac{525 - 500}{100/\sqrt{n}}; n = 44$$

2. A. $z_L = \dfrac{4.0 - 5.4}{1.0/\sqrt{4}} = -2.80$; $z_U = \dfrac{7.0 - 5.4}{1.0/\sqrt{4}} = 3.20$

The chance is $.003 + .000 = .003$.

    B. The range 4.9 to 5.9 mg per 100 ml is symmetrical about the mean, 5.4 mg per 100 ml, so one can use the two-tailed normal table (Appendix Table A2). Hence,

$$1.96 = \frac{0.5}{1.0/\sqrt{n}}; n = 16$$

3. A. $z = 3.00$; the chance, from Appendix Table A1, is .001.

    B. Yes, the result, as is determined in part A, is very unlikely to occur by chance variation. Some possibilities to be investigated further might include diet, lack of exercise, and a different age and race composition of prisoners compared with the general population.

4. A. A supply of 2 mg of drug is sufficient for a total of $2/0.004 = 500$ g of body weight. With a sample of 25 mice, a total of 500 g of weight corresponds with a mean weight of $500/25 = 20$ g.

$$z = \frac{20 - 19}{4/\sqrt{25}} = 1.25$$

The chance of running short, from Appendix Table A1, is .106.

B. From Appendix Table A1, $z = 2.33$. Thus, the mean weight to make provision for is:

$$2.33 = \frac{\bar{x} - 19}{4/\sqrt{25}}$$

or $\bar{x} = 20.864$ g. This corresponds with a total weight in the sample of 25 mice of $20.864 \times 25 = 521.6$ g, which then requires $521.6 \times .004 = 2.09$ mg of the drug.

5. $\bar{x} + 1.96\, \sigma/\sqrt{49} = 4.94$
$\bar{x} - 1.96\, \sigma/\sqrt{49} = 4.62$
$\bar{x} = 4.78$ liters

Therefore, $\sigma = 0.57$ liters. From Appendix Table A2, $z = \pm 1.65$ encompasses 90 percent of the standard normal distribution. The upper limit for 90 percent of the distribution of vital capacities is $\mu + 1.65\sigma$ and the lower limit is $\mu - 1.65\sigma$, and so the range is $(\mu + 1.65\sigma) - (\mu - 1.65\sigma) = 2 \times 1.65\sigma = 2 \times 1.65 \times .57 = 1.88$ liters.

6. A. $1.96 \times 1.03/\sqrt{n} = 0.20$; $n = 102$ men.

B. (1) More, (2) less, and (3) one cannot tell by inspection; the interval is wider than that in part A, but the confidence is also greater than that in A. The actual number of men is derived from $2.58 \times 1.03/\sqrt{n} = .26$; thus $n = 104$ men, which is about the same result as in Part A.

7. A. 10.61 mm Hg mean decrease

B. $z = \dfrac{10.61 - 15}{17/\sqrt{25}} = -1.29$

The chance, from Appendix Table A1, is .099.

C. Increase the sample size.

D. $2.33 = \dfrac{c - 5}{17/\sqrt{n}}$

$-1.65 = \dfrac{c - 15}{17/\sqrt{n}}$

The solution of the two equations gives $n = 46$ and $c = 10.85$ mm Hg.

E. (1) More, (2) more, (3) less, and (4) the same number of patients

8. A. The results of the tests of significance are tabulated below:

Paired or independent	t ratio	df	P
(1) Paired	0.31	21	$> .10$
(2) Paired	2.27	15	$< .05$
(3) Independent	0.81	36	$> .10$
(4) Independent	-1.34	36	$> .10$
(5) Independent	1.51	36	$> .10$

B. (1) -2.3 to 3.1 beats per minute, (2) 0.2 to 6.6 beats per minute

C. 143 coffee drinkers, 138 noncoffee drinkers

9. A. SD for boys is $\sqrt{5.27/19} = 0.53$; $\pm 1.96 \times 0.53/\sqrt{n} = \pm 0.10$; therefore $n = 108$ boys.

B. From Appendix Table A3, "just significant at the 2 percent level" with $20 + 5 - 2 = 23$ df means $t = 2.500$. Hence,

$$2.500 = \frac{3.195 - 2.575}{\sqrt{s^2 \left(\frac{1}{20} + \frac{1}{5}\right)}}$$

so $s^2 = 0.246$. For the pooled s^2,

$$0.246 = \frac{5.27 + \Sigma (x_G - \bar{x}_G)^2}{20 + 5 - 2}$$

Thus, $\Sigma(x_G - \bar{x}_G)^2 = 0.388$. Finally, the SD for the girls is $\sqrt{0.388/4} = 0.31$ liters.

10. A. Yes. One should perform the independent-samples t test. From the SD of seven hypertensive women, the sum of squares about the mean is $19.7^2 \times 6 = 2,329$. From the SD of seven normotensive women, the sum of squares about the mean is $28.4^2 \times 6 = 4,839$. Hence, the pooled $s^2 = (2,329 + 4,839)/(7 + 7 - 2) = 597.3$. Thus, $t_{12} = 0.77$ $(P > .10)$.

B. No. One must perform the paired-samples t test; one therefore needs to know the differences over the six-month period for each of the seven hypertensive female's sodium-intake values.

C. The mean would remain unchanged (i.e., the mean of all 49 values is the same as the mean of seven means of seven values). The SDs will differ, but one is unable to speculate exactly how the SDs would differ. However, there would likely be a large variation among the daily values for each woman. Hence, the SD of all 49 values would be greatly influenced by such variation, whereas the SD of seven weekly means would not be much influenced by the day-to-day variation. Thus, one might expect the SD of all 49 observations to be larger than the SD of seven weekly mean values.

   The key number for conducting inferences to a larger population of hypertensive women in parts A and B is the seven women and the variation from woman to woman. The results based on all 49 observations indiscriminately lump together the daily variation and the variation between women. (See the discussion on pp. 39–43.)

Chapter 5

1. A. $z_c = \dfrac{|35 - (144)(.36)| - \frac{1}{2}}{\sqrt{(144)(.36)(.64)}} = 2.84$

From Appendix Table A1, $P = .002$. There is the possibility that some may actually not be susceptible and have acquired immunity; there is also the possibility that not all members of the group had uniform exposure to the agent.

B.   Neglecting the continuity correction,

$$2.58 = \frac{.28 - .36}{\sqrt{(.36)(.64)/n}}$$

Therefore, $n = 240$.

2. A.   Neglecting the continuity correction,

$$2.58 = \frac{.03}{\sqrt{\pi(1 - \pi)/n}}$$

Therefore, $n = 7{,}396\pi(1 - \pi)$. When $\pi = .7$, $n = 1{,}553$; when $\pi = .8$, $n = 1{,}183$. Hence, he will need somewhere between 1,200 and 1,500 in his sample.

B.   He will need more persons. Families will tend to have a similar immunization status. This contradicts the basic assumption in the binomial distribution of independent trials.

C.   One might consider the use of decennial census data, city directories, aerial photographs, or listings of areas of housing demolition and the construction of new housing.

3. A. $\pm 1.96 = \dfrac{|x - (100)(.20)| - \frac{1}{2}}{\sqrt{(100)(.20)(.80)}}$

Using the lower-tail equation, $x = 11.66$, or 11 or fewer complications with the new technique.

B.   Using the answer in part A,

$$z_c = \frac{|11 - (100)(.10)| - \frac{1}{2}}{\sqrt{(100)(.10)(.90)}} = 0.17$$

Thus, when $\pi = .10$, the chance of failing to reject the null hypothesis that $\pi = .20$ is, from Appendix Table A1, .433.

C. $n = \left[\dfrac{1.96\sqrt{(.20)(.80)} + 1.65\sqrt{(.10)(.90)}}{.10 - .20} \right]^2 = 164$

D. Lack of simultaneous controls is the problem. The investigator is using historical controls, and the study is open to criticisms analogous to those discussed on pages 119–120.

4. With $\pi = \text{Pr(Preference of new)}$, the null hypothesis is $\pi = .5$. Since

$$25 = \left[\frac{z_\alpha \sqrt{(.5)(.5)} + 1.65\sqrt{(.8)(.2)}}{.8 - .5} \right]^2$$

$z_\alpha = 1.68$. Since it was a two-sided test, Appendix Table A2 indicates the type I error or significance level was 9.3 percent, or approximately 10 percent.

5. A.

		New treatment		
		Improvement	No improvement	Total
Standard Treatment	Improvement	13	2	15
	No improvement	7	3	10
	Total	20	5	25

B. Discarding the tied pairs, the untied pairs for analysis are the 7 and 2 in the table in part A. Since there are $n = 9$ total untied pairs and the null hypothesis is $\pi = \frac{1}{2}$, the criterion for the use of the normal distribution becomes $9(\frac{1}{2}) = 4.5 < 5$. It thus cannot be used safely. One must then use the exact binomial, namely, the chance of 0, 1, or 2 successes when $n = 9$ and $\pi = \frac{1}{2}$: $\text{Pr}(0, 1, \text{or } 2 \text{ successes}) = (1 + 9 + 36)/2^9 = 46/512$. In performing a two-tailed test, one must consider the probability of such a result at the other extreme. By symmetry, the probability is the same, so the total probability under the null hypothesis is $2 \times 46/512 = .180$. The conclusion is: not statistically significant $(P = .180)$.

6. A. There is a total of 99 untied pairs. Using the normal approximation to the binomial distribution,

$$z_c = \frac{|69 - (99)(.5)| - \frac{1}{2}}{\sqrt{(99)(.5)(.5)}} = 3.82$$

For a two-sided test, $P < .001$, which is highly statistically significant.

Alternatively, by chi-square, the expected number of untied pairs of each kind is $(99)(0.5) = 49.5$. Thus,

$$\chi_c^2 = \frac{(|69 - 49.5| - 0.5)^2}{49.5} + \frac{(|30 - 49.5| - 0.5)^2}{49.5} = 14.59$$

From Appendix Table A4 with 1 df, $P < .001$.

B. In a retrospective study of this kind, one would want to explore the limitations and possible biases analogous to those discussed on pages 279–284.

7. The results can be summarized in the following table:

		Treatment group		
		Gamma-globulin	Controls	Total
Posttransfusion Hepatitis	Yes	12	33	45
	No	762	783	1,545
	Total	774	816	1,590

A. By the test for the comparison of independent proportions, $p = 45/1{,}590 = .0283$ and $q = 1 - p = 1 - .0283 = .9717$. Since each of $n_T p$, $n_T q$, $n_C p$, and $n_C q$ is obviously greater than 5, one can perform the approximate test using the normal distribution:

$$z_c = \frac{\dfrac{33 - 0.5}{816} - \dfrac{12 + 0.5}{774}}{\sqrt{(.0283)(.9717)\left(\dfrac{1}{816} + \dfrac{1}{774}\right)}} = \frac{.0237}{.0083} = 2.85$$

From Appendix Table A2, $P = .004$.

Alternatively, by chi-square, the following expected quantities are obtained for the four entries in the body of the above table:

		Treatment group	
		Gamma-globulin	Control
Posttransfusion Hepatitis	Yes	21.9	23.1
	No	752.1	792.9

For each quantity, $(|O - E| - \frac{1}{2}) = 9.9 - 0.5 = 9.4$. Thus,

$$\chi_c^2 \ (1 \ \text{df}) = 9.4^2 \left(\frac{1}{21.9} + \frac{1}{23.1} + \frac{1}{752.1} + \frac{1}{792.9}\right) = 8.09$$

and, from Appendix Table A4 with 1 df, $P < .01$.

The conclusion is that there is a statistically significant difference in the rates of posttransfusion hepatitis ($P < .01$).

B. There was the lack of random assignment. Alternate assignment can lead to bias, and, particularly, with alternate weeks in one city, it may be that the variation in sources of blood and the possibilities of contamination with hepatitis are in phase with the weekly assignments to treatment groups. (See the discussion on pp. 259–260.)

There was also the lack of a uniform period of follow-up. Were the durations of follow-up similar in the two groups? With monthly tests of liver function, there would be a difference between someone followed for 3 months and someone followed for 6 months in meeting the criterion for hepatitis of "two abnormal monthly liver function values." It might be preferable to attempt to calculate the rates on a person-months basis or with life-table methods, as discussed in Chapter 9.

In addition, the study was not blind. The use of placebo controls might be preferable. (See the discussion on pp. 262–264.)

C. One would first calculate the following expected quantities for calculation of chi-square:

City	Cases of hepatitis		No hepatitis		Total
	Observed (O)	Expected (E)	Observed (O)	Expected (E)	
A	22	23.7	565	563.3	587
B	9	5.9	137	140.1	146
C	2	3.4	81	79.6	83
Total	33		783		816

$$\chi^2(2 \text{ df}) = \Sigma(O - E)^2/E = 1.7^2/23.7 + 1.7^2/563.4$$
$$+ 3.1^2/5.9 + 3.1^2/140.1$$
$$+ 1.4^2/3.4 + 1.4^2/79.6$$
$$= 0.12 + 0.01 + 1.63 + 0.07 + 0.58 + 0.02 = 2.43$$

No statistically significant difference occurs by city for the hepatitis rates among the controls.

D. If there had been a significant difference, one might have investigated and compared the sources of blood in the three cities. One might have examined the characteristics of patients to see if, for any reason, the patients in one city were more susceptible toward hepatitis infection.

8. A. Disagree. The calculation presented consists only of the contribution to chi-square for the women developing disease; the proper calculation must add to this the contribution for the women who did *not* develop disease. In the total group of 210 women, the

proportion not developing disease was obviously $1 - .100 = .900$. Thus,

	Castrate group	Control group
Observed without disease (O):	$100 - 17 = 83$	$110 - 4 = 106$
Expected without disease (E):	$(100)(.90) = 90$	$(110)(.90) = 99$

One must then add to the previous chi-square,

$$\frac{6.5^2}{90} + \frac{6.5^2}{99} = .90$$

This gives a total chi-square of $8.07 + 0.90 = 8.97$, which actually does not differ much from the incomplete result stated in the question.

B.   No. As presented, there are too many possibilities for selection or bias to explain the results. The following criticisms are relevant:

Comparability of groups at the time of operation.   Perhaps those in the castrate group had this operation because they were in poorer health. Hence, one might expect them to develop subsequent cardiovascular disease more frequently. Actually, for all one knows, the castrate group may have had more cardiovascular disease at the time of operation (the question states nothing concerning their cardiovascular status at time of operation).

Deaths are not considered.   Many women would not be available for examination because they had died. Further, among the deaths it is exceedingly plausible that many died from or with cardiovascular diseases.

Even if there were no deaths, there are very low response rates. These rates are $100/424 = 24$ percent in the castrate group and $110/462 = 24$ percent in the control group. Why did some women respond while others did not? One might suggest plausible reasons why women with cardiovascular disease might be either more willing or less willing to come in for an examination. In any event, these very low response rates signify the possibility of selective factors influencing the results.

No account is made for the variation in the length of the follow-up interval since operation.   Women who had their operations early in the 20-year period would have a much longer follow-up interval than women who had their operations toward the end of the 20-year period.

9.   Let x denote the number of successes among the 20 treatment patients.

Then $p = (x + 12)/40$ and $q = 1 - p = (28 - x)/40$. Using the formula for the comparison of two independent proportions,

$$1.96 = \frac{\dfrac{x - 0.5}{20} - \dfrac{12 + 0.5}{20}}{\sqrt{\left(\dfrac{x + 12}{40}\right)\left(\dfrac{28 - x}{40}\right)\left(\dfrac{1}{20} + \dfrac{1}{20}\right)}} = \frac{(x - 13)}{\sqrt{(12 + x)(28 - x)/40}}$$

Squaring both sides gives:

$$3.84 = \frac{40(x - 13)^2}{(12 + x)(28 - x)}$$

Trial and error indicates that $x = 19$ is the smallest integral value of x that will produce a statistically significant difference.

Chapter 6

1. A. Perform the paired-samples t test on y data:

   $\bar{y} = 18.1$ lb
   $\Sigma(y - \bar{y})^2 = 8{,}636 - 290^2/16 = 3{,}380$
   $s_y^2 = 3{,}380/15 = 225.33$
   $t_{15} = 18.1/\sqrt{225.33/16} = 4.82$

   The change in weight was statistically significant ($P < .001$).
   B. Reader provides.
   C. $\Sigma xy = 58{,}385$
   $\Sigma(x - \bar{x})(y - \bar{y}) = 58{,}385 - (2{,}902)(290)/16 = 5{,}786$
   $\Sigma(x - \bar{x})^2 = 546{,}542 - 2{,}902^2/16 = 20{,}192$
   $\bar{x} = 181.4$ lb

   $b = 5{,}786/20{,}192 = 0.287$ lb of weight loss per initial weight in lb
   $a = 18.1 - (0.287)(181.4) = 34.0$

   Least-squares regression line: $Y = -34.0 + 0.287x$ or $Y = 18.1 + 0.287(x - 181.4)$
   D. $s_{y \cdot x} = \dfrac{1}{14}(3{,}380 - 5{,}786^2/20{,}192) = 123.00$

   $SE(b) = \sqrt{123.00/20{,}192} = 0.0780$
   $t_{14} = 0.287/0.0780 = 3.68$
   $P < .001$

   The slope of the regression line is significantly different from zero.
   E. This author's weight is 185 lb. The predicted mean weight loss at one year for diabetics weighing 185 lb initially is $Y_0 = 18.1 + 0.287(185 - 181.4) = 19.13$ lb. The width of the 95 percent confidence limits (using $t_{14, .05} = 2.145$) is:

$$\pm 2.145 \sqrt{123.00\left(\frac{1}{16} + \frac{3.6^2}{20{,}192}\right)} = \pm 5.98 \text{ lb}$$

The 95 percent confidence interval on the mean weight loss at one year for diabetics with an initial weight of 185 lb is 19.13 ± 5.98, or 13.2 to 25.1 lb.

F.   The width of the 95 percent limits (using $t_{14, .05} = 2.145$) is:

$$\pm 2.145 \sqrt{123.00 \left(1 + \frac{1}{16} + \frac{3.6^2}{20,192}\right)} = \pm 24.53 \text{ lb}$$

The 95 percent limits on weight loss at one year for diabetics with an initial weight of 185 lb is 19.13 ± 24.53, or -5.4 to 43.7 lb.

G.   The limits in part E are the confidence limits on the *mean* weight loss of a group of diabetics with a specified initial weight; the limits in part F are the limits on an *individual's* weight loss among a large group of diabetics with a specified initial weight.

2.   A.   Reader provides.
     B.   The sums of squares and the cross-products about the means are:

$$\Sigma(w - \bar{w})^2 = 3.15 \qquad \Sigma(w - \bar{w})(x - \bar{x}) = 1.46$$
$$\Sigma(x - \bar{x})^2 = 1.87 \qquad \Sigma(y - \bar{y})(z - \bar{z}) = 194$$
$$\Sigma(y - \bar{y})^2 = 267 \qquad \Sigma(w - \bar{w})(y - \bar{y}) = 25.5$$
$$\Sigma(z - \bar{z})^2 = 226 \qquad \Sigma(x - \bar{x})(z - \bar{z}) = 10.5$$

Thus the correlation coefficients are:

(1) w and y: .88   (3) w and x: .60
(2) x and z: .51   (4) y and z: .79

C.   From Appendix Table A5, with 10 df, correlations of .576, .708, and .823 are necessary to achieve significance at the 5, 1, and 0.1 percent levels, respectively. Thus,

Correlation	Statistically significant	P value
w with y	yes	$<.001$
x with z	no	$>.05$
w with x	yes	$<.05$
y with z	yes	$<.001$

A statistically significant correlation means that, if the null hypothesis of no correlation in the underlying population were true, a correlation as large as or larger than that observed in the sample would be unlikely to occur by chance alone. Therefore, one rejects the null hypothesis and concludes there is a correlation in the underlying population.

Chapter 7

1. A. For null hypotheses (1) and (2), use the signed rank test:

16 DBI patients		9 Diabinese patients	
Weight loss at 1 yr (lb)	Signed rank	Weight loss at 1 yr (lb)	Signed rank
15	8	25	7
44	15.5	13	6
31	13	41	8
39	14	−11	−4.5
6	4	−8	−3
16	9	4	1.5
21	11	0	
44	15.5	11	4.5
5	3	−4	−1.5
12	7		
−3	−1.5		
19	10		
10	5.5		
24	12		
−3	−1.5		
10	5.5		
Sum of positive signed ranks	133		27
Sum of negative signed ranks	3		9

(1) From Appendix Table A6, with 16 differences 19 and 117 are required for the sums of signed ranks to be significant at the 1 percent level. The sample result is 3 and 133, which is more extreme. Therefore, there is a statistically significant weight loss at one year following DBI treatment ($P < .01$).

(2) From Appendix Table A6, with 8 differences 3 and 33 are required for the sums of signed ranks to be significant at the 5 percent level. The sample result of 9 and 27 is clearly not that extreme. Therefore, there is no statistically significant weight loss at one year following Diabinese therapy ($P > .05$).

Initial weight

9 Diabinese patients		16 DBI patients	
Actual value in lb	Rank in total sample	Actual value in lb	Rank in total sample
202	21	225	23
177	14	235	24
179	15	173	12
167	11	223	22
162	9	200	19.5
150	5.5	199	18
200	19.5	129	1
174	13	242	25
163	10	140	2
		156	8
		146	3
		195	17
		155	7
		185	16
		150	5.5
		149	4
Sum of ranks 118		207	

One-year weight change

9 Diabinese patients		16 DBI patients	
Actual loss in lb	Rank in total sample	Actual loss in lb	Rank in total sample
25	20	15	15
13	14	44	24.5
41	23	31	21
−11	1	39	22
−8	2	6	9
4	7	16	16
0	6	21	18
11	12	44	24.5
−4	3	5	8
		12	13
		−3	4.5
		19	17
		10	11
		24	19
		−3	4.5
		10	10
Sum of ranks 88		237	

For null hypotheses (3) and (4), use the rank sum test:

(3) From Appendix Table A7, with $n_1 = 9$ and $n_2 = 16$, significance at the 5 percent level is achieved when the sum of the ranks in the sample with 9 patients is 82 or lower or 152 or higher. The observed sum of ranks is 118, which is not this extreme. Hence, there is no statistically significant difference in the initial weight of Diabinese patients and DBI patients ($P > .05$).

(4) As in (3), the sum of ranks in the sample of 9 patients must be 82 or less to achieve significance at the 5 percent level. The observed value of 88 falls just short of being this extreme. Thus, there is not a statistically significant difference in weight loss at one year among Diabinese-treated patients compared with DBI-treated patients ($P > .05$). The results, however, approach this level of statistical significance.

B. Results of the analogous t test:

Paired or independent	df	t ratio	P value
(1) Paired	15	4.82[a]	<.001
(2) Paired	8	1.41	>.05
(3) Independent	23	0.50	>.05
(4) Independent	23	1.57	>.05

[a] From the answer to question 1.A for Chapter 6.

2. Ranks for the data in question 2 of Chapter 6:

	w	x	y	z
	Grade-point average		National Board scores	
Student	Preclinical	Clinical	Part I	Part II
a	2	3	1	4.5
b	9	6	6.5	9
c	3	9	2	1
d	10.5	12	11	11
e	12	11	12	12
f	5	2	3.5	6
g	7.5	4.5	8.5	8
h	7.5	7.5	6.5	7
i	1	7.5	3.5	2
j	10.5	10	10	10
k	5	1	5	4.5
l	5	4.5	8.5	3

	Σd^2	Rank correlation
(1) w and y	31.5	.89
(2) x and z	150.5	.47
(3) w and x	126	.56
(4) y and z	59	.79

Chapter 9

A. Death rate per person-months of observation:

	Potential recipients	Transplant patients	
		Including waiting time	Excluding waiting time
Person-months observation	104.0	56.5	44.5
Deaths per 100 person-months observation	26.0	23.0	29.2

B. Life table for the data of part A:

x to $x+1$ (mo)	O_x	d_x	w_x	q_x	p_x	P_x
Potential Recipients:						
0–1	42	19	2	.4634	.5366	1
1–2	21	4	1	.1951	.8049	.5366
2–3	16	2	–	.1250	.8750	.4319
3–4	14	2	2	.1538	.8462	.3779
4–5	10	–	1	0	1	.3198
5–6	9	–	2	0	1	.3198
6–7	7	–	2	0	1	.3198
7–8	5	–	4	0	1	.3198
8–9	1	–	1	0	1	.3198
Transplant Patients – Including Waiting Time:						
0–1	15	3	–	.2000	.8000	1
1–2	12	2	–	.1667	.8333	.8000
2–3	10	2	–	.2000	.8000	.6667
3–4	8	1	–	.1250	.8750	.5333
4–5	7	1	–	.1429	.8571	.4667
5–6	6	2	–	.3333	.6667	.4000

x to $x+1$ (mo)	O_x	d_x	w_x	q_x	p_x	P_x
6–7	4	2	1	.5714	.4286	.2667
7–8	1	—	—	0	1	.1143
8–9	1	—	1	0	1	.1143
Transplant Patients – Excluding Waiting Time:						
0–1	15	5	—	.3333	.6667	1
1–2	10	2	—	.2000	.8000	.6667
2–3	8	1	—	.1250	.8750	.5333
3–4	7	—	1	0	1	.4667
4–5	6	3	—	.5000	.5000	.4667
5–6	3	1	—	.3333	.6667	.2333
6–7	2	1	—	.5000	.5000	.1556
7–8	1	—	1	0	1	.0778
8–9	—	—	—	—	—	—

C. The set of data in which waiting time is excluded (see the discussion on p. 302).

D. Since this was not a controlled clinical trial with random assignment to treatment groups, one would want to investigate the comparability of the two groups regarding the factors related to the prognosis with the disease under study. Are the groups comparable with respect to age, sex, previous history, the stage of disease, and so forth? In particular, one would investigate the possibility that patients with a better prognosis are more likely to receive cardiac allografts, whereas those with poorer prognoses wind up in the "potential" recipient group (see Chapter 10).

Chapter 12

1. *Lack of denominators.* One would want to know the *underlying* population for the two age groups in the area served by the hospital over the three five-year intervals. For all one knows, the population composition in the area served by the hospital may have changed in a manner similar to the changes in the numerator figures presented.

2. *Similar problem with lack of denominators.* Also, these data do not deal with incidence; even if one had proper denominators, "prevalence" and not "incidence" would be the more appropriate word for any rates that were calculated. In addition, there is the issue of the extremely selective nature of an autopsy group.

   The second statement highlights how far out on a limb an investigator might go with an inference drawn from an autopsy study (see the discussion on pp. 6–7).

3. *Lack of a comparison group.* One would want to know the sizes of the lesions that did *not* involute spontaneously. The proper method for assessing the chance of spontaneous involution is to calculate, for each size category, the ratio of the number of lesions involuting divided by the total number of lesions of that size.

4. *Lack of a standard of comparison.* For all one knows, two-thirds of the general population may have been at some time 11 percent or more overweight. In addition, without further specification, the phrase "at some time" is much too vague. Could this even refer to infancy? Another point of difficulty is the statement concerning the availability of data on maximum weight. For what proportion of diabetics were the data not available? There is also the possible selective factor that patients who appeared to be obese tended to be queried regarding their maximum weight, while others with a non-obese appearance tended not to be asked the question. Thus, the data may have tended to be available *because* the patient was obese.

5. *Incomplete follow-up.* A meaningful mean survival figure must await the mortality of the 30 who were still alive at time of study completion.

6. *Lack of accounting for age distributions of the underlying populations.* Specialty practice is relatively new, and therefore the age distribution of specialists will tend to be weighted to the younger age groups whereas the age distribution of general practitioners will tend to group at the higher ages. Specialists and general practitioners may die at identical age-specific rates, but the younger age distribution of all specialists will give, among their deaths, a lower mean age compared with general practitioners.

7. *Lack of a denominator.* Granted that one accepts 45 years of age or older as a crude criterion for women being menopausal and post-menopausal, the data presented are only the numerator data for the hospital. One must consider the menopausal-postmenopausal age composition of the population served by the hospital.

8. *It is not clear how the restriction that both parents be dead avoids the bias of wives being younger than their husbands.* It is well known that wives outlive their husbands. No doubt, among the diabetic patients there are many whose fathers have died but their mothers are still alive. The restriction that both parents be dead deliberately selects for those instances of early death among mothers.

9. *Selective nature of autopsy group.* One can more readily determine coronary heart disease in an autopsy group than in total deaths, mostly without autopsy, in the United States. In addition, even though the study was restricted to patients over age 40, age adjustment would be helpful.

10 and 11. *Possibility of Berkson's fallacy.* There may be differential ad-

mission rates to the study groups for the diseases in question that may explain the observed associations.

12. *Lack of accounting for the extremely small proportion of time spent in strenuous activity compared with the extremely large proportion spent sleeping or resting.* A more meaningful figure would be the number stricken with heart attacks during a time of strenuous activity *per man-hours* of involvement in strenuous activity compared with the same rate for sleeping and resting.

13. *One must account for the relative number of hospital admissions for appendectomy and gastrectomy.* If there were 2.5 more appendectomies than gastrectomies, then the utilization of hospital resources in terms of total days of hospitalization would be identical. No doubt, the ratio of appendectomy to gastrectomy patients is more than 2.5 to 1, so appendectomy is a more important operation in terms of utilization of resources.

14. *Lack of age adjustment.* Alaskans are younger than Bay Staters.

15. *Lack of standard of comparison.* What are the food histories of those who attended the luau and did not become ill? With the addition of these data, the appropriate technique to implicate a particular food in a foodborne epidemic is to calculate, for each food served, the disease attack rates among those who ate the food compared with those who did not eat the food. The largest such difference relative to its standard error will most often implicate the contaminated food. The following table presents, for each of the foods consumed at the luau, the missing data on the food histories of 144 persons attending the luau who did not become ill, the attack rates for each food, the

	a	b	c	d	$\dfrac{a}{a+c}$	$\dfrac{b}{b+d}$			Diff.
			144 Persons not ill		Illness attack rates (%)				
	38 Persons ill						Difference in attack rates	SE of diff.	divided by SE of diff.
Food	Ate food	Did not eat food	Ate food	Did not eat food	Ate food	Did not eat food			
Kalua pig	38	0	137	7	21.7	0	21.7	15.7	1.39
Chicken long rice	37	1	125	19	22.8	5.0	17.8	9.6	1.85
Squid luau	36	2	108	36	25.0	5.3	19.7	7.4	2.66
Lomi salmon	36	2	118	26	23.4	7.1	16.3	8.4	1.95
Poki aku	34	4	89	55	27.6	6.8	20.8	6.4	3.73
Crab	31	7	46	98	40.3	6.7	33.6	6.1	5.51
Opihi	34	4	105	39	24.5	9.3	15.2	7.1	2.14
Liver	19	19	54	90	26.0	17.4	8.6	6.1	1.40
Poi	34	4	130	14	20.7	22.2	−1.5	10.1	−0.15
Sweet potato	34	4	125	19	21.4	17.4	4.0	9.1	0.44
Haupia	28	10	110	34	20.3	22.7	−2.4	7.0	−0.34
Cake	31	7	121	23	20.4	23.3	−2.9	8.1	−0.36
Kulolo	30	8	103	41	22.6	16.3	6.3	6.8	0.93

difference in attack rates for those who ate and did not eat the food, the standard errors of these differences, and the resulting critical ratios (the difference divided by the standard error of the difference).

Looking at the last column of the table, the one food that clearly stands out as suspect is crab. Although food specimens from the luau had not been retained, the investigation of crabs caught at the same locale as those served at the luau yielded positive cultures for the organism suspected of producing the illness.

Appendix Tables

Table A1. Areas in one tail of the standard normal curve

This table shows the shaded area

z	.00	.01	.02	.03	.04	.05	.06	.07	.08	.09
0.0	.500	.496	.492	.488	.484	.480	.476	.472	.468	.464
0.1	.460	.456	.452	.448	.444	.440	.436	.433	.429	.425
0.2	.421	.417	.413	.409	.405	.401	.397	.394	.390	.386
0.3	.382	.378	.374	.371	.367	.363	.359	.356	.352	.348
0.4	.345	.341	.337	.334	.330	.326	.323	.319	.316	.312
0.5	.309	.305	.302	.298	.295	.291	.288	.284	.281	.278
0.6	.274	.271	.268	.264	.261	.258	.255	.251	.248	.245
0.7	.242	.239	.236	.233	.230	.227	.224	.221	.218	.215
0.8	.212	.209	.206	.203	.200	.198	.195	.192	.189	.187
0.9	.184	.181	.179	.176	.174	.171	.169	.166	.164	.161
1.0	.159	.156	.154	.152	.149	.147	.145	.142	.140	.138
1.1	.136	.133	.131	.129	.127	.125	.123	.121	.119	.117
1.2	.115	.113	.111	.109	.107	.106	.104	.102	.100	.099
1.3	.097	.095	.093	.092	.090	.089	.087	.085	.084	.082
1.4	.081	.079	.078	.076	.075	.074	.072	.071	.069	.068
1.5	.067	.066	.064	.063	.062	.061	.059	.058	.057	.056
1.6	.055	.054	.053	.052	.051	.049	.048	.048	.046	.046
1.7	.045	.044	.043	.042	.041	.040	.039	.038	.038	.037
1.8	.036	.035	.034	.034	.033	.032	.031	.031	.030	.029
1.9	.029	.028	.027	.027	.026	.026	.025	.024	.024	.023
2.0	.023	.022	.022	.021	.021	.020	.020	.019	.019	.018
2.1	.018	.017	.017	.017	.016	.016	.015	.015	.015	.014
2.2	.014	.014	.013	.013	.013	.012	.012	.012	.011	.011
2.3	.011	.010	.010	.010	.010	.009	.009	.009	.009	.008
2.4	.008	.008	.008	.008	.007	.007	.007	.007	.007	.006
2.5	.006	.006	.006	.006	.006	.005	.005	.005	.005	.005
2.6	.005	.005	.004	.004	.004	.004	.004	.004	.004	.004
2.7	.003	.003	.003	.003	.003	.003	.003	.003	.003	.003
2.8	.003	.002	.002	.002	.002	.002	.002	.002	.002	.002
2.9	.002	.002	.002	.002	.002	.002	.002	.001	.001	.001
3.0	.001									

Adapted from Croxton [25].

Table A2. Areas in two tails of the standard normal curve

This table shows
the shaded areas

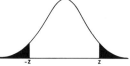

z	.00	.01	.02	.03	.04	.05	.06	.07	.08	.09
0.0	1.000	.992	.984	.976	.968	.960	.952	.944	.936	.928
0.1	.920	.912	.904	.897	.889	.881	.873	.865	.857	.849
0.2	.841	.834	.826	.818	.810	.803	.795	.787	.779	.772
0.3	.764	.757	.749	.741	.734	.726	.719	.711	.704	.697
0.4	.689	.682	.674	.667	.660	.653	.646	.638	.631	.624
0.5	.617	.610	.603	.596	.589	.582	.575	.569	.562	.555
0.6	.549	.542	.535	.529	.522	.516	.509	.503	.497	.490
0.7	.484	.478	.472	.465	.459	.453	.447	.441	.435	.430
0.8	.424	.418	.412	.407	.401	.395	.390	.384	.379	.373
0.9	.368	.363	.358	.352	.347	.342	.337	.332	.327	.322
1.0	.317	.312	.308	.303	.298	.294	.289	.285	.280	.276
1.1	.271	.267	.263	.258	.254	.250	.246	.242	.238	.234
1.2	.230	.226	.222	.219	.215	.211	.208	.204	.201	.197
1.3	.194	.190	.187	.184	.180	.177	.174	.171	.168	.165
1.4	.162	.159	.156	.153	.150	.147	.144	.142	.139	.136
1.5	.134	.131	.129	.126	.124	.121	.119	.116	.114	.112
1.6	.110	.107	.105	.103	.101	.099	.097	.095	.093	.091
1.7	.089	.087	.085	.084	.082	.080	.078	.077	.075	.073
1.8	.072	.070	.069	.067	.066	.064	.063	.061	.060	.059
1.9	.057	.056	.055	.054	.052	.051	.050	.049	.048	.047
2.0	.046	.044	.043	.042	.041	.040	.039	.038	.038	.037
2.1	.036	.035	.034	.033	.032	.032	.031	.030	.029	.029
2.2	.028	.027	.026	.026	.025	.024	.024	.023	.023	.022
2.3	.021	.021	.020	.020	.019	.019	.018	.018	.017	.017
2.4	.016	.016	.016	.015	.015	.014	.014	.014	.013	.013
2.5	.012	.012	.012	.011	.011	.011	.010	.010	.010	.010
2.6	.009	.009	.009	.009	.008	.008	.008	.008	.007	.007
2.7	.007	.007	.007	.006	.006	.006	.006	.006	.005	.005
2.8	.005	.005	.005	.005	.005	.004	.004	.004	.004	.004
2.9	.004	.004	.004	.003	.003	.003	.003	.003	.003	.003
3.0	.003									

Adapted from Croxton [25].

Table A3. Percentage points of the t distribution (this table gives the values of t for differing df that cut off specified proportions of the area in one and in two tails of the t distribution)

df	Area in two tails				
	.10	.05	.02	.01	.001
	Area in one tail				
	.05	.025	.01	.005	.0005
1	6.314	12.706	31.821	63.657	636.619
2	2.920	4.303	6.965	9.925	31.598
3	2.353	3.182	4.541	5.841	12.941
4	2.132	2.776	3.747	4.604	8.610
5	2.015	2.571	3.365	4.032	6.859
6	1.943	2.447	3.143	3.707	5.959
7	1.895	2.365	2.998	3.499	5.405
8	1.860	2.306	2.896	3.355	5.041
9	1.833	2.262	2.821	3.250	4.781
10	1.812	2.228	2.764	3.169	4.587
11	1.796	2.201	2.718	3.106	4.437
12	1.782	2.179	2.681	3.055	4.318
13	1.771	2.160	2.650	3.012	4.221
14	1.761	2.145	2.624	2.977	4.140
15	1.753	2.131	2.602	2.947	4.073
16	1.746	2.120	2.583	2.921	4.015
17	1.740	2.110	2.567	2.898	3.965
18	1.734	2.101	2.552	2.878	3.922
19	1.729	2.093	2.539	2.861	3.883
20	1.725	2.086	2.528	2.845	3.850
21	1.721	2.080	2.518	2.831	3.819
22	1.717	2.074	2.508	2.819	3.792
23	1.714	2.069	2.500	2.807	3.767
24	1.711	2.064	2.492	2.797	3.745
25	1.708	2.060	2.485	2.787	3.725
26	1.706	2.056	2.479	2.779	3.707
27	1.703	2.052	2.473	2.771	3.690
28	1.701	2.048	2.467	2.763	3.674
29	1.699	2.045	2.462	2.756	3.659
30	1.697	2.042	2.457	2.750	3.646
40	1.684	2.021	2.423	2.704	3.551
60	1.671	2.000	2.390	2.660	3.460
120	1.658	1.980	2.358	2.617	3.373
∞	1.645	1.960	2.326	2.576	3.291

From Pearson and Hartley [86].

Table A4. Percentage points of the chi-square distribution (this table gives the values of χ^2 for differing df that cut off specified proportions of the upper tail of the chi-square distribution)

df	Area in upper tail			
	.10	.05	.01	.001
1	2.71	3.84	6.63	10.83
2	4.61	5.99	9.21	13.82
3	6.25	7.81	11.34	16.27
4	7.78	9.49	13.28	18.47
5	9.24	11.07	15.09	20.52
6	10.64	12.59	16.81	22.46
7	12.02	14.07	18.48	24.32
8	13.36	15.51	20.09	26.13
9	14.68	16.92	21.67	27.88
10	15.99	18.31	23.21	29.59
11	17.28	19.68	24.73	31.26
12	18.55	21.03	26.22	32.91
13	19.81	22.36	27.69	34.53
14	21.06	23.68	29.14	36.12
15	22.31	25.00	30.58	37.70
16	23.54	26.30	32.00	39.25
17	24.77	27.59	33.41	40.79
18	25.99	28.87	34.81	42.31
19	27.20	30.14	36.19	43.82
20	28.41	31.41	37.57	45.32
21	29.62	32.67	38.93	46.80
22	30.81	33.92	40.29	48.27
23	32.01	35.17	41.64	49.73
24	33.20	36.42	42.98	51.18
25	34.38	37.65	44.31	52.62

From Pearson and Hartley [86].

Table A5. Critical values of sample correlation coefficient, r, for test of null hypothesis that population correlation is zero (this table gives the values of r required to achieve statistical significance at the specified level)

df	Significance level for two-tail test		
	.05	.01	.001
1	.997	—	—
2	.950	.990	.999
3	.878	.959	.991
4	.811	.917	.974
5	.754	.875	.951
6	.707	.834	.925
7	.666	.798	.898
8	.632	.765	.872
9	.602	.735	.847
10	.576	.708	.823
11	.553	.684	.801
12	.532	.661	.780
13	.514	.641	.760
14	.497	.623	.742
15	.482	.606	.725
16	.468	.590	.708
17	.456	.575	.693
18	.444	.561	.679
19	.433	.549	.665
20	.423	.537	.652
25	.381	.487	.597
30	.349	.449	.554
35	.325	.418	.519
40	.304	.393	.490
45	.288	.372	.465
50	.273	.354	.443
60	.250	.325	.408
70	.232	.302	.380
80	.217	.283	.357
90	.205	.267	.338
100	.195	.254	.321

From Pearson and Hartley [86].

Table A6. Critical values for the signed rank test in the comparison of two groups in paired samples (this table gives the values of the sum of the signed ranks required to achieve statistical significance in a test of the null hypothesis of no difference in the population)

Number of differences	Significance level for two-tail test		
	.05	.02	.01
6	0, 21	——	——
7	2, 26	0, 28	——
8	3, 33	1, 35	0, 36
9	5, 40	3, 42	1, 44
10	8, 47	5, 50	3, 52
11	10, 56	7, 59	5, 61
12	13, 65	9, 69	7, 71
13	17, 74	12, 79	9, 82
14	21, 84	15, 90	12, 93
15	25, 95	19, 101	15, 105
16	29, 107	23, 113	19, 117
17	34, 119	28, 125	23, 130
18	40, 131	32, 139	27, 144
19	46, 144	37, 153	32, 158
20	52, 158	43, 167	37, 173
21	58, 173	49, 182	42, 189
22	66, 187	55, 198	48, 205
23	73, 203	62, 214	54, 222
24	81, 219	69, 231	61, 239
25	89, 236	76, 249	68, 257

Adapted from Tukey [107].

Table A7. Critical values for the rank sum test in the comparison of two groups in independent samples (this table gives, for the sum of the ranks in the smaller of two independent samples, the values required to achieve statistical significance in a test of the null hypothesis of no difference between the populations)

n_1, n_2	Significance level, two-tail			n_1, n_2	Significance level, two-tail		
	.05	.01	.001		.05	.01	.001
2, 8	3, 19			4, 9	15, 41	11, 45	
2, 9	3, 21			4, 10	15, 45	12, 48	
2, 10	3, 23			4, 11	16, 48	12, 52	
2, 11	4, 24			4, 12	17, 51	13, 55	
2, 12	4, 26			4, 13	18, 54	14, 58	10, 62
2, 13	4, 28			4, 14	19, 57	14, 62	10, 66
2, 14	4, 30			4, 15	20, 60	15, 65	10, 70
2, 15	4, 32			4, 16	21, 63	15, 69	11, 73
2, 16	4, 34			4, 17	21, 67	16, 72	11, 77
2, 17	5, 35			4, 18	22, 70	16, 76	11, 81
2, 18	5, 37			4, 19	23, 73	17, 79	12, 84
2, 19	5, 39	3, 41		4, 20	24, 76	18, 82	12, 88
2, 20	5, 41	3, 43		4, 21	25, 79	18, 86	12, 92
2, 21	6, 42	3, 45		4, 22	26, 82	19, 89	13, 95
2, 22	6, 44	3, 47		4, 23	27, 85	19, 93	13, 99
2, 23	6, 46	3, 49		4, 24	28, 88	20, 96	13, 103
2, 24	6, 48	3, 51		4, 25	28, 92	20, 100	14, 106
2, 25	6, 50	3, 53					
				5, 5	17, 38	15, 40	
3, 5	6, 21			5, 6	18, 42	16, 44	
3, 6	7, 23			5, 7	20, 45	17, 48	
3, 7	7, 26			5, 8	21, 49	17, 53	
3, 8	8, 28			5, 9	22, 53	18, 57	15, 60
3, 9	8, 31	6, 33		5, 10	23, 57	19, 61	15, 65
3, 10	9, 33	6, 36		5, 11	24, 61	20, 65	16, 69
3, 11	9, 36	6, 39		5, 12	26, 64	21, 69	16, 74
3, 12	10, 38	7, 41		5, 13	27, 68	22, 73	17, 78
3, 13	10, 41	7, 44		5, 14	28, 72	22, 78	17, 83
3, 14	11, 43	7, 47		5, 15	29, 76	23, 82	18, 87
3, 15	11, 46	8, 49		5, 16	31, 79	24, 86	18, 92
3, 16	12, 48	8, 52		5, 17	32, 83	25, 90	19, 96
3, 17	12, 51	8, 55		5, 18	33, 87	26, 94	19, 101
3, 18	13, 53	8, 58		5, 19	34, 91	27, 98	20, 105
3, 19	13, 56	9, 60		5, 20	35, 95	28, 102	20, 110
3, 20	14, 58	9, 63		5, 21	37, 98	29, 106	21, 114
3, 21	14, 61	9, 66	6, 69	5, 22	38, 102	29, 111	21, 119
3, 22	15, 63	10, 68	6, 72	5, 23	39, 106	30, 115	22, 123
3, 23	15, 66	10, 71	6, 75	5, 24	40, 110	31, 119	23, 127
3, 24	16, 68	10, 74	6, 78	5, 25	42, 113	32, 123	23, 132
3, 25	19, 71	11, 76	6, 81				
				6, 6	26, 52	23, 55	
4, 4	10, 26			6, 7	27, 57	24, 60	
4, 5	11, 29			6, 8	29, 61	25, 65	21, 69
4, 6	12, 32	10, 34		6, 9	31, 65	26, 70	22, 74
4, 7	13, 35	10, 38		6, 10	32, 70	27, 75	23, 79
4, 8	14, 38	11, 41		6, 11	34, 74	28, 80	23, 85

Adapted from White [114].

n_1, n_2	Significance level, two-tail			n_1, n_2	Significance level, two-tail		
	.05	.01	.001		.05	.01	.001
6, 12	35, 79	30, 84	24, 90	9, 12	71, 127	63, 135	55, 143
6, 13	37, 83	31, 89	25, 95	9, 13	73, 134	65, 142	56, 151
6, 14	38, 88	32, 94	26, 100	9, 14	76, 140	67, 149	58, 158
6, 15	40, 92	33, 99	26, 106	9, 15	79, 146	70, 155	60, 165
6, 16	42, 96	34, 104	27, 111	9, 16	82, 152	72, 162	61, 173
6, 17	43, 101	36, 108	28, 116	9, 17	84, 159	74, 169	63, 180
6, 18	45, 105	37, 113	29, 121	9, 18	87, 165	76, 176	65, 187
6, 19	46, 110	38, 118	29, 127	9, 19	90, 171	78, 183	66, 195
6, 20	48, 114	39, 123	30, 132	9, 20	93, 177	81, 189	68, 202
6, 21	50, 118	40, 128	31, 137	9, 21	95, 184	83, 196	70, 209
6, 22	51, 123	42, 132	32, 142				
6, 23	53, 127	43, 137	33, 147	10, 10	78, 132	71, 139	63, 147
6, 24	55, 131	44, 142	34, 152	10, 11	81, 139	74, 146	65, 155
				10, 12	85, 145	76, 154	67, 163
				10, 13	88, 152	79, 161	69, 171
7, 7	36, 69	32, 73	28, 77	10, 14	91, 159	81, 169	71, 179
7, 8	38, 74	34, 78	29, 83	10, 15	94, 166	84, 176	73, 187
7, 9	40, 79	35, 84	30, 89	10, 16	97, 173	86, 184	75, 195
7, 10	42, 84	37, 89	31, 95	10, 17	100, 180	89, 191	77, 203
7, 11	44, 89	38, 95	32, 101	10, 18	103, 187	92, 198	79, 211
7, 12	46, 94	40, 100	33, 107	10, 19	107, 193	94, 206	81, 219
7, 13	48, 99	41, 106	34, 113	10, 20	110, 200	97, 213	83, 227
7, 14	50, 104	43, 111	35, 119				
7, 15	52, 109	44, 117	36, 125	11, 11	96, 157	87, 166	78, 175
7, 16	54, 114	46, 122	37, 131	11, 12	99, 165	90, 174	81, 183
7, 17	56, 119	47, 128	38, 137	11, 13	103, 172	93, 182	83, 192
7, 18	58, 124	49, 133	39, 143	11, 14	106, 180	96, 190	85, 201
7, 19	60, 129	50, 139	41, 148	11, 15	110, 187	99, 198	87, 210
7, 20	62, 134	52, 144	42, 154	11, 16	114, 194	102, 206	90, 218
7, 21	64, 139	53, 150	43, 160	11, 17	117, 202	105, 214	92, 227
7, 22	66, 144	55, 155	44, 166	11, 18	121, 209	108, 222	94, 236
7, 23	68, 149	57, 160	45, 172	11, 19	124, 217	111, 230	97, 244
8, 8	49, 87	43, 93	38, 98	12, 12	115, 185	106, 194	95, 205
8, 9	51, 93	45, 99	40, 104	12, 13	119, 193	109, 203	98, 214
8, 10	53, 99	47, 105	41, 111	12, 14	123, 201	112, 212	100, 224
8, 11	55, 105	49, 111	42, 118	12, 15	127, 209	115, 221	103, 233
8, 12	58, 110	51, 117	43, 125	12, 16	131, 217	119, 229	105, 243
8, 13	60, 116	53, 123	45, 131	12, 17	135, 225	122, 238	108, 252
8, 14	63, 121	54, 130	46, 138	12, 18	139, 233	125, 247	111, 261
8, 15	65, 127	56, 136	47, 145				
8, 16	67, 133	58, 142	49, 151	13, 13	137, 214	125, 226	114, 237
8, 17	70, 138	60, 148	50, 158	13, 14	141, 223	129, 235	116, 248
8, 18	72, 144	62, 154	51, 165	13, 15	145, 232	133, 244	119, 258
8, 19	74, 150	64, 160	53, 171	13, 16	150, 240	137, 253	122, 268
8, 20	77, 155	66, 166	54, 178	13, 17	154, 249	140, 263	125, 278
8, 21	79, 161	68, 172	56, 184				
8, 22	82, 166	70, 178	57, 191	14, 14	160, 246	147, 259	134, 272
				14, 15	164, 256	151, 269	137, 283
9, 9	63, 108	56, 115	50, 121	14, 16	169, 265	155, 279	140, 294
9, 10	65, 115	58, 122	52, 128				
9, 11	68, 121	61, 128	53, 136	15, 15	185, 280	171, 294	156, 309

Table A8. Critical values of sample rank correlation coefficient, r_s, for test of null hypothesis that population correlation is zero (this table gives the values of r_s required to achieve statistical significance at the specified level)

Number of observation pairs	Significance level for two-tail test	
	.05	.01
6	.886	—
7	.786	—
8	.738	.881
9	.683	.833
10	.648	.794
11	.623	.818
12	.591	.780
13	.566	.745
14	.545	.716
15	.525	.689
16	.507	.666
17	.490	.645
18	.476	.625
19	.462	.608
20	.450	.591
21	.438	.576
22	.428	.562
23	.418	.549
24	.409	.537
25	.400	.526
26	.392	.515
27	.385	.505
28	.377	.496
29	.370	.487
30	.364	.478

From Beyer [11].

References

1. Anscombe, F. J. Sequential medical trials. *J. Am. Stat. Assoc.* 58:365, 1963.
2. Armitage, P. *Statistical Methods in Medical Research.* New York: Wiley, 1971.
3. Armitage, P. *Sequential Medical Trials.* Springfield, Ill.: Thomas, 1960.
4. Atkins, H. Conduct of a controlled clinical trial. *Br. Med. J.* 2:377, 1966.
5. Balcon, R., Jewitt, D. E., Davies, J. P. H., and Oram, S. A controlled trial of propranolol in acute myocardial infarction. *Lancet* 2:917, 1966.
6. Beecher, H. K. Ethics and clinical research. *N. Engl. J. Med.* 274:1354, 1966.
7. Beecher, H. K. Pain, placebos and physicians. *Practitioner* 189:141, 1962.
8. Berkow, J. W., Shugarman, R. G., Maumenee, E., and Patz, A. A retrospective study of blind diabetic patients. *J.A.M.A.* 193:867, 1965.
9. Berkson, J. The statistical study of association between smoking and lung cancer. *Mayo Clin. Proc.* 30:319, 1955.
10. Berkson, J. Limitations of the application of fourfold table analysis to hospital data. *Biometrics* 2:47, 1946.
11. Beyer, W. H. (Ed.). *Handbook of Tables for Probability and Statistics.* Cleveland: Chemical Rubber Co., 1966.
12. Bliss, C. I. *Statistics in Biology.* New York: McGraw-Hill, 1967. Vol. 1.
13. Boles, R. S., and Westerman, M. P. Seasonal incidence and precipitating causes of hemorrhage from peptic ulcer. *J.A.M.A.* 156:1379, 1954.
14. Brown, A., Mohamed, S. D., Montgomery, R. D., Armitage, P., and Laurence, D. R. Value of a large dose of antitoxin in clinical tetanus. *Lancet* 2:227, 1960.
15. Bruce, R. A., and Yarnall, S. R. Computer-aided diagnosis of cardiovascular disorders. *J. Chronic Dis.* 19:473, 1966.
16. Chalmers, T. C. When should randomization begin? *Lancet* 1:858, 1968.
17. Clausen, J., Felsby, M., Schønau Jørgensen, F., Lyager Nielsen, B., Rain, J., and Strange, B. Absence of prophylactic effect of propranolol in myocardial infarction. *Lancet* 2:920, 1966.
18. Cochran, W. G., and Cox, G. M. *Experimental Designs* (2d ed.). New York: Wiley, 1957.
19. Colton, T. A rebuttal of "Statistical ward rounds 4." *Clin. Pharmacol. Ther.* 9:113, 1968.
20. Colton, T., and Buxbaum, R. C. Motor vehicle inspection and motor vehicle accident mortality. *Am. J. Public Health* 58:1090, 1968.
21. Colton, T., Gosselin, R. E., and Smith, R. P. The tolerance of coffee drinkers to caffeine. *Clin. Pharmacol. Ther.* 9:31, 1968.
22. Cooper, E. S., Cooper, J. W., and Schnabel, T. G., Jr. Pitfalls in the diagnosis of bacterial endocarditis. *Arch. Intern. Med.* 118:55, 1966.
23. Cornfield, J. Sequential trials, sequential analysis and the likelihood principle. *Am. Stat.* 20(2):18, 1966.
24. Cresswell, W. L., and Froggatt, P. *The Causation of Bus Driver Accidents.* New York: Oxford University Press, 1963.
25. Croxton, F. E. *Elementary Statistics with Applications in Medicine.* New York: Prentice-Hall, 1953.

26. D'Arcy Hart, P. History of randomised control trials. *Lancet* 1:965, 1972.
27. Dawber, T. R., Meadors, G. F., and Moore, F. E., Jr. Epidemiological approaches to heart disease: the Framingham Study. *Am. J. Public Health* 41:279, 1951.
28. Dawber, T. R., Moore, F. E., Jr., and Mann, G. V. Coronary heart disease in the Framingham Study. *Am. J. Public Health* 47:4, 1957.
29. Dixon, W. J., and Massey, F. J., Jr. *Introduction to Statistical Analysis* (3d ed.). New York: McGraw-Hill, 1969.
30. Doll, R., and Hill, A. B. Lung cancer and other causes of death in relation to smoking. *Br. Med. J.* 2:1071, 1956.
31. Dorland, W. A. N. *Dorland's Illustrated Medical Dictionary* (24th ed.). Philadelphia: Saunders, 1967.
31a. Dorland, W. A. N. *Dorland's Illustrated Medical Dictionary* (25th ed.). Philadelphia: Saunders, 1974.
32. Dorland, W. A. N. *The American Illustrated Medical Dictionary* (20th ed.). Philadelphia: Saunders, 1945.
33. Editorial. A pillar of medicine. *J.A.M.A.* 195:1145, 1966.
34. Editorial. Propranolol and myocardial infarction. *Lancet* 2:950, 1966.
35. Editorial. Bias, the Achilles heel of the therapeutic trial. *N. Engl. J. Med.* 272:915, 1965.
36. Editorial. Significance of significant. *N. Engl. J. Med.* 278:1232, 1968.
37. Elveback, L., Guillier, C. L., and Keating, F. R., Jr. Health, normality and the ghost of Gauss. *J.A.M.A.* 211:69, 1970.
38. "Even at home, drinkers run risk of getting smashed." *Medical World News* 10(48):5, 1969.
39. Finn, R., Jones, P. O., Tweedie, M. C. K., Hall, S. M., Dinsdale, O. F., and Bourdillon, R. E. Frequency distribution curve of uric acid in the general population. *Lancet* 2:185, 1966.
40. Fisher, R. A. *The Design of Experiments*. London: Oliver and Boyd, 1935.
41. Fisher, R. A., and Yates, F. *Statistical Tables for Biological, Agricultural and Medical Research* (6th ed.). New York: Hafner, 1964.
42. Forrester, J. C., and Ury, H. K. The signed-rank (Wilcoxon) test in the rapid analysis of biological data. *Lancet* 1:239, 1969.
43. Freedman, M. J., and Frajola, W. G. Serum lipid patterns in men under 45 years with myocardial infarction. *Am. J. Med. Sci.* 246:277, 1963.
44. Gifford, R. H., and Feinstein, A. R. A critique of methodology in studies of anticoagulant therapy for acute myocardial infarction. *N. Engl. J. Med.* 280:351, 1969.
45. Gold, H., Mehta, D., Golfinos, A., and Kwit, N. T. A method for the assay of antihypertensive activity of drugs in ambulant patients with hypertension. *Am. J. Med. Sci.* 246:1, 1963.
46. Grant, A. P. Sequential trial of isocarboxazid in angina pectoris. *Br. Med. J.* 1:513, 1962.
47. Graubard, S. R. (Ed.). Ethical aspects of experimentation with human subjects. *Daedalus* 98, 1969.
48. Greenwod, M. The errors of sampling of the survivorship tables. Appendix 1 in *Reports on Public Health and Statistical Subjects,* No. 33. London: His Majesty's Stationery Office, 1926.
49. Gregg, N. Congenital cataract following German measles in the mother. *Trans. Ophthalmol. Soc. Aust.* 111:35, 1941.
50. Hall, G. H. The clinical application of Bayes' theorem. *Lancet* 2:555, 1967.
51. Hamilton, M. Propranolol in myocardial infarction. *Lancet* 2:643, 1965.
52. Hansen, H., Marolla, F., and Stein, Z. Survival-times after cardiac allografts. *Lancet* 1:1266, 1969.

53. Harris, E. L., and Fitzgerald, J. D. (Eds.). *The Principles and Practice of Clinical Trials.* Edinburgh: Livingstone, 1970.

54. Harvald, B., Hilden, T., and Lund, E. Long-term anticoagulant therapy after myocardial infarction. *Lancet* 2:626, 1962.

55. Herring, R. A. The relationship of marital status in females to mortality from cancer of the breast, female genital organs and other sites. *Am. Soc. Control Cancer* 18:4, 1936.

56. Hill, A. B. *Principles of Medical Statistics* (9th ed.). New York: Oxford University Press, 1971.

57. Hill, A. B. Medical ethics and controlled trials. *Br. Med. J.* 1:1043, 1963.

58. Hill, A. B. *Statistical Methods in Clinical and Preventive Medicine.* New York: Oxford University Press, 1962.

59. Jennett, W. B., and Cross, J. N. Influence of pregnancy and oral contraception on the incidence of strokes in women of childbearing age. *Lancet* 1:1019, 1967.

60. Jick, H., Slone, D., Westerholm, B., Inman, W. H. W., Vessey, M. P., Shapiro, S., Lewis, G. P., and Worcester, J. Venous thromboembolic disease and ABO blood types. *Lancet* 1:539, 1969.

61. Johnson, O. D., Ruchelman, H., and Ford, R. V. Diuretics and hypertension: effect of sodium balance. *N. Engl. J. Med.* 267:336, 1962.

62. Kannel, W. B., Castelli, W. P., McNamara, P. M., McKee, P. A., and Feinleib, M. Role of blood pressure in the development of congestive heart failure. *N. Engl. J. Med.* 287:781, 1972.

63. Kendall, M. G. *Rank Correlation Methods* (2d ed.). New York: Hafner, 1955.

64. LeShan, L. An emotional life-history pattern associated with neoplastic disease. *Ann. N.Y. Acad. Sci.* 125(Art. 3):780, 1966.

65. LeVay, S. Survival-times after cardiac allografts. *Lancet* 1:1048, 1969.

66. Levine, S. A. Elusive errors in coronary statistics. *J.A.M.A.* 195:860, 1966.

67. Lusted, L. B. *Introduction to Medical Decision Making.* Springfield, Ill.: Thomas, 1968.

68. Mahon, W. A., and Daniel, E. E. A method for the assessment of reports of drug trials. *Can. Med. Assoc. J.* 90:565, 1964.

69. Mainland, D. Statistical ward rounds 4. *Clin. Pharmacol. Ther.* 8:615, 1967.

70. Mainland, D. *Elementary Medical Statistics* (2d ed.). Philadelphia: Saunders, 1963.

71. Mainland, D. The risk of fallacious conclusions from autopsy data on the incidence of diseases with applications to heart disease. *Am. Heart J.* 45:644, 1953.

72. Mainland, D., Herrera, L., and Sutcliffe, M. I. *Tables for Use with Binomial Samples.* New York: Dept. of Medical Statistics, New York University College of Medicine, 1956.

73. Martin, S. P., Donaldson, M. C., London, C. D., Peterson, O. L., and Colton, T. Inputs into coronary care during thirty years: a cost effectiveness study. *Ann. Intern. Med.* 81:289, 1974.

74. Mathur, K. S. Environmental factors in coronary heart disease. *Circulation* 21:684, 1960.

75. McKissock, W., Richardson, A., and Walsh, L. "Posterior-communicating" aneurysms: a controlled trial of conservative and surgical treatment. *Lancet* 1:1203, 1960.

76. Medical Research Council. Streptomycin treatment of pulmonary tuberculosis. *Br. Med. J.* 2:769, 1948.

77. Messmer, B. J., Nora, J. J., Leachman, R. D., and Cooley, D. A. Survival-times after cardiac allografts. *Lancet* 1:954, 1969.

78. Miall, W. E., Kass, E. H., Ling, J., and Stuart, K. L. Factors influencing arterial pressure in the general population in Jamaica. *Br. Med. J.* 2:497, 1962.

79. Mosteller, F., Rourke, R. E. K., and Thomas, G. B., Jr. *Probability with Statistical Applications* (2d ed.). Reading, Mass.: Addison-Wesley, 1970.

80. Nader, R. *Unsafe at Any Speed: the Designed-in Dangers of the American Automobile.* New York: Grossman, 1965.

81. National Bureau of Standards. *Tables of the Binomial Probability Distribution.* Washington, D.C.: U.S. Govt. Printing Office, 1950.

82. Oldham, P. D. *Measurement in Medicine: the Interpretation of Numerical Data.* Philadelphia: Lippincott, 1968.

83. Papadrianos, E., Haagensen, C. D., and Cooley, E. Cancer of the breast as a familial disease. *Ann. Surg.* 165:10, 1967.

84. Pearl, R. Cancer and tuberculosis. *Am. J. Hyg.* 9:97, 1929.

85. Pearl, R., Sutton, A. C., and Howard, W. T., Jr. Experimental treatment of cancer with tuberculin. *Lancet* 1:1078, 1929.

86. Pearson, E. S., and Hartley, H. O. *Biometrika Tables for Statisticians* (3d ed.). Cambridge, England: Cambridge University Press, 1966. Vol. 1.

87. Pillard, R. C. Book review of "Marihuana Reconsidered." *N. Engl. J. Med.* 285:416, 1971.

88. Prince, A. M., and Gershon, R. K. The use of serum enzyme determinations to detect anicteric hepatitis. *Transfusion* 5:120, 1965.

89. Public Health Service. *Vital Statistics of the United States, 1968.* Vol. II, Part A, Section 5. Washington, D.C.: U.S. Govt. Printing Office, 1971.

90. Public Health Service. *Vital Statistics of the United States, 1967.* Vol. II, Part A, Section 1. Washington, D.C.: U.S. Govt. Printing Office, 1969.

91. Public Health Service. *Vital Statistics of the United States, 1965.* Vol. II, Part A, Section 2. Washington, D.C.: U.S. Govt. Printing Office, 1967.

92. Public Health Service. *Smoking and Health: Report of the Advisory Committee to the Surgeon General.* Washington, D.C.: U.S. Govt. Printing Office, 1964.

93. Rossiter, C. E. Propranolol in myocardial infarction. *Lancet* 2:852, 1965.

94. Ruffin, J. M., Grizzle, J. E., Hightower, N. C., McHardy, G., Shull, H., and Kirsner, J. B. A cooperative double-blind evaluation of gastric "freezing" in the treatment of duodenal ulcer. *N. Engl. J. Med.* 281:16, 1969.

95. Rutstein, D. D. *The Coming Revolution in Medicine.* Cambridge, Mass.: M.I.T. Press, 1967.

96. Sartwell, P. E. The distribution of incubation periods of infectious disease. *Am. J. Hyg.* 51:310, 1950.

97. Sartwell, P. E., Masi, A. T., Arthes, F. G., Greene, G. R., and Smith, H. E. Thromboembolism and oral contraceptives: an epidemiologic case control study. *Am. J. Epidemiol.* 90:365, 1969.

98. Schoolman, H. M. Statistics in medical research. *N. Engl. J. Med.* 280:218, 1969.

99. Schor, S., and Karten, I. Statistical evaluation of medical journal manuscripts. *J.A.M.A.* 195:1123, 1966.

100. Seltser, R., and Sartwell, P. E. The effect of occupational exposure to radiation on the mortality of physicians. *J.A.M.A.* 190:1046, 1964.

101. Snedecor, G. W., and Cochran, W. G. *Statistical Methods* (6th ed.). Ames, Iowa: Iowa State University Press, 1967.

102. Snow, P. J. D. Effect of propranolol in myocardial infarction. *Lancet* 2:551, 1965.

103. Snow, P. J. D., and Clarke, C. Propranolol in myocardial infarction. *Lancet* 2:852, 1965.

104. Sokal, R. R., and Rohlf, F. J. *Biometry: the Principles and Practice of Sta-*

tistics in Biological Research. San Francisco: Freeman, 1969.

105. Stephen, S. A. Propranolol in acute myocardial infarction: a multicentre trial. *Lancet* 2:1435, 1966.

106. Strong, J. P., McGill, H. C., Jr., Tejada, C., and Holman, R. L. The natural history of atherosclerosis: comparison of the early aortic lesions in New Orleans, Guatemala, and Costa Rica. *Am. J. Pathol.* 34:731, 1958.

107. Tukey, J. W. The simplest signed rank tests. Memorandum report 17. Princeton, N.J.: Statistical Research Group, Princeton University, 1949.

108. Vessey, M. D., and Doll, R. Investigation of relation between use of oral contraceptives and thromboembolic disease: a further report. *Br. Med. J.* 2:651, 1969.

109. Waife, S. O., and Shapiro, A. P. (Eds.). *The Clinical Evaluation of New Drugs.* New York: Hoeber, 1959.

110. Wald, A. *Sequential Analysis.* New York: Wiley, 1947.

111. Wallis, W. A., and Roberts, H. V. *Statistics—A New Approach.* Glencoe, Ill.: Free Press, 1956.

112. Warren, S. Longevity and causes of death from irradiation in physicians. *J.A.M.A.* 162:464, 1956.

113. West, E. D. The signed rank (Wilcoxon) test. *Lancet* 1:526, 1969.

114. White, C. The use of ranks in a test of significance for comparing two treatments. *Biometrics* 8:33, 1952.

115. Wilcoxon, F. Individual comparisons by ranking methods. *Biometrics Bull.* 1:80, 1945.

116. Williams, S. V., Munford, R. S., Colton, T., Murphy, D. A., and Poskanzer, D. C. Mortality among physicians: a cohort study. *J. Chronic Dis.* 24:393, 1971.

117. Winer, B., Lubbe, W. F., and Colton, T. Antihypertensive actions of diuretics. *J.A.M.A.* 204:775, 1969.

118. Witts, L. O. (Ed.). *Medical Surveys and Clinical Trials* (2d ed.). New York: Oxford University Press, 1964.

119. World Health Organization. *Manual of the International Statistical Classifications of Diseases, Injuries, and Causes of Death* (8th revision). Geneva: World Health Organization, 1967.

Index